Production Credits

Chief Executive Officer: Clayton Jones
Chief Operating Officer: Don W. Jones, Jr.
President, Higher Education and Professional Publishing: Robert W. Holland, Jr.
V.P., Sales and Marketing: William J. Kane
V.P., Design and Production: Anne Spencer
V.P., Manufacturing and Inventory Control: Therese Connell
Publisher: Christopher Davis

Senior Acquisitions Editor: Nancy Anastasi Duffy
Editorial Assistant: Jessica Acox
Production Editor: Wendy Swanson
Associate Marketing Manager: Ilana Goddess
Composition: Newgen
Cover Design: Anne Spencer
Printing and Binding: Cenveo
Cover Printing: Cenveo

If you obtained your Pocket Pharmacopoeia from a bookstore, please send your address to info@tarascon.com. This allows you to be the first to hear of updates! (We don't sell or distribute our mailing lists, by the way.) To order extra copies, please go the the last page of this book.

The cover woodcut is *The Apothecary* by Jost Amman, Frankfurt, 1574. Many of you knew that The Well of Souls were the dark continent walls adorned with otherworldly caricatures of protocol and cleverness, hearkening to far away and long ago. We will send a free copy of next year's edition to the first 25 who can solve this puzzle: A pill bottle contains one pill, either clonazepam or clonidine. A clonidine pill is placed into the bottle, the bottle is shaken, and a clonidine pill is removed. What are the chances that a clonazepam pill remains? Pretty easy, right? Think, think, think, think.

W9-AXZ-421

CONTENTS

Tarascon Pocket Pharmacopoeia®

2009 Classic Shirt-Pocket Edition

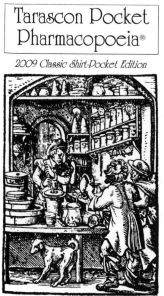

23ʳᴰ EDITION

"Desire to take medicines ... distinguishes man from animals."
—Sir William Osler

Editor in Chief
Richard J. Hamilton, MD, FAAEM, FACMT
Chair, Department of Emergency Medicine
Drexel University College of Medicine
Philadelphia, PA

JONES AND BARTLETT PUBLISHERS
Sudbury, Massachusetts
BOSTON   TORONTO   LONDON   SINGAPORE

World Headquarters

Jones and Bartlett
Publishers
40 Tall Pine Drive
Sudbury, MA 01776
978-443-5000
info@jbpub.com
www.jbpub.com

Jones and Bartlett
Publishers Canada
6339 Ormindale Way
Mississauga, Ontario
L5V 1J2 Canada

Jones and Bartlett
Publishers International
Barb House, Barb Mews
London W6 7PA
United Kingdom

Jones and Bartlett's books and products are available through most bookstores and
online booksellers. To contact Jones and Bartlett Publishers directly, call 800-832-
0034, fax 978-443-8000, or visit our website www.jbpub.com.

Substantial discounts on bulk quantities of Jones and Bartlett's publications
are available to corporations, professional associations, and other qualified
organizations. For details and specific discount information, contact the special
sales department at Jones and Bartlett via the above contact information or send
an email to specialsales@jbpub.com.

The information in the *Pocket Pharmacopoeia* is compiled from sources believed to
be reliable, and exhaustive efforts have been put forth to make the book as accurate
as possible. The *Pocket Pharmacopoeia* is edited by a panel of drug information ex-
perts with extensive peer review and input from more than 50 practicing clinicians of
multiple specialties. Our goal is to provide health professionals focused, core prescribing
information in a convenient, organized, and concise fashion. We include FDA-approved
dosing indications and those off-label uses that have a reasonable basis to support
their use. *However the accuracy and completeness of this work cannot be guaranteed.*
Despite our best efforts this book may contain typographical errors and omissions. The
Pocket Pharmacopoeia is intended as a quick and convenient reminder of information you
have already learned elsewhere. The contents are to be used as a guide only, and health
care professionals should use sound clinical judgment and individualize therapy to each
specific patient care situation. This book is not meant to be a replacement for training,
experience, continuing medical education, or studying the latest drug prescribing
literature. This book is sold without warranties of any kind, express or implied, and the
publisher and editors disclaim any liability, loss, or damage caused by the contents.
Although drug companies purchase and distribute our books as promotional items, the
Tarascon editorial staff alone determines all book content.

ISSN 1945-9076

ISBN-13: 978-0-7637-7419-6

6048

Printed in the United States of America

13 12 11 10 09   10 9 8 7 6 5 4 3 2

PAGE INDEX FOR TABLES

TARASCON POCKET PHARMACOPOEIA EDITORIAL STAFF*

PREFACE TO THE TARASCON POCKET PHARMACOPOEIA®

The *Tarascon Pocket Pharmacopoeia* arranges drugs by clinical class with a comprehensive index in the back. Trade names are italicized and capitalized. Drug doses shown in mg/kg are generally intended for children, while fixed doses represent typical adult recommendations. Brackets indicate currently available formulations, although not all pharmacies stock all formulations. The availability of generic, over-the-counter, and scored formulations are mentioned. Codes are as follows:

▶ **METABOLISM & EXCRETION:** L = primarily liver, K = primarily kidney, LK = both, but liver > kidney, KL = both, but kidney > liver.

♀ **SAFETY IN PREGNANCY:** A = Safety established using human studies, B = Presumed safety based on animal studies, C = Uncertain safety; no human studies and animal studies show an adverse effect, D = Unsafe - evidence of risk that may in certain clinical circumstances be justifiable, X = Highly unsafe - risk of use outweighs any possible benefit. For drugs which have not been assigned a category: + Generally accepted as safe, ? Safety unknown or controversial, – Generally regarded as unsafe.

▶ **SAFETY IN LACTATION:** + Generally accepted as safe, ? Safety unknown or controversial, – Generally regarded as unsafe. Many of our "+" listings are from the AAP policy "The Transfer of Drugs and Other Chemicals Into Human Milk" (see www.aap.org) and may differ from those recommended by the manufacturer.

© **DEA CONTROLLED SUBSTANCES:** I = High abuse potential, no accepted use (eg, heroin, marijuana), II = High abuse potential and severe dependence liability (eg, morphine, codeine, hydromorphone, cocaine, amphetamines, methylphenidate, secobarbital). Some states require triplicates. III = Moderate dependence liability (eg, *Tylenol #3, Vicodin*), IV = Limited dependence liability (benzodiazepines, propoxyphene, phentermine), V = Limited abuse potential (eg, *Lomotil*).

$ **RELATIVE COST:** Cost codes used are "per month" of maintenance therapy (eg, antihypertensives) or "per course" of short-term therapy (eg, antibiotics). Codes are calculated using average wholesale prices (at press time in US dollars) for the most common indication and route of each drug at a typical adult dosage. For maintenance therapy, costs are calculated based upon a 30 day supply or the quantity that might typically be used in a given month. For short-term therapy (ie, 10 days or less), costs are calculated on a single treatment course. When multiple forms

Code	Cost
$	< $25
$$	$25 to $49
$$$	$50 to $99
$$$$	$100 to $199
$$$$$	≥ $200

are available (eg, generics), these codes reflect the least expensive generally available product. When drugs don't neatly fit into the classification scheme above, we have assigned codes based upon the relative cost of other similar drugs. *These codes should be used as a rough guide only,* as (1) they reflect cost, not charges, (2) pricing often varies substantially from location to location and time to time, and (3) HMOs, Medicaid, and buying groups often negotiate quite different pricing. Check with your local pharmacy if you have any questions.

🍁 CANADIAN TRADE NAMES: Unique common Canadian trade names not used in the US are listed after a maple leaf symbol. Trade names used in both nations or only in the US are displayed without such notation.

ABBREVIATIONS IN TEXT

AAP - American Academy of Pediatrics	CrCl - creatinine clearance	IU - international units
ac - before meals	CVA - stroke	IV - intravenous
ADHD - attention deficit & hyperactivity disorder	d - day	JRA - juvenile rheumatoid arthritis
	D5W - 5% dextrose	kg - kilogram
	DPI - dry powder inhaler	LFTs - liver fxn tests
AHA - American Heart Association	ET - endotracheal	LV - left ventricular
ANC - absolute neutrophil count	EPS - extrapyramidal symptoms	mcg - microgram
ASA - aspirin	g - gram	mEq - milliequivalent
AUC - area under curve	gtts - drops	mg - milligram
bid - twice per day	GERD - gastroesophageal reflux dz	MI - myocardial infarction
BP - blood pressure	GU - genitourinary	min - minute
BPH - benign prostatic hyperplasia	h - hour	mL - milliliter
CAD - coronary artery disease	HAART - highly active antiretroviral therapy	mo - months old
		ng - nanogram
cap - capsule	HCTZ - hydrochlorothiazide	NHLBI - National Heart, Lung, and Blood Institute
CMV - cytomegalovirus	HSV - herpes simplex virus	NS - normal saline
CNS - central nervous system	HTN - hypertension	NYHA - New York Heart Association
COPD - chronic obstructive pulmonary disease	IM - intramuscular	N/V - nausea/vomiting
	INR - international normalized ratio	OA - osteoarthritis
		pc - after meals

PO - by mouth	
PR - by rectum	
prn - as needed	
q - every	
qhs - at bedtime	
qid - four times/day	
qod - every other day	
q pm - every evening	
RA - rheumatoid arthritis	
SC - subcutaneous	
soln - solution	
supp - suppository	
susp - suspension	
tab - tablet	
TB - tuberculosis	
TCAs - tricyclic antidepressants	
tid - 3 times/day	
tiw - 3 times/week	
TNF - tumor necrosis factor	
UTI - urinary tract infection	
wk - week	
yo - years old	

THERAPEUTIC DRUG LEVELS

Drug	Level	Optimal Timing
amikacin peak	20-35 mcg/ml	30 minutes after infusion
amikacin trough	<5 mcg/ml	Just prior to next dose
carbamazepine trough	4-12 mcg/ml	Just prior to next dose
cyclosporine trough	50-300 ng/ml	Just prior to next dose
digoxin	0.8-2.0 ng/ml	Just prior to next dose
ethosuximide trough	40-100 mcg/ml	Just prior to next dose
gentamicin peak	5-10 mcg/ml	30 minutes after infusion
gentamicin trough	<2 mcg/ml	Just prior to next dose
lidocaine	1.5-5 mcg/ml	12-24 hours after start of infusion
lithium trough	0.6-1.2 meq/l	Just prior to first morning dose
NAPA	10-30 mcg/ml	Just prior to next procainamide dose
phenobarbital trough	15-40 mcg/ml	Just prior to next dose
phenytoin trough	10-20 mcg/ml	Just prior to next dose
primidone trough	5-12 mcg/ml	Just prior to next dose
procainamide	4-10 mcg/ml	Just prior to next dose
quinidine	2-5 mcg/ml	Just prior to next dose
theophylline	5-15 mcg/ml	8-12 hrs after once daily dose
tobramycin peak	5-10 mcg/ml	30 minutes after infusion
tobramycin trough	<2 mcg/ml	Just prior to next dose
valproate trough (epilepsy)	50-100 mcg/ml	Just prior to next dose
valproate trough (mania)	45-125 mcg/ml	Just prior to next dose
vancomycin trough	5-20 mcg/ml	Just prior to next dose

PEDIATRIC DRUGS		Age	2m	4m	6m	9m	12m	15m	2y	3y	5y
		Kg	5	6½	8	9	10	11	13	15	19
		Lbs	11	15	17	20	22	24	28	33	42
med	***strength***	***freq***	***teaspoons of liquid per dose*** *(1 tsp= 5 ml)*								
Tylenol (mg)		q4h	80	80	120	120	160	160	200	240	280
Tylenol (tsp)	160/t	q4h	½	½	¾	¾	1	1	1¼	1½	1¾
ibuprofen (mg)		q6h	-	-	75†	75†	100	100	125	150	175
ibuprofen (tsp)	100/t	q6h	-	-	¾†	¾†	1	1	1¼	1½	1¾
amoxicillin or	125/t	bid	1	1¼	1½	1¾	1¾	2	2¼	2¾	3½
Augmentin	200/t	bid	½	¾	1	1	1¼	1¼	1½	1¾	2¼
(not otitis media)	250/t	bid	½	½	¾	¾	1	1	1¼	1¼	1¾
	400/t	bid	¼	½	½	½	¾	¾	¾	1	1
amoxicillin,	200/t	bid	1	1¼	1¾	2	2	2¼	2¾	3	4
(otitis media)‡	250/t	bid	¾	1¼	1½	1½	1¾	1¾	2¼	2½	3¼
	400/t	bid	½	¾	¾	1	1	1¼	1½	1½	2
Augmentin ES‡	600/t	bid	⅜	½	½	¾	¾	¾	1	1¼	1½
azithromycin*§	100/t	qd	¼†	½†	½	½	½	½	¾	¾	1
(5-day Rx)	200/t	qd	--	¼†	¼	¼	¼	¼	½	½	½
Bactrim/Septra	---	bid	½	¾	1	1	1	1¼	1½	1½	2
cefaclor*	125/t	bid	1	1	1¼	1½	1½	1¾	2	2½	3
"	250/t	bid	½	½	¾	¾	¾	1	1	1¼	1½
cefadroxil	125/t	bid	½	¾	1	1	1¼	1¼	1½	1¾	2¼
"	250/t	bid	¼	½	½	½	¾	¾	¾	1	1
cefdinir	125/t	qd	--	¾†	1	1	1	1¼	1½	1¾	2
cefixime	100/t	qd	½	½	¾	¾	¾	1	1	1¼	1½
cefprozil*	125/t	bid	--	¾†	1	1	1¼	1½	1½	2	2¼
"	250/t	bid	--	½†	½	½	¾	¾	¾	1	1¼
cefuroxime	125/t	bid	--	¾	¾	1	1	1	1½	1¾	2¼
cephalexin	125/t	qid	--	½	¾	¾	1	1	1¼	1½	1¾
"	250/t	qid	--	¼	¼	½	½	½	¾	¾	1
clarithromycin	125/t	bid	½†	½†	½	½	¾	¾	¾	1	1¼
"	250/t	bid	--	--	--	¼	½	½	½	½	¾
dicloxacillin	62½/t	qid	½	¾	1	1	1¼	1¼	1½	1¾	2
nitrofurantoin	25/t	qid	¼	½	½	½	½	¾	¾	¾	1
Pediazole	---	tid	½	½	¾	¾	1	1	1	1¼	1½
penicillin V**	250/t	bid-tid	--	1	1	1	1	1	1	1	1
cetirizine	5/t	qd	-	-	½	½	½	½	½	½	½
Benadryl	12.5/t	q6h	½	½	¾	¾	1	1	1¼	1½	2
prednisolone	15/t	qd	¼	½	½	¾	¾	¾	1	1	1¼
prednisone	5/t	qd	1	1¼	1½	1¾	2	2¼	2½	3	3¾
Robitussin	---	q4h	-	-	¼†	¼†	½	½	¾	¾	1
Tylenol w/ codeine		q4h	-	-	-	-	-	-	-	1	1

* Dose shown is for otitis media only; see dosing in text for alternative indications.

† Dosing at this age/weight not recommended by manufacturer.

‡ AAP now recommends high dose (80-90 mg/kg/d) for all otitis media in children; with Augmentin used as ES only.

§Give a double dose of azithromycin the first day.

**AHA dosing for streptococcal pharyngitis. Treat for 10 days.

PEDIATRIC VITAL SIGNS AND INTRAVENOUS DRUGS

Age		Pre-matr	New-born	2m	4m	6m	9m	12m	15m	2y	3y	5y
Weight	(Kg)	2	3½	5	6½	8	9	10	11	13	15	19
	(Lbs)	4½	7½	11	15	17	20	22	24	28	33	42
Maint fluids	(ml/h)	8	14	20	26	32	36	40	42	46	50	58
ET tube	(mm)	2½	3/3½	3½	3½	3½	4	4	4½	4½	4½	5
Defib	(Joules)	4	7	10	13	16	18	20	22	26	30	38
Systolic BP	(high)	70	80	85	90	95	100	103	104	106	109	114
	(low)	40	60	70	70	70	70	70	70	75	75	80
Pulse rate	(high)	145	145	180	180	180	160	160	160	150	150	135
	(low)	100	100	110	110	110	100	100	100	90	90	65
Resp rate	(high)	60	60	50	50	50	46	46	30	30	25	25
	(low)	35	30	30	30	24	24	20	20	20	20	20
adenosine	(mg)	0.2	0.3	0.5	0.6	0.8	0.9	1	1.1	1.3	1.5	1.9
atropine	(mg)	0.1	0.1	0.1	0.13	0.16	0.18	0.2	0.22	0.26	0.30	0.38
Benadryl	(mg)	-	-	5	6½	8	9	10	11	13	15	19
bicarbonate	(meq)	2	3½	5	6½	8	9	10	11	13	15	19
dextrose	(g)	1	2	5	6½	8	9	10	11	13	15	19
epinephrine	(mg)	.02	.04	.05	.07	.08	.09	0.1	0.11	0.13	0.15	0.19
lidocaine	(mg)	2	3½	5	6½	8	9	10	11	13	15	19
morphine	(mg)	0.2	0.3	0.5	0.6	0.8	0.9	1	1.1	1.3	1.5	1.9
mannitol	(g)	2	3½	5	6½	8	9	10	11	13	15	19
naloxone	(mg)	.02	.04	.05	.07	.08	.09	0.1	0.11	0.13	0.15	0.19
diazepam	(mg)	0.6	1	1.5	2	2.5	2.7	3	3.3	3.9	4.5	5
fosphenytoin*	(PE)	40	70	100	130	160	180	200	220	260	300	380
lorazepam	(mg)	0.1	0.2	0.3	0.35	0.4	0.5	0.5	0.6	0.7	0.8	1.0
phenobarb	(mg)	30	60	75	100	125	125	150	175	200	225	275
phenytoin*	(mg)	40	70	100	130	160	180	200	220	260	300	380
ampicillin	(mg)	100	175	250	325	400	450	500	550	650	750	1000
ceftriaxone	(mg)	-	-	250	325	400	450	450	550	650	750	1000
cefotaxime	(mg)	100	175	250	325	400	450	500	550	650	750	1000
gentamicin	(mg)	5	8	12	16	20	22	25	27	32	37	47

*Loading doses; fosphenytoin dosed in "phenytoin equivalents".

CONVERSIONS		
Temperature:	Liquid:	Weight:
F = (1.8) C + 32	1 fluid ounce = 30ml	1 kilogram = 2.2 lbs
C = (F - 32)/(1.8)	1 teaspoon = 5ml	1 ounce = 30 g
	1 tablespoon = 15ml	1 grain = 65 mg

Alveolar-arterial oxygen gradient = A-a = 148 - 1.2($PaCO_2$) - PaO_2
[normal = 10-20 mmHg, breathing room air at sea level]

Calculated osmolality = 2Na + glucose/18 + BUN/2.8 + ethanol/4.6
[normal 280-295 meq/L. Na in meq/L; all others in mg/dL]

Pediatric IV maintenance fluids (see table on page 7)
4 ml/kg/hr **or** 100 ml/kg/day for first 10 kg, plus
2 ml/kg/hr **or** 50 ml/kg/day for second 10 kg, plus
1 ml/kg/hr **or** 20 ml/kg/day for all further kg

$$mcg/kg/min = \frac{16.7 \times drug\ conc\ [mg/ml] \times infusion\ rate\ [ml/h]}{weight\ [kg]}$$

$$Infusion\ rate\ [ml/h] = \frac{desired\ mcg/kg/min \times weight\ [kg] \times 60}{drug\ concentration\ [mcg/ml]}$$

Fractional excretion of sodium =
[Pre-renal, etc <1%; ATN, etc >1%]
$$\left[\frac{urine\ Na\ /\ plasma\ Na}{urine\ creat\ /\ plasma\ creat} \right] \times 100\%$$

Anion gap = Na − (Cl + HCO_3)   [normal = 10-14 meq/L]

$$Creatinine\ clearance = \frac{(lean\ kg)(140 - age)(0.85\ if\ female)}{(72)(stable\ creatinine\ [mg/dL])}$$
[normal >80]

Glomerular filtration rate using MDRD equation (ml/min/1.73 m²)
= 186 × (creatinine)$^{-1.154}$ × (age)$^{-0.203}$ × (0.742 if ♀) × (1.210 if African American)

Body surface area (BSA) = square root of: $\left[\dfrac{height\ (cm) \times weight\ (kg)}{3600} \right]$
[in m²]

DRUG THERAPY REFERENCE WEBSITES (selected)

Professional societies or governmental agencies with drug therapy guidelines		
AHRQ	Agency for Healthcare Research and Quality	www.ahcpr.gov
AAP	American Academy of Pediatrics	www.aap.org
ACC	American College of Cardiology	www.acc.org
ACCP	American College of Chest Physicians	www.chestnet.org
ACCP	American College of Clinical Pharmacy	www.accp.com
AHA	American Heart Association	www.americanheart.org
ADA	American Diabetes Association	www.diabetes.org
AMA	American Medical Association	www.ama-assn.org
ATS	American Thoracic Society	www.thoracic.org
ASHP	Amer. Society Health-Systems Pharmacists	www.ashp.org
CDC	Centers for Disease Control & Prevention	www.cdc.gov
CDC	CDC bioterrorism and radiation exposures	www.bt.cdc.gov
IDSA	Infectious Diseases Society of America	www.idsociety.org
MHA	Malignant Hyperthermia Association	www.mhaus.org
NHLBI	National Heart, Lung, & Blood Institute	www.nhlbi.nih.gov
Other therapy reference sites		
Cochrane library		www.cochrane.org
Emergency Contraception Website		www.not-2-late.com
Immunization Action Coalition		www.immunize.org
Int'l Registry for Drug-Induced Arrhythmias		www.qtdrugs.org
Managing Contraception		www.managingcontraception.com
Nephrology Pharmacy Associates		www.nephrologypharmacy.com

ANALGESICS

Antirheumatic Agents—Biologic Response Modifiers

NOTE *Death, sepsis, and serious infections (eg, TB) have been reported.*

ADALIMUMAB (Humira) RA, psoriatic arthritis, ankylosing spondylitis: 40 mg SC q2 wk, alone or in combination with methotrexate or other disease-modifying antirheumatic drugs (DMARDs). May increase frequency to q wk if not on methotrexate. Crohn's disease: 160 mg SC at wk 0, 80 mg at wk 2, then 40 mg every other wk starting with wk 4. [Trade only: 40 mg pre-filled glass syringes or vials with needles, 2 per pack.] ▶Serum ♀B ▶- $$$$$

ANAKINRA (Kineret) RA: 100 mg SC daily. [Trade only: 100 mg pre-filled glass syringes with needles, 7 or 28 per box. ▶K ♀B ▶? $$$$$

ETANERCEPT (Enbrel) RA, psoriatic arthritis, ankylosing spondylitis: 50 mg SC q wk. Plaque psoriasis: 50 mg SC twice weekly × 3 mo, then 50 mg SC q wk. JRA 4–17 yo: 0.8 mg/kg SC q wk, to max single dose of 50 mg. Max dose per injection site is 25 mg. [Supplied in a carton containing four dose trays and as single-use prefilled syringes. Each dose tray contains one 25 mg single-use vial of etanercept, one syringe (1 mL sterile bacteriostatic water for injection, containing 0.9% benzyl alcohol), one plunger, and two alcohol swabs. Single-use syringes contain 50 mg/mL.] ▶Serum ♀B ▶- $$$$$

INFLIXIMAB (Remicade) RA: 3 mg/kg IV in combination with methotrexate at 0, 2, and 6 wk. Ankylosing spondylitis: 5 mg/kg IV at 0, 2, and 6 wk. Plaque psoriasis; psoriatic arthritis; moderately to severely active Crohn's disease, ulcerative colitis, or fistulizing disease: 5 mg/kg IV infusion at 0, 2, and 6 wk, then every 8 wk. ▶Serum ♀B ▶? $$$$$

Antirheumatic Agents—Disease Modifying Antirheumatic Drugs (DMARDs)

AZATHIOPRINE (Azasan, Imuran, ✦Immunoprin, Oprisine) RA: Initial dose 1 mg/kg (50–100 mg) PO daily or divided bid. Increase after 6–8 wk. [Generic/Trade: Tabs 50 mg, scored. Trade only (Azasan): 75, 100 mg, scored.] ▶LK ♀D ▶- $$$

HYDROXYCHLOROQUINE (Plaquenil) RA: start 400–600 mg PO daily, then taper to 200–400 mg daily. SLE: 400 PO daily-bid to start, then taper to 200–400 mg daily. [Generic/Trade: Tabs 200 mg, scored.] ▶K ♀C ▶+ $

LEFLUNOMIDE (Arava) RA: 100 mg PO daily × 3 d. Maintenance: 10–20 mg PO daily. ▶LK ♀X ▶- $$$$$ [Generic/Trade: Tabs 10, 20 mg. Trade only: Tab 100 mg.]

METHOTREXATE (Rheumatrex, Trexall) RA, psoriasis: Start with 7.5 mg/wk PO single dose or 2.5 mg PO q12h × 3 doses given as a course once weekly. Max dose 20 mg/wk. Supplement with 1 mg/d of folic acid. Chemotherapy doses vary by indication. [Trade only (Trexall): Tabs 5, 7.5, 10, 15 mg. Dose Pak (Rheumatrex) 2.5 mg (#8,12,16,20,24s). Generic/Trade: Tabs 2.5 mg, scored.] ▶LK ♀X ▶- $$

Muscle Relaxants

BACLOFEN (Lioresal, Kemstro)   Spasticity related to MS or spinal cord disease/injury: Start 5 mg PO tid, then increase by 5 mg/dose q3d until 20 mg PO tid. Max dose 20 mg qid. [Generic only: Tabs 10, 20 mg. Trade only: (Kemstro) Tabs-orally disintegrating 10, 20 mg.] ▶K ♀C ▶+ $$

CARISOPRODOL (Soma)   Acute musculoskeletal pain: 350 mg PO tid-qid. Abuse potential. [Generic/Trade: Tabs 350 mg. Trade only: Tabs 250 mg.] ▶LK ♀? ▶- $

CHLORZOXAZONE (Parafon Forte DSC)   Musculoskeletal pain: 500–750 mg PO tid-qid to start. Decrease to 250 mg tid-qid. [Generic/Trade: Tabs 250 & 500 mg (Parafon Forte DSC 500 mg tabs scored).] ▶LK ♀C ▶? $

CYCLOBENZAPRINE (Amrix, Flexeril, Fexmid)   Musculoskeletal pain: Start 5–10 mg PO tid, max 30 mg/d or 15–30 mg (extended release) PO daily. Not recommended in elderly. [Generic/Trade: Tab 5, 10 mg. Generic only: Tab 7.5 mg. Trade only: (Amrix) Extended-release caps 15, 30 mg.] ▶LK ♀B ▶? $

DANTROLENE (Dantrium)   Chronic spasticity related to spinal cord injury, stroke, cerebral palsy, MS: 25 mg PO daily to start, up to max of 100 mg bid-qid if necessary. Malignant hyperthermia: 2.5 mg/kg rapid IV push q 5–10 min continuing until symptoms subside or to a max 10 mg/kg dose. [Generic/Trade: Caps 25, 50, 100 mg.] ▶LK ♀C ▶- $$$$

METAXALONE (Skelaxin)   Musculoskeletal pain: 800 mg PO tid-qid. [Trade only: Tabs 800 mg, scored.] ▶LK ♀? ▶? $$$

METHOCARBAMOL (Robaxin, Robaxin-750)   Acute musculoskeletal pain: 1500 mg PO qid or 1000 mg IM/IV tid × 48–72h. Maintenance: 1000 mg PO qid, 750 mg PO q4h, or 1500 mg PO tid. Tetanus: specialized dosing. [Generic/Trade: Tabs 500 & 750 mg. OTC in Canada.] ▶LK ♀C ▶? $$

ORPHENADRINE (Norflex)   Musculoskeletal pain: 100 mg PO bid. 60 mg IV/IM bid. [Generic only: 100 mg extended release. OTC in Canada.] ▶LK ♀C ▶? $$

TIZANIDINE (Zanaflex)   Muscle spasticity due to MS or spinal cord injury: 4–8 mg PO q6–8h prn, max 36 mg/d. [Generic/Trade: Tabs 4 mg, scored. Trade only: Caps 2, 4, 6 mg. Generic only: Tabs 2 mg.] ▶LK ♀C ▶? $$$$

Non-Opioid Analgesic Combinations

ASCRIPTIN (aspirin + aluminum hydroxide + magnesium hydroxide + calcium carbonate) (Aspir-Mox)   Multiple strengths. 1–2 tabs PO q4h. [OTC: Trade only: Tabs 325 mg ASA/50 mg Mg hydroxide/50 mg Al hydroxide/50 mg Ca carbonate (Ascriptin & Aspir-Mox). 500 mg ASA/33 mg Mg hydroxide/33 mg Al hydroxide/237 mg Ca carbonate (Ascriptin Max Strength).] ▶K ♀D ▶? $

BUFFERIN (aspirin + calcium carbonate + magnesium oxide + magnesium carbonate)   1–2 tabs/caplets PO q4h. Max 12 in 24h. [OTC: Trade only: Tabs/caplets 325 mg ASA/158 mg Ca carbonate/63 mg of Mg oxide/34 mg of Mg carbonate. Bufferin ES: 500 mg ASA/222.3 mg Ca carbonate/88.9 mg of Mg oxide/55.6 mg of Mg carbonate ▶K ♀D ▶? $

ESGIC (acetaminophen + butalbital + caffeine) 1–2 tabs or caps PO q4h. Max 6 in 24 h. [Generic only: Tabs/caps, 325 mg acetaminophen/50 mg butalbital/40 mg caffeine. Oral soln 325/50/40 mg per 15 mL. Generic/Trade: Tabs, Esgic Plus is 500/50/40 mg.] ▶LK ♀C ▶? $

EXCEDRIN MIGRAINE (acetaminophen + aspirin + caffeine) 2 tabs/caps/geltabs PO q6h while symptoms persist. Max 8 in 24 h. [OTC/Generic/Trade: Tabs/caplets/geltabs acetaminophen 250 mg/ASA 250 mg/caffeine 65 mg.] ▶LK ♀D ▶? $

FIORICET (acetaminophen + butalbital + caffeine) 1–2 tabs PO q4h. Max 6 in 24 h. [Generic/Trade: Tab 325 mg acetaminophen/50 mg butalbital/40 mg caffeine.] ▶LK ♀C ▶? $

FIORINAL (aspirin + butalbital + caffeine) (✚Tecnal, Trianal) 1–2 tabs PO q4h. Max 6 tabs in 24 h. [Generic/Trade: Cap 325 mg aspirin/50 mg butalbital/40 mg caffeine.] ▶KL ♀D ▶– ©III $

GOODY'S EXTRA STRENGTH HEADACHE POWDER (acetaminophen + aspirin + caffeine) One powder PO followed with liquid, or stir powder into a glass of water or other liquid. Repeat in 4–6 h prn. Max 4 powders in 24 h. [OTC trade only: 260 mg acetaminophen/520 mg ASA/32.5 mg caffeine per powder paper.] ▶LK ♀D ▶? $

NORGESIC (orphenadrine + aspirin + caffeine) Multiple strengths; write specific product on Rx. Norgesic: 1–2 tabs PO tid-qid. Norgesic Forte, 1 tab PO tid-qid. [Generic/Trade: Tabs Norgesic 25 mg orphenadrine/385 mg aspirin/30 mg caffeine. Norgesic Forte 50/770/60 mg.] ▶KL ♀D ▶? $

PHRENILIN (acetaminophen + butalbital) Tension or muscle contraction headache: 1–2 tabs PO q4h. Max 6 in 24 h. [Generic/Trade: Tabs, Phrenilin 325 mg acetaminophen/50 mg butalbital. Caps, Phrenilin Forte 650/50 mg.] ▶LK ♀C ▶? $

SEDAPAP (acetaminophen + butalbital) 1–2 tabs PO q4h. Max 6 tabs in 24 h. [Generic only: Tab 650 mg acetaminophen/50 mg butalbital.] ▶LK ♀C ▶? $

SOMA COMPOUND (carisoprodol + aspirin) 1–2 tabs PO qid. Abuse potential. [Generic/Trade: Tab 200 mg carisoprodol/325 mg ASA.] ▶LK ♀D ▶– $$$

ULTRACET (tramadol + acetaminophen) (✚Tramacet) Acute pain: 2 tabs PO q4–6h prn, max 8 tabs/d for ≤5 d. Adjust dose in elderly & renal dysfunction. Avoid in opioid-dependent patients. Seizures may occur if concurrent antidepressants or seizure disorder. [Generic/Trade: Tab 37.5 mg tramadol/325 mg acetaminophen.] ▶KL ♀C ▶– $$

Nonsteroidal Anti-Inflammatories—COX-2 Inhibitors

CELECOXIB (Celebrex) OA, ankylosing spondylitis: 200 mg PO daily or 100 mg PO bid. RA: 100–200 mg PO bid. Familial adenomatous polyposis: 400 mg PO bid with food. Acute pain, dysmenorrhea: 400 mg × 1, then 200 bid prn. An additional 200 mg dose may be given on d 1 if needed. JRA: 2–17 yo: 10–25 kg: 50 mg PO bid. >25 kg: 100 mg PO bid. Contraindicated in sulfonamide allergy. [Trade only: Caps 50, 100, 200, 400 mg.] ▶L ♀C (D in 3rd trimester) ▶? $$$$$

Nonsteroidal Anti-Inflammatories—Salicylic Acid Derivatives

ASPIRIN (*Ecotrin, Empirin, Halfprin, Bayer, Anacin, Zorprin, ASA*) (♣*Asaphen,* Entrophen, Novasen)   Analgesia: 325–650 mg PO/PR q4–6h. Platelet aggregation inhibition: 81–325 mg PO daily. [Generic/Trade: (OTC): tabs, 325, 500 mg; chewable 81 mg; enteric-coated 81,162 mg (Halfprin), 81, 325, 500 mg (Ecotrin), 650, 975 mg. Trade only: tabs, controlled-release 650, 800 mg (ZORprin, Rx). Generic only (OTC): supp 60, 120, 200, 300, 600 mg.] ▶K ♀D ▶? $

CHOLINE MAGNESIUM TRISALICYLATE (*Trilisate*)   1500 mg PO bid. [Generic only: Tabs 500, 750, 1000 mg. Solution 500 mg/5 mL.] ▶K ♀C (D in 3rd trimester) ▶? $$

DIFLUNISAL (*Dolobid*)   Pain: 500–1000 mg initially, then 250–500 mg PO q8–12h. RA/OA: 500 mg-1 g PO divided bid. [Generic/Trade: Tabs 250 & 500 mg.] ▶K ♀C (D in 3rd trimester) ▶- $$$

SALSALATE (*Salflex, Disalcid, Amigesic*)   3000 mg/d PO divided q8–12h. [Generic only: Tabs 500 & 750 mg, scored.] ▶K ♀C (D in 3rd trimester) ▶? $$

Nonsteroidal Anti-Inflammatories—Other

ARTHROTEC (diclofenac + misoprostol)   OA: one 50/200 tab PO tid. RA: one 50/200 tab PO tid-qid. If intolerant, may use 50/200 or 75/200 PO bid. Misoprostol is an abortifacient. [Trade only: Tabs 50/200, 75/200 mg diclofenac/mcg misoprostol.] ▶LK ♀X ▶- $$$$$

DICLOFENAC (*Voltaren, Voltaren XR, Cataflam, Flector, ♣Voltaren Rapide*)   Multiple strengths; write specific product on Rx. Immediate or delayed release 50 mg PO bid-tid or 75 mg PO bid. Extended release (Voltaren XR): 100–200 mg PO daily. Patch (Flector): Apply one patch to painful area bid. Gel: 2–4 g to affected area qid. [Generic/Trade: Tabs, immediate-release (Cataflam) 50 mg, extended-release (Voltaren XR) 100 mg. Generic only: Tabs, delayed-release 25, 50, 75 mg. Trade only: Patch (Flector) 1.3% diclofenac epolamine. Topical gel (Voltaren) 1% 100 g tube.] ▶L ♀B (D in 3rd trimester) ▶- $$$

ETODOLAC (♣*Ultradol*)   Multiple strengths; write specific product on Rx. Immediate release 200–400 mg PO bid-tid. Extended release: 400–1200 mg PO daily. [Generic only: Caps immediate-release 200, 300 mg, Tabs immediate-release 400, 500 mg, Tabs extended-release 400, 500, 600 mg.] ▶L ♀C (D in 3rd trimester) ▶- $$$

FLURBIPROFEN (*Ansaid, ♣Froben, Froben SR*)   200–300 mg/d PO divided bid-qid. [Generic/Trade: Tabs immediate-release 50 & 100 mg.] ▶L ♀B (D in 3rd trimester) ▶+ $$$

IBUPROFEN (*Motrin, Advil, Nuprin, Rufen, Neoprofen*)   200–800 mg PO tid-qid. Peds >6 mo: 5–10 mg/kg PO q6–8h. [OTC: Cap/Liqui-Gel Cap 200 mg. Tabs 100, 200 mg. Chewable tabs 50, 100 mg. Susp (infant drops) 50 mg/1.25 mL (with calibrated dropper) & 100 mg/5 mL. Rx Generic/Trade: Tabs 300, 400, 600, 800 mg.] ▶L ♀B (D in 3rd trimester) ▶+ $

INDOMETHACIN (*Indocin, Indocin SR, Indocin IV, ✦Indocid-P.D.A.*) Multiple strengths; write specific product on Rx. Immediate release preparations 25–50 mg cap PO tid. Sustained release: 75 mg cap PO daily-bid. [Generic/Trade: Cap, sustained-release 75 mg. Generic only: Caps, immediate-release 25, 50 mg, Supp 50 mg. Trade only: Oral susp 25 mg/5 mL (237 mL).] ▶L ♀B (D in 3rd trimester) ▶+ $

KETOPROFEN (*Orudis, Orudis KT, Actron, Oruvail, ✦Orudis SR*) Immediate release: 25–75 mg PO tid-qid. Extended release: 100–200 mg cap PO daily. [OTC: Tab, immediate-release 12.5 mg. Rx Generic only: Caps, extended-release 100, 150, 200 mg, Caps, immediate-release 25, 50, 75 mg.] ▶L ♀B (D in 3rd trimester) ▶- $$$

KETOROLAC (*Toradol*) Moderately severe acute pain: 15–30 mg IV/IM q6h or 10 mg PO q4–6h prn. Combined duration IV/IM and PO is not to exceed 5 d. [Generic only: Tab 10 mg.] ▶L ♀C (D in 3rd trimester) ▶+ $

MEFENAMIC ACID (*Ponstel, ✦Ponstan*) Mild to moderate pain, primary dysmenorrhea: 500 mg PO initially, then 250 mg PO q6h prn for ≤1 wk. [Trade only: Cap 250 mg.] ▶L ♀D ▶- $$$$

MELOXICAM (*Mobic, ✦Mobicox*) RA/OA: 7.5 mg PO daily. JRA, ≥2 yo: 0.125 mg/kg PO daily. [Generic/Trade: Tabs 7.5, 15 mg. Trade only: Susp 7.5 mg/5 mL (1.5 mg/mL).] ▶L ♀C (D in 3rd trimester) ▶? $

NABUMETONE (*Relafen*) RA/OA: Initial: two 500 mg tabs (1000 mg) PO daily. May increase to 1500–2000 mg PO daily or divided bid. [Generic only: Tabs 500 & 750 mg.] ▶L ♀C (D in 3rd trimester) ▶- $$$

NAPROXEN (*Naprosyn, Aleve, Anaprox, EC-Naprosyn, Naprelan*) Immediate release: 250–500 mg PO bid. Delayed release: 375–500 mg PO bid (do not crush or chew). Controlled release: 750–1000 mg PO daily. JRA ≤13 kg: 2.5 mL PO bid. 14–25 kg: 5 mL PO bid. 26–38 kg: 7.5 mL PO bid. 500 mg naproxen = 550 mg naproxen sodium. [OTC Generic/Trade (Aleve): Tab immediate-release 200 mg. OTC Trade only (Aleve): Caps & Gelcaps immediate-release 200 mg. Rx Generic/Trade: Tabs immediate-release (Naprosyn) 250, 375, 500 mg, (Anaprox) 275 mg, 550 mg. Tabs delayed-release enteric coated (EC-Naprosyn) 375, 500 mg. Tabs, controlled-release (Naprelan) 375, 500 mg. Susp (Naprosyn) 125 mg/5 mL.] ▶L ♀B (D in 3rd trimester) ▶+ $$$

OXAPROZIN (*Daypro*) 1200 mg PO daily. [Generic/Trade: Tabs 600 mg, trade scored.] ▶L ♀C (D in 3rd trimester) ▶- $$$

PIROXICAM (*Feldene, Fexicam*) 20 mg PO daily. [Generic/Trade: Caps 10 & 20 mg.] ▶L ♀B (D in 3rd trimester) ▶+ $$$

SULINDAC (*Clinoril*) 150–200 mg PO bid. [Generic/Trade: Tabs 200 mg. Generic only: Tabs 150 mg.] ▶L ♀C (D in 3rd trimester) ▶- $$$

NSAIDs — If one class fails, consider another. *Salicylic acid derivatives*: aspirin, diflunisal, salsalate, Trilisate. *Propionic acids*: flurbiprofen, ibuprofen, ketoprofen, naproxen, oxaprozin. *Acetic acids*: diclofenac, etodolac, indomethacin, ketorolac, nabumetone, sulindac, tolmetin. *Fenamates*: meclofenamate. *Oxicams*: meloxi-cam, piroxicam. *COX-2 inhibitors*: celecoxib.

TIAPROFENIC ACID (✚*Surgam, Surgam SR*)　Canada only. 600 mg PO daily of sustained release, or 300 mg PO bid of regular release. [Generic/Trade: Tab 300 mg. Trade only: Cap, sustained-release 300 mg. Generic only: Tab 200 mg.] ▶K ♀C (D in 3rd trimester) ▶- $$

TOLMETIN (*Tolectin*)　200–600 mg PO tid. [Generic/Trade: Tabs 200 (trade scored) & 600 mg. Cap 400 mg.] ▶L ♀C (D in 3rd trimester) ▶+ $$$$

Opioid Agonist-Antagonists

BUPRENORPHINE (*Buprenex, Subutex*)　Analgesia: 0.3–0.6 mg IV/IM q6h prn. Treatment of opioid dependence: Induction 8 mg SL on d 1, 16 mg SL on d 2. Maintenance: 16 mg SL daily. Can individualize to range of 4–24 mg SL daily. [Trade only (Subutex): SL tabs 2, 8 mg.] ▶L ♀C ▶- ©III $ IV, $$$$$ ©IV

BUTORPHANOL (*Stadol, Stadol NS*)　0.5–2 mg IV or 1–4 mg IM q3–4h prn. Nasal spray (Stadol NS): 1 spray (1 mg) in 1 nostril q3–4h. Abuse potential. [Generic only: Nasal spray 1 mg/spray, 2.5 mL bottle (14–15 doses/bottle).] ▶LK ♀C ▶+ ©IV $$$

NALBUPHINE (*Nubain*)　10–20 mg IV/IM/SC q3–6h prn. ▶LK ♀? ▶? $

PENTAZOCINE (*Talwin NX*)　30 mg IV/IM q3–4h prn (Talwin). 1 tab PO q3–4h. (Talwin NX = 50 mg pentazocine/0.5 mg naloxone). [Generic/Trade: Tab 50 mg with 0.5 mg naloxone, trade scored.] ▶LK ♀C ▶? ©IV $$$

Opioid Agonists

CODEINE　0.5–1 mg/kg up to 15–60 mg PO/IM/IV/SC q4–6h. Do not use IV in children. [Generic only: Tabs 15, 30, & 60 mg. Oral soln: 15 mg/5 mL.] ▶LK ♀C ▶- ©II $$

FENTANYL (*Duragesic, Actiq, Fentora, Sublimaze, IONSYS*)　Transdermal (Duragesic): 1 patch q72 h (some with chronic pain may require q48h dosing). May wear more than one patch to achieve the correct analgesic effect. Transmucosal lozenge (Actiq) for breakthrough cancer pain: 200–1600 mcg, goal is 4 lozenges on a stick/d in conjunction with long-acting opioid. Buccal tab (Fentora) for breakthrough cancer pain: 100–800 mcg, titrated to pain relief. Adult analgesia/procedural sedation: 50–100 mcg slow IV over 1–2 min; carefully titrate to effect. Analgesia: 50–100 mcg IM q1–2h prn. [Generic only: Transdermal patches 12.5, 25, 50, 75, 100 mcg/h. Actiq lozenges on a stick, berry flavored 200, 400, 600, 800, 1,200, 1,600 mcg. Trade only: IONSYS: Iontophoretic transdermal system: 40 mcg fentanyl per activation; max 6 doses per h. Max per system is eighty 40 mcg doses over 24 h. Trade only: (Fentora) buccal tab 100, 200, 300, 400, 600, 800 mcg.] ▶L ♀C ▶+ ©II $$$$$

HYDROMORPHONE (*Dilaudid, Dilaudid-5, ✚Hydromorph Contin*)　Adults: 2–4 mg PO q4–6h. Titrate dose as high as necessary to relieve cancer pain or other types of non-malignant pain where chronic opioids are used. 0.5–2 mg IM/SC or slow IV q4–6h. 3 mg PR q6–8h. Peds ≤12 yo: 0.03–0.08 mg/kg PO q4–6h prn. 0.015 mg/kg/dose IV q4–6h prn. [Generic only: Tabs 2, 4 mg. Generic/Trade: Tabs 8 mg (8 mg trade scored). Oral solution 5 mg/5 mL. Supp 3 mg.] ▶L ♀C ▶? ©II $$

Analgesics: Opioid Equivalency—Recommended starting dose - Adults >50 kg

	IV/SC/IM	PO		IV/SC/IM	PO
Opioid Agonists					
morphine	10 mg q3–4h	30 mg q3–4h	oxycodone	n.a.	10 mg q3–4h
codeine	60 mg q2h	60 mg q3–4h	oxymorphone	1 mg q3–4h	n.a.
fentanyl	0.1 mg q1h	n.a.	**Opioid Agonist-Antagonist and Partial Agonist**		
hydromor-phone	1.5 mg q3–4h	6 mg q3–4h	buprenorphine	0.4 mg q6–8h	n.a.
hydrocodone	n.a.	10 mg q3–4h	butorphanol	2 mg q3–4h	n.a.
levorphanol	2 mg q6–8h	4 mg q6–8h	nalbuphine	10 mg q3–4h	n.a.
meperidine§	100 mg q3h	n.r.	pentazocine	n.r.	50 mg q4–6h

§Doses should be limited to <600 mg/24 h and total duration of use <48 h; not for chronic pain. *Approximate dosing, adapted from 1992 AHCPR guidelines, www.ahcpr.gov. IV doses should be titrated slowly with appropriate monitoring. All PO dosing is with immediate-release preparations. Use lower doses initially in those not currently taking opioids. Individualize all dosing, especially in the elderly, children, and patients with chronic pain, opioid tolerance, or hepatic/renal insufficiency. Many recommend initially using lower than equivalent doses when switching between different opioids. Not available = n.a. Not recommended = n.r. Methadone is excluded due to poor consensus on equivalence.

LEVORPHANOL (Levo-Dromoran) 2 mg PO q6–8h prn. [Generic only: Tabs 2 mg, scored.] ▶L ♀C ▶? ©II $$$$

MEPERIDINE (Demerol, pethidine) 1–1.8 mg/kg up to 150 mg IM/SC/PO or slow IV q3–4h. 75 mg meperidine IV,IM,SC = 300 mg meperidine PO. [Generic/Trade: Tabs 50 (trade scored) & 100 mg. Syrup 50 mg/5 mL (trade banana flavored).] ▶LK ♀C but + ▶+ ©II $$$

METHADONE (Diskets, Dolophine, Methadose, ◆Metadol) Severe pain in opioid-tolerant patients: 2.5–10 mg IM/SC/PO q3–4h prn. Titrate dose as high as necessary to relieve cancer pain or other types of non-malignant pain where chronic opioids are necessary. Opioid dependence: 20–100 mg PO daily. Treatment >3 wk is maintenance and only permitted in approved treatment programs. [Generic/Trade: Tabs 5, 10 mg, Dispersible tabs 40 mg (for opioid dependence only). Oral concentrate (intensol): 10 mg/mL. Generic only: Oral soln 5 & 10 mg/5 mL.] ▶L ♀C ▶? ©II $

FENTANYL TRANSDERMAL DOSE (Dosing based on ongoing morphine requirement.)

Morphine* (IV/IM)	Morphine* (PO)	Transdermal fentanyl*
10–22 mg/d	60–134 mg/d	25 mcg/h
23–37 mg/d	135–224 mg/d	50 mcg/h
38–52 mg/d	225–314 mg/d	75 mcg/h
53–67 mg/d	315–404 mg/d	100 mcg/h

*For higher morphine doses see product insert for transdermal fentanyl equivalencies.

MORPHINE (*MS Contin, Kadian, Avinza, Roxanol, Oramorph SR, MSIR, DepoDur, ✦Statex, M.O.S., Doloral*)   Controlled-release tabs (MS Contin, Oramorph SR): Start at 30 mg PO q8–12h. Controlled-release caps (Kadian): 20 mg PO q12–24h. Extended-release caps (Avinza): Start at 30 mg PO daily. Do not break, chew, or crush MS Contin or Oramorph SR. Kadian & Avinza caps may be opened & sprinkled in applesauce for easier administration, however the pellets should not be crushed or chewed. 0.1–0.2 mg/kg up to 15 mg IM/SC or slow IV q4h. Titrate dose as high as necessary to relieve cancer pain or other types of non-malignant pain where chronic opioids are necessary. [Generic/Trade: Tabs, immediate-release 15 & 30 mg. Oral soln: 10 mg/5 mL, 20 mg/5 mL, 20 mg/mL (concentrate). Rectal suppositories 5, 10, 20 & 30 mg. Controlled-release tabs (MS Contin) 15, 30, 60, 100, 200 mg. Trade only: Controlled-release caps (Kadian) 10, 20, 30, 50, 60, 80, 100, 200 mg., Controlled-release caps (Oramorph SR) 15, 30, 60, 100 mg. Extended-release caps (Avinza) 30, 60, 90 & 120 mg. Generic only: Tabs, immediate-release 10 mg.] ▶LK ♀C ▶+ ⊚II $$$$
OXYCODONE (*Roxicodone, OxyContin, Percolone, OxyIR, OxyFAST, ✦Endocodone, Supeudol*)   Immediate-release preparations: 5 mg PO q4–6h prn. Controlled-release (OxyContin): 10–40 mg PO q12h (No supporting data for shorter dosing intervals for controlled-release tabs.) Titrate dose as high as necessary to relieve cancer pain or other types of non-malignant pain where chronic opioids are necessary. Do not break, chew, or crush controlled release preparations. [Generic/Trade: Immediate-release: Tabs (scored) & caps 5 mg. Tabs 15, 30 mg. Oral soln 5 mg/5 mL. Oral concentrate 20 mg/mL. Generic only: Immediate release tabs 10, 20 mg. Trade only: Controlled-release tabs: 10, 15, 20, 30, 40, 60, 80 mg.] ▶L ♀C ▶– ⊚II $$$$$
OXYMORPHONE (*Opana*)   10–20 mg PO q4–6h (immediate release) or 5 mg q12h (extended release) in opioid-naive patients, 1 h before or 2 h after meals. 1–1.5 mg IM/SC q4–6h prn. 0.5 mg IV q4–6h prn, increase dose until pain adequately controlled. [Trade only: Extended release tabs (Opana ER) 5, 7.5, 10, 15, 20, 30, 40 mg, Immediate release tabs (Opana IR) 5, 10 mg.] ▶L ♀C ▶? ⊚II $$$$
PROPOXYPHENE (*Darvon-N, Darvon Pulvules*)   65–100 mg PO q4h prn. [Generic/Trade: Caps 65 mg. Trade only: Tabs 100 mg (Darvon-N).] ▶L ♀C ▶+ ⊚IV $$

Opioid Analgesic Combinations

NOTE See individual components for more information. May cause drowsiness and/or sedation, which may be enhanced by alcohol & other CNS depressants. Opioids, carisoprodol, butalbital may be habit-forming. Avoid exceeding 4 g/d of acetaminophen in combination products. Caution people who drink ≥ 3 alcoholic drinks/d to limit acetaminophen to 2.5 g/d due to additive liver toxicity. Opioids commonly cause constipation - concurrent laxatives recommended. All are pregnancy class D if used for prolonged periods or in high doses at term.

ANEXSIA (hydrocodone + acetaminophen)   Multiple strengths; write specific product on Rx. 1 tab PO q4–6h prn. [Generic/Trade: Tabs 5/325, 5/500,

(cont.)

7.5/325, 7.5/650, 10/750 mg hydrocodone/mg acetaminophen, scored.] ▶LK ♀C ▶- ©III $$

CAPITAL WITH CODEINE SUSP (acetaminophen + codeine) 15 mL PO q4h prn. >12 yo use adult dose. 7–12 yo 10 mL/dose q4–6h prn. 3–6 yo 5 mL/dose q4–6h prn. [Generic = oral soln. Trade = susp. Both codeine 12 mg and acetaminophen 120 mg per 5 mL (trade, fruit punch flavor).] ▶LK ♀C ▶? ©V $

COMBUNOX (oxycodone + ibuprofen) 1 tab PO q6h prn for ≤7 d. Max 4 tabs/24h. [Generic/Trade: Tab 5 mg oxycodone/400 mg ibuprofen.] ▶L ♀C (D in 3rd trimester) ▶? ©II $$

DARVOCET (propoxyphene + acetaminophen) Multiple strengths; write specific product on Rx. 50/325, 2 tabs PO q4h prn. 100/500 or 100/650, 1 tab PO q4h prn. [Generic/Trade: Tabs 50/325 (Darvocet N-50), 100/650 (Darvocet N-100), & 100/500 (Darvocet A500), mg propoxyphene/mg acetaminophen.] ▶L ♀C ▶+ ©IV $$

EMPIRIN WITH CODEINE (aspirin + codeine) (➧ *292 tab*) Multiple strengths; write specific product on Rx.1–2 tabs PO q4h prn. [Generic only: Tabs 325/30 & 325/60 mg ASA/mg codeine. Empirin brand no longer made.] ▶LK ♀D ▶- ©III $

FIORICET WITH CODEINE (acetaminophen + butalbital + caffeine + codeine) 1–2 caps PO q4h prn. Max 6 caps/24h. [Generic/Trade: Cap 325 mg acetaminophen/50 mg butalbital/40 mg caffeine/30 mg codeine.] ▶LK ♀C ▶- ©III $$$

FIORINAL WITH CODEINE (aspirin + butalbital + caffeine + codeine) (➧ *Fiorinal C-1/4, Fiorinal C-1/2, Tecnal C-1/4, Tecnal C-1/2*) 1–2 caps PO q4h prn. Max 6 caps/24h. [Generic/Trade: Cap 325 mg ASA/50 mg butalbital /40 mg caffeine/30 mg codeine.] ▶LK ♀D ▶- ©III $$$

IBUDONE (hydrocodone + ibuprofen) 1 tab PO q4–6h prn, max dose 5 tabs/d. [Generic/Trade: Tab 5/200 mg and 10/200 mg hydrocodone/ ibuprofen.] ▶LK ♀- ▶? ©III $$$

LORCET (hydrocodone + acetaminophen) 1–2 caps (5/500) PO q4–6h prn, max dose 8 caps/d. 1 tab PO q4–6h prn (7.5/650 & 10/650), max dose 6 tabs/d. [Generic/Trade: Caps 5/500 mg, Tabs 7.5/650, 10/650 mg hydrocodone/acetaminophen.] ▶LK ♀C ▶- ©III $

LORTAB (hydrocodone + acetaminophen) 1–2 tabs 2.5/500 & 5/500 PO q4–6h prn, max dose 8 tabs/d. 1 tab 7.5/500 & 10/500 PO q4–6h prn, max dose 5 tabs/d. Elixir 15 mL PO q4–6h prn, max 6 doses/d. [Generic/ Trade: Lortab 5/500 (scored), Lortab 7.5/500 (trade scored) & Lortab 10/500 mg hydrocodone/ mg acetaminophen. Elixir: 7.5/500 mg hydrocodone/mg acetaminophen/15 mL. Trade only: Tabs 2.5/500 mg.] ▶LK ♀C ▶- ©III $$

MAXIDONE (hydrocodone + acetaminophen) 1 tab PO q4–6h prn, max dose 5 tabs/d. [Trade only: Tab 10/750 mg hydrocodone/mg acetaminophen.] ▶LK ♀C ▶- ©III $$$

MERSYNDOL WITH CODEINE (acetaminophen + codeine + doxylamine) Canada only. 1–2 tabs PO q4–6h prn. Max 12 tabs/24 h. [Trade only: OTC tab acetaminophen 325 mg + codeine phosphate 8 mg + doxylamine 5 mg.] ▶LK ♀C ▶? $

NORCO (hydrocodone + acetaminophen) 1–2 tabs PO q4–6h prn (5/325), max dose 12 tabs/d. 1 tab (7.5/325 & 10/325) PO q4–6h prn, max dose 8 & 6 tabs/d, respectively. [Trade only: Tabs 5/325, 7.5/325 & 10/325 mg hydrocodone/acetaminophen, scored.] ▶L ♀C ▶? ©III $$$

PERCOCET (oxycodone + acetaminophen) (✦*Percocet-demi, Oxycocet, Endocet*) Multiple strengths; write specific product on Rx. 1–2 tabs PO q4–6h prn (2.5/325 & 5/325). 1 tab PO q4–6 prn (7.5/500 & 10/650). [Trade only: Tabs 2.5/325 oxycodone/acetaminophen. Generic/Trade: Tabs 5/325, 7.5/325, 7.5/500, 10/325, 10/650 mg. Generic only: 2.5/300, 5/300, 7.5/300, 10/300, 2.5/400, 5/400, 7.5/400, 10/400, 10/500 mg.] ▶L ♀C ▶– ©II $

PERCODAN (oxycodone + aspirin) (✦*Oxycodan, Endodan*) 1 tab PO q6h prn. [Generic/Trade: Tab 4.88/325 mg oxycodone/ASA (trade scored).] ▶LK ♀D ▶– ©II $$

ROXICET (oxycodone + acetaminophen) Multiple strengths; write specific product on Rx. 1 tab PO q6h prn. Soln: 5 mL PO q6h prn. [Generic/Trade: Tab 5/325 mg. Cap/Caplet 5/500 mg. Soln 5/325 per 5 mL, mg oxycodone/acetaminophen.] ▶L ♀C ▶– ©II $

SOMA COMPOUND WITH CODEINE (carisoprodol + aspirin + codeine) Moderate to severe musculoskeletal pain:1–2 tabs PO qid prn. [Generic/Trade: Tab 200 mg carisoprodol/325 mg ASA/16 mg codeine.] ▶L ♀D ▶– ©III $$$

SYNALGOS-DC (dihydrocodeine + aspirin + caffeine) 2 caps PO q4h prn. [Trade only: Cap 16 mg dihydrocodeine/356.4 mg ASA/30 mg caffeine. "Painpack"=12 caps.] ▶L ♀C ▶– ©III $

TALACEN (pentazocine + acetaminophen) 1 tab PO q4h prn. [Generic/Trade: Tab 25 mg pentazocine/650 mg acetaminophen, trade scored.] ▶L ♀C ▶? ©IV $$$

TYLENOL WITH CODEINE (codeine + acetaminophen) (✦*Lenoltec, Emtec, Triatec*) Multiple strengths; write specific product on Rx. 1–2 tabs PO q4h prn. Elixir 3–6 yo 5 mL/dose. 7–12 yo 10 mL/dose q4–6h prn. [Generic only: Tabs Tylenol #2 (15/300). Tylenol with Codeine Elixir 12/120 per 5 mL, mg codeine/mg acetaminophen. Generic/Trade: Tabs Tylenol #3 (30/300), Tylenol #4 (60/300). Canadian forms come with (Lenoltec, Tylenol) or without (Empracet, Emtec) caffeine.] ▶LK ♀C ▶– ©III $

TYLOX (oxycodone + acetaminophen) 1 cap PO q6h prn. [Generic/Trade: Cap 5 mg oxycodone/500 mg acetaminophen.] ▶L ♀C ▶– ©II $

VICODIN (hydrocodone + acetaminophen) 5/500 (max dose 8 tabs/d) & 7.5/750 (max dose of 5 tabs/d): 1–2 tabs PO q4–6h prn. 10/660: 1 tab PO q4–6h prn (max of 6 tabs/d). [Generic/Trade: Tabs Vicodin (5/500), Vicodin ES (7.5/750), Vicodin HP (10/660), scored, mg hydrocodone/mg acetaminophen.] ▶LK ♀C ▶? ©III $

VICOPROFEN (hydrocodone + ibuprofen) 1 tab PO q4–6h prn, max dose 5 tabs/d. [Generic/Trade: Tab 7.5/200 mg hydrocodone/ibuprofen. Generic only: Tab 2.5/200, 5/200, 10/200 mg.] ▶LK ♀– ▶? ©III $$$

WYGESIC (propoxyphene + acetaminophen) 1 tab PO q4h prn. [Generic only: Tab 65 mg propoxyphene/650 mg acetaminophen.] ▶L ♀C ▶– ©IV $

XODOL (hydrocodone + acetaminophen)   1 tab PO q4–6 prn, max 6 doses/d. [Trade only: Tabs 5/300, 7.5/300, 10/300 mg hydrocodone/acetaminophen.] ▶LK ♀C ▶- ©III $$

ZYDONE (hydrocodone + acetaminophen)   1–2 tabs (5/400) PO q4–6h prn, max dose 8 tabs/d. 1 tab (7.5/400, 10/400) q4–6h prn, max dose 6 tabs/d. [Trade only: Tabs 5/400, 7.5/400, & 10/400 mg hydrocodone/mg acetaminophen.] ▶LK ♀C ▶? ©III $$

Opioid Antagonists

NALOXONE (Narcan)   Adult opioid overdose: 0.4–2 mg q2–3 min prn. Adult post-op reversal 0.1–0.2 mg q2–3 min prn. Peds opioid overdose 0.01 mg/kg IV; may give 0.1 mg/kg if inadequate response. Peds post-op reversal: 0.005–0.01 mg q2–3 min prn. May use IM/SC/ET if IV not available.   ▶LK ♀B ▶? $

Other Analgesics

ACETAMINOPHEN (Tylenol, Panadol, Tempra, Paracetamol, ✦Abenol, Atasol, Pediatrix)   325–650 mg PO/PR q4–6h prn. Max dose 4 g/d. OA: 2 extended release caplets (ie, 1300 mg) PO q8h around the clock. Peds: 10–15 mg/kg/dose PO/PR q4–6h prn. [OTC: Tabs 325, 500, 650 mg. Chewable Tabs 80 mg. Oral disintegrating Tabs 80, 160 mg. Caps/Gelcaps/Caplet 500 mg. Extended-release caplets 650 mg. Liquid 160 mg/5 mL & 500 mg/15 mL. Infant drops 80 mg/0.8 mL. Suppositories 80, 120, 325, & 650 mg.] ▶LK ♀B ▶+ $

TRAMADOL (Ultram, Ultram ER)   Moderate to moderately severe pain: 50–100 mg PO q4–6h prn, max 400 mg/d. Chronic pain, extended release: 100–300 mg PO daily. Adjust dose in elderly, renal & hepatic dysfunction. Avoid in opioid-dependent patients. Seizures may occur with concurrent antidepressants or seizure disorder. [Generic/Trade: Tab, immediate-release 50 mg. Trade only: Extended release tabs 100, 200, 300 mg.] ▶KL ♀C ▶- $$$

WOMEN'S TYLENOL MENSTRUAL RELIEF (acetaminophen + pamabrom)   2 caplets PO q4–6h. [OTC: Caplet 500 mg acetaminophen/25 mg pamabrom (diuretic).] ▶LK ♀B ▶+ $

ANESTHESIA

Anesthetics & Sedatives

DEXMEDETOMIDINE (Precedex)   ICU sedation <24h: Load 1 mcg/kg over 10 min followed by infusion 0.2–0.7 mcg/kg/h titrated to desired sedation endpoint. Beware of bradycardia and hypotension. ▶LK ♀C ▶? $$$$

ETOMIDATE (Amidate)   Induction 0.3 mg/kg IV. ▶L ♀C ▶? $

KETAMINE (Ketalar)   1–2 mg/kg IV over 1–2 min or 4 mg/kg IM induces 10–20 min dissociative state. Concurrent atropine minimizes hypersalivation. ▶L ♀? ▶? ©III $

METHOHEXITAL (*Brevital*) Induction 1–1.5 mg/kg IV, duration 5 min. ▶L ♀B ▶? ©IV $

MIDAZOLAM (*Versed*) Adult sedation/anxiolysis: 5 mg or 0.07 mg/kg IM; or 1 mg IV slowly q2–3 min up to 5 mg. Peds: 0.25–1.0 mg/kg to max of 20 mg PO, or 0.1–0.15 mg/kg IM. IV route (6 mo to 5 yo): Initial dose 0.05–0.1 mg/kg IV, then titrated to max 0.6 mg/kg. IV route (6–12 yo): Initial dose 0.025–0.05 mg/kg IV, then titrated to max 0.4 mg/kg. Monitor for respiratory depression. [Oral liquid 2 mg/mL.] ▶LK ♀D ▶- ©IV $

PENTOBARBITAL (*Nembutal*) Pediatric sedation: 1–6 mg/kg IV, adjusted in increments of 1–2 mg/kg to desired effect, or 2–6 mg/kg IM, max 100 mg. ▶LK ♀D ▶? ©II $$

PROPOFOL (*Diprivan*) 40 mg IV q10sec until induction (2–2.5 mg/kg). ICU ventilator sedation: infusion 5–50 mcg/kg/min. ▶L ♀B ▶- $$$

THIOPENTAL (*Pentothal*) Induction 3–5 mg/kg IV, duration 5 min. ▶L ♀C ▶? ©III $

Local Anesthetics

ARTICAINE (*Septocaine, Zorcaine*) 4% injection (includes epinephrine). [4% (includes epinephrine 1:100,000) ▶LK ♀C ▶? $

BUPIVACAINE (*Marcaine, Sensorcaine*) Local and regional anesthesia. [0.25%, 0.5%, 0.75%, all with or without epinephrine.] ▶LK ♀C ▶? $

DUOCAINE (bupivacaine + lidocaine—local anesthetic) Local anesthesia, nerve block for eye surgery. [Vials contain bupivacaine 0.375% + lidocaine 1%.] ▶LK ♀C ▶? $

LIDOCAINE—LOCAL ANESTHETIC (*Xylocaine*) 0.5–1% injection with and without epinephrine. [0.5,1,1.5,2%. With epi: 0.5,1,1.5,2%.] ▶LK ♀B ▶? $

MEPIVACAINE (*Carbocaine, Polocaine*) 1–2% injection. [1,1.5,2,3%.] ▶LK ♀C ▶? $

Neuromuscular Blockers

ROCURONIUM (*Zemuron*) 0.6 mg/kg IV. Duration 30 min. ▶L ♀B ▶? $$

SUCCINYLCHOLINE (*Anectine, Quelicin*) 0.6–1.1 mg/kg IV. Peds: 2 mg/kg IV. ▶Plasma ♀C ▶? $

VECURONIUM (*Norcuron*) 0.08–0.1 mg/kg IV. Duration 15–30 min. ▶LK ♀C ▶? $

ANTIMICROBIALS

Aminoglycosides

NOTE *See also dermatology and ophthalmology.*

AMIKACIN (*Amikin*) 15 mg/kg up to 1500 mg/d IM/IV divided q8–12h. Peak 20–35 mcg/mL, trough <5 mcg/mL. Alternative 15 mg/kg IV q24h. ▶K ♀D ▶? $$$

GENTAMICIN (*Garamycin*) Adults: 3–5 mg/kg/d IM/IV divided q8h. Peak 5–10 mcg/mL, trough <2 mcg/mL. Alternative 5–7 mg/kg IV q24h. Peds: 2–2.5 mg/kg q8h. ▶K ♀D ▶+ $

STREPTOMYCIN Combo therapy for TB: 15 mg/kg up to 1 g IM daily. 10 mg/kg up to 750 mg if >59 yo. Peds: 20–40 mg/kg up to 1 g IM daily. Nephrotoxicity, ototoxicity. ▶K ♀D ▶+ $$$$$

TOBRAMYCIN (*Nebcin, TOBI*) Adults: 3–5 mg/kg/d IM/IV divided q8h. Peak 5–10 mcg/mL, trough <2 mcg/mL. Alternative 5–7 mg/kg IV q24h. Peds: 2–2.5 mg/kg q8h. Cystic fibrosis (TOBI): 300 mg neb bid 28 d on, then 28 d off. [Trade only: TOBI 300 mg ampules for nebulizer.] ▶K ♀D ▶? $$

Antifungal Agents—Azoles

CLOTRIMAZOLE (*Mycelex, ✦Canesten, Clotrimaderm*) Oral troches 5 ×/d × 14 d. [Generic/Trade: Oral troches 10 mg.] ▶L ♀C ▶? $$$$$

FLUCONAZOLE (*Diflucan*) Vaginal candidiasis: 150 mg PO single dose ($). All other dosing regimens IV/PO. Oropharyngeal/ esophageal candidiasis: 200 mg first d, then 100 mg daily. Systemic candidiasis, cryptococcal meningitis: 400 mg daily. Peds: Oropharyngeal/esophageal candidiasis: 6 mg/kg first d, then 3 mg/kg daily. Systemic candidiasis: 6–12 mg/kg daily. Cryptococcal meningitis: 12 mg/kg on first d, then 6 mg/kg daily. [Generic/Trade: Tabs 50, 100, 150, 200 mg. 150 mg tab in single-dose blister pack. Susp 10 & 40 mg/mL (35 mL).] ▶K ♀C ▶+ $$$$

ITRACONAZOLE (*Sporanox*) Oral caps for onychomycosis "pulse dosing": 200 mg PO bid for 1st wk of mo × 2 mo (fingernails) or 3–4 mo (toenails). Oral soln for oropharyngeal or esophageal candidiasis: 100–200 mg PO daily or 100 mg bid swish & swallow in 10 mL increments on empty stomach. For life-threatening infections, load with 200 mg PO tid × 3 d. Contraindicated with cisapride, dofetilide, ergot alkaloids, lovastatin, PO midazolam, pimozide, quinidine, simvastatin, triazolam. Negative inotrope; do not use for onychomycosis if ventricular dysfunction. [Generic/Trade: Cap 100 mg. Trade only: Oral soln 10 mg/mL (150 mL).] ▶L ♀C ▶- $$$$$

KETOCONAZOLE (*Nizoral*) 200–400 mg PO daily. Hepatotoxicity. Contraindicated with cisapride, midazolam, pimozide, triazolam. H2 blockers, proton pump inhibitors, antacids impair absorption. [Generic/Trade: Tabs 200 mg.] ▶L ♀C ▶? + $$$

POSACONAZOLE (*Noxafil*) Prevention of invasive Aspergillus or Candida infection, ≥13 yo: 200 mg (5 mL) PO tid. Take with full meal or liquid nutritional supplement. CYP 3A4 inhibitor. [Trade only: Oral susp 40 mg/mL, 105 mL bottle.] ▶Glucuronidation ♀C ▶- $$$$$

VORICONAZOLE (*Vfend*) IV: 6 mg/kg q12h × 2, then 3–4 mg/kg IV q12h (use 4 mg/kg for non-candidal infections). Infuse over 2 h. PO: 200 mg q12h if >40 kg, 100 mg PO q12 h if <40 kg. Take 1 h before/after meals. With efavirenz: Use voriconazole 400 mg PO bid & efavirenz 300 mg PO once daily. Treat esophageal candidiasis with oral regimen for ≥2 wk & continuing for >1 wk past symptom resolution. Treat systemic candidal infections for ≥2 wk past symptom resolution or last positive culture, whichever is longer. Treat invasive pulmonary aspergillosis for ≥6–12 wk; treat immunosuppressed patients throughout immunosuppression and until lesions resolved. Many drug interactions. [Trade only: Tabs 50,200 mg (contains lactose), susp 40 mg/mL (75 mL).] ▶L ♀D ▶? $$$$$

Antifungal Agents—Echinocandins

ANIDULAFUNGIN (*Eraxis*) Candidemia: 200 mg IV load on d 1, then 100 mg IV once daily. Esophageal candidiasis: 100 mg IV load on d 1, then 50 mg IV once daily. Max infusion rate of 1.1 mg/min to prevent histamine reactions. ▶Degraded chemically ♀C ▶? $$$$$

CASPOFUNGIN (*Cancidas*) Infuse over 1 h. 70 mg loading dose on d 1, then 50 mg once daily. Peds: 70 mg/m2 loading dose on d 1, then 50 mg/m2 once daily (max of 70 mg/d). ▶KL ♀C ▶? $$$$$

MICAFUNGIN (*Mycamine*) Infuse IV over 1 h. Esophageal candidiasis: 150 mg once daily. Prevention of candidal infections in bone marrow transplant patients: 50 mg once daily. Candidemia, acute disseminated candidiasis, Candida peritonitis/ abscess: 100 mg once daily. ▶L, feces ♀C ▶? $$$$$

Antifungal Agents—Polyenes

AMPHOTERICIN B DEOXYCHOLATE (*Fungizone*) Test dose 0.1 mg/kg up to 1 mg slow IV. Wait 2–4 h, and if tolerated then begin 0.25 mg/kg IV daily and advance to 0.5–1.5 mg/kg/d depending on fungal type. Max dose 1.5 mg/kg/d. ▶Tissues ♀B ▶? $$$$

AMPHOTERICIN B LIPID FORMULATIONS (*Amphotec, Abelcet, AmBisome*) Abelcet: 5 mg/kg/d IV at 2.5 mg/kg/h. AmBisome: 3–5 mg/kg/d IV over 2 h. Amphotec: Test dose of 10 mL over 15–30 min, observe for 30 min, then 3–4 mg/kg/d IV at 1 mg/kg/h. ▶? ♀B ▶? $$$$$

Antifungal Agents—Other

FLUCYTOSINE (*Ancobon*) 50–150 mg/kg/d PO divided qid. Myelosuppression. [Trade only: Caps 250, 500 mg.] ▶K ♀C ▶- $$$$$

GRISEOFULVIN (*Grifulvin V, ✦Fulvicin*) Tinea capitis: 500 mg PO daily in adults; 15–20 mg/kg up to 1 g PO daily in peds. Treat × 4–6 wk, continuing for 2 wk past symptom resolution. [Generic/Trade: Susp 125 mg/5 mL (120 mL), Tabs 500 mg.] ▶Skin ♀C ▶? $$$$

NYSTATIN (*Mycostatin, ✦Nilstat, Nyaderm, Candistatin*) Thrush: 4–6 mL PO swish & swallow qid. Infants: 2 mL/dose with 1 mL in each cheek qid. [Generic only: Susp 100,000 units/mL (60 & 480 mL).] ▶Not absorbed ♀B ▶? $$

TERBINAFINE (*Lamisil*) Onychomycosis: 250 mg PO daily × 6 wk for fingernails, × 12 wk for toenails. "Pulse dosing": 500 mg PO daily for first wk of mo × 2 mo (fingernails) or 4 mo (toenails). Tinea capitis, ≥4 yo: Give granules once daily with food × 6 wk: 125 mg if <25 kg, 187.5 mg if 25–35 kg, 250 mg if >35 kg. [Generic/Trade: Tabs 250 mg. Trade only: Oral granules 125 & 187.5 mg/packet.] ▶LK ♀B ▶- $

Antimalarials

NOTE For help treating malaria or getting antimalarials, see www.cdc.gov/malaria or call the CDC "malaria hotline" (770) 488–7788 Monday-Friday 8 am to 4:30 pm EST; after h / weekend (770) 488–7100. Pediatric doses of antimalarials should never exceed adult doses.

CHLOROQUINE (*Aralen*) Malaria prophylaxis, chloroquine-sensitive areas: 8 mg/kg up to 500 mg PO q wk from 1–2 wk before exposure to 4 wk after. Chloroquine resistance widespread. [Generic only: Tabs 250 mg. Generic/Trade: Tabs 500 mg (500 mg phosphate equivalent to 300 mg base).] ▶KL ♀C but + ▶+ $

MALARONE (atovaquone + proguanil) Prevention of malaria: 1 adult tab PO daily from 1–2 d before exposure until 7 d after. Treatment of malaria: 4 adult tabs PO daily × 3 d. Take with food or milky drink. [Trade only: Adult tabs atovaquone 250 mg + proguanil 100 mg; pediatric tabs 62.5 mg + 25 mg.] ▶Fecal excretion; LK ♀C ▶? $$$$

MEFLOQUINE (*Lariam*) Malaria prophylaxis for chloroquine-resistant areas: 250 mg PO q wk from 1 wk before exposure to 4 wk after. Treatment: 1250 mg PO single dose. Peds. Malaria prophylaxis: Give PO once weekly starting 1 wk before exposure to 4 wk after: <15 kg, 5 mg/kg (prepared by pharmacist); 15–19 kg, ¼ tab; 20–30 kg, ½ tab; 31–45 kg, ¾ tab; >45 kg, 1 tab. Treatment: 20–25 mg/kg PO; can divide into 2 doses given 6–8 h apart. Take on full stomach. [Generic/Trade: Tabs 250 mg.] ▶L ♀C ▶? $$

PRIMAQUINE (Prevention of relapse): P vivax/ovale malaria: 0.5 mg/kg up to 30 mg base PO daily × 14 d. Do not use unless normal G6PD level. [Generic only: Tabs 26.3 mg (equiv to 15 mg base).] ▶L ♀- ▶- $$

QUININE (*Qualaquin*) Malaria: 648 mg PO tid. Peds: 25–30 mg/kg/d up to 2 g/d PO divided q8h. Treat for 3 d (Africa/South America) or 7 d (Southeast Asia). Also give 7-d course of doxycycline, tetracycline or clindamycin. Commonly prescribed for nocturnal leg cramps, but not FDA approved for this indication: 260–325 mg PO qhs. FDA believes risks outweigh benefits for this indication. Can cause life-threatening adverse effects: Cinchonism with overdose; hemolysis with G6PD deficiency; hypersensitivity; thrombocytopenia; QT interval prolongation possible; many drug interactions. [Trade only: Caps 324 mg. Unapproved quinine products removed from US market by Feb 2007 with interstate shipment to cease by June 2007.] ▶L ♀C ▶+? $

Antimycobacterial Agents

NOTE *Two or more drugs are needed for the treatment of active mycobacterial infections. See guidelines at http://www.thoracic.org/sections/publications/statements/.*

DAPSONE (*Aczone*) Pneumocystis prophylaxis, leprosy: 100 mg PO daily. Pneumocystis treatment: 100 mg PO daily with trimethoprim 5 mg/kg PO tid × 21 d. Acne (Aczone): Apply bid. [Generic only: Tabs 25,100 mg. Trade only (Aczone): gel 5% 30 g.] ▶LK ♀C ▶- $

ETHAMBUTOL (*Myambutol*, ◆*Etibi*) 15–20 mg/kg PO daily. Dose with whole tabs: Give PO daily 800 mg if 40–55 kg, 1200 mg if 56–75 kg, 1600 mg if 76–90 kg. Base dose on estimated lean body weight. Peds: 15–20 mg/kg up to 1 g PO daily. [Generic/Trade: Tabs 100, 400 mg.] ▶LK ♀C but + ▶+ $$$$

ISONIAZID (*INH*, ◆*Isotamine*) Adults: 5 mg/kg up to 300 mg PO daily. Peds: 10–15 mg/kg up to 300 mg PO daily. Hepatotoxicity. Consider supplemental pyridoxine 10–50 mg PO daily. [Generic only: Tabs 100,300 mg, syrup 50 mg/5 mL.] ▶LK ♀C but + ▶+ $

PYRAZINAMIDE (*PZA*, ✦*Tebrazid*) 20–25 mg/kg up to 2000 mg PO daily. Dose with whole tabs: Give PO daily 1000 mg if 40–55 kg, 1500 mg if 56–75 kg, 2000 mg if 76–90 kg. Base dose on estimated lean body weight. Peds: 15–30 mg/kg up to 2000 mg PO daily. Hepatotoxicity. [Generic only: Tabs 500 mg.] ▶LK ♀C ▶? $$$$

RIFABUTIN (*Mycobutin*) 300 mg PO daily or 150 mg PO bid. [Trade only: Caps 150 mg.] ▶L ♀B ▶? $$$$$

RIFAMATE (isoniazid + rifampin) 2 caps PO daily on empty stomach. [Generic/Trade: Caps isoniazid 150 mg + rifampin 300 mg.] ▶LK ♀C but + ▶+ $$$$

RIFAMPIN (*Rimactane, Rifadin*, ✦*Rofact*) TB: 10 mg/kg up to 600 mg PO/IV daily. Peds: 10–20 mg/kg up to 600 mg PO/IV daily. IV and PO doses are the same. Take oral doses on empty stomach. Neisseria meningitidis carriers: 600 mg PO bid × 2 d. Peds: age ≥1 mo, 10 mg/kg up to 600 mg PO bid × 2 d. Age <1 mo, 5 mg/kg PO bid × 2 d. IV & PO doses are the same. [Generic/Trade: Caps 150,300 mg. Pharmacists can make oral susp.] ▶L ♀C but + ▶+ $$$

RIFAPENTINE (*Priftin*) 600 mg PO twice weekly × 2 mo, then once weekly × 4 mo. Use for continuation therapy only in selected HIV-negative patients. [Trade only: Tabs 150 mg.] ▶Esterases, fecal ♀C ▶? $$$$

RIFATER (isoniazid + rifampin + pyrazinamide) 6 tabs PO daily if ≥55 kg, 5 daily if 45–54 kg, 4 daily if ≤44 kg. [Trade only: Tab Isoniazid 50 mg + rifampin 120 mg + pyrazinamide 300 mg.] ▶LK ♀C ▶? $$$$$

Antiparasitics

ALBENDAZOLE (*Albenza*) Hydatid disease, neurocysticercosis: 400 mg PO bid. 15 mg/kg/d up to 800 mg/d if <60 kg. [Trade only: Tabs 200 mg.] ▶L ♀C ▶? $$$

ATOVAQUONE (*Mepron*) Pneumocystis treatment: 750 mg PO bid × 21 d. Pneumocystis prevention: 1500 mg PO daily. Take with meals. [Trade only: Susp 750 mg/5 mL (210 mL), foil pouch 750 mg/5 mL (5 & 10 mL).] ▶Fecal ♀C ▶? $$$$$

IVERMECTIN (*Stromectol*) Single PO dose of 200 mcg/kg for strongyloidiasis, scabies (not for children <15 kg), 150 mcg/kg for onchocerciasis. Take on empty stomach with water. [Trade only: Tab 3 mg.] ▶L ♀C ▶+ $$

MEBENDAZOLE (*Vermox*) Pinworm: 100 mg PO × 1; repeat in 2 wk. Roundworm, whipworm, hookworm: 100 mg PO bid × 3d. [Generic only: Chew tab 100 mg.] ▶L ♀C ▶? $$

NITAZOXANIDE (*Alinia*) Cryptosporidial or Giardial diarrhea: 100 mg bid for 1–3 yo, 200 mg bid for 4–11 yo, 500 mg bid for adults and children ≥12 yo. Give PO with food ×7 d. Use susp for <12 yo. [Trade only: Oral susp 100 mg/5 mL 60 mL bottle, tab 500 mg.] ▶L ♀B ▶? $$$$

PAROMOMYCIN 25–35 mg/kg/d PO divided tid with or after meals. [Generic only: Caps 250 mg.] ▶Not absorbed ♀C ▶- $$$$

PENTAMIDINE (*Pentam, NebuPent*) Pneumocystis treatment: 4 mg/kg IM/IV daily × 21 d. Pneumocystis prevention: 300 mg nebulized q 4 wk. [Trade only: Aerosol 300 mg.] ▶K ♀C ▶- $$$

PRAZIQUANTEL (*Biltricide*) Schistosomiasis: 20 mg/kg PO q4–6h × 3 doses. Neurocysticercosis: 50 mg/kg/d PO divided tid × 15 d (up to 100 mg/kg/d for peds). [Trade only: Tabs 600 mg.] ▶LK ♀B ▶- $$$

PYRANTEL (*Antiminth, Pin-X, Pinworm, ♣Combantrin*) Pinworm and roundworm: 11 mg/kg up to 1 g PO single dose. [OTC Trade only (Pin-X): Susp 144 mg/mL (equivalent to 50 mg/mL of pyrantel base) 30, 60 mL. Tab 720.5 mg (equivalent to 250 mg of pyrantel base). OTC Generic only: Cap 180 mg (equivalent to 62.5 mg of pyrantel base).] ▶Not absorbed ♀- ▶? $

PYRIMETHAMINE (*Daraprim*) CNS toxoplasmosis in AIDS. Acute therapy: 200 mg PO × 1, then 50 mg (<60 kg) to 75 mg (≥60 kg) PO once daily + sulfadiazine + leucovorin 10–20 mg PO once daily (can increase to ≥50 mg/d) for ≥6 wk. Secondary prevention: Pyrimethamine 25–50 mg PO once daily + sulfadiazine + leucovorin 10–25 mg PO once daily. [Trade only: Tabs 25 mg.] ▶L ♀C ▶+ $$

THIABENDAZOLE (*Mintezol*) Helminths: 22 mg/kg/dose up to 1500 mg PO bid after meals. Treat × 2 d for strongyloidiasis, cutaneous larva migrans. [Trade only: Chew tab 500 mg, susp 500 mg/5 mL (120 mL).] ▶LK ♀C ▶? $

TINIDAZOLE (*Tindamax*) Adults: 2 g PO daily × 1 d for trichomoniasis or giardiasis, × 3 d for amebiasis. Bacterial vaginosis: 2 g PO once daily × 2 d or 1 g PO once daily × 5 d. Peds, >3 yo: 50 mg/kg (up to 2 g) PO daily × 1 d for giardiasis, × 3 d for amebiasis. Take with food. [Trade only: Tabs 250,500 mg. Pharmacists can compound oral susp.] ▶KL ♀C ▶?- $

Antiviral Agents—Anti-CMV

CIDOFOVIR (*Vistide*) CMV retinitis in AIDS: 5 mg/kg IV q wk × 2, then 5 mg/kg q2 wk. Severe nephrotoxicity. ▶K ♀C ▶- $$$$$

FOSCARNET (*Foscavir*) CMV retinitis: 60 mg/kg IV (over 1 h) q8h or 90 mg/kg IV (over 1.5–2 h) q12h × 2–3 wk, then 90–120 mg/kg/d IV over 2h. HSV infection: 40 mg/kg (over 1 h) q8–12h. Nephrotoxicity, seizures. ▶K ♀C ▶? $$$$$

GANCICLOVIR (*DHPG*) CMV retinitis: Induction 5 mg/kg IV q12h for 14–21 d. Maintenance 6 mg/kg IV daily for 5 d per wk. Myelosuppression. Potential carcinogen, teratogen. May impair fertility. [Generic only: Caps 250, 500 mg.] ▶K ♀C ▶- $$$$$

VALGANCICLOVIR (*Valcyte*) CMV retinitis: 900 mg PO bid × 21 d, then 900 mg PO daily. Prevention of CMV disease in high-risk kidney, kidney-pancreas, heart transplant patients: 900 mg PO daily from within 10 d after transplant until 100 d post-transplant. Greater bioavailability than oral ganciclovir. Give with food. Impaired fertility, myelosuppression, potential carcinogen & teratogen. [Trade only: Tabs 450 mg.] ▶K ♀C ▶- $$$$$

Antiviral Agents—Anti-Herpetic

ACYCLOVIR (*Zovirax*) Genital herpes: 400 mg PO tid × 7–10 d for first episode, × 5 d for recurrent episodes. Chronic suppression of genital herpes: 400 mg PO bid, 400–800 mg PO bid-tid in HIV infection. Zoster: 800 mg PO 5 times/d × 7–10 d. Chickenpox: 20 mg/kg up to 800 mg PO qid × 5 d. Adult IV: 5–10 mg/kg

(cont.)

IV q8h, each dose over 1h. Peds, herpes encephalitis: 20 mg/kg IV q8h × 10 d for 3 mo–12 yo, adult dose for ≥12 yo. Neonatal herpes: 20 mg/kg IV q8h × 21 d for disseminated/CNS disease, × 14 d for skin/mucous membranes. [Generic/Trade: Caps 200 mg, tabs 400,800 mg. Susp 200 mg/5 mL.] ▶K ♀B ▶+ $

FAMCICLOVIR (Famvir) First-episode genital herpes: 250 mg PO tid × 7–10 d. Recurrent genital herpes: 1000 mg PO bid × 2 doses; 500 bid × 7 d if HIV-infected. Chronic suppression of genital herpes: 250 mg PO bid; 500 mg PO bid if HIV infected. Recurrent herpes labialis: 1500 mg PO single dose; 500 bid × 7 d if HIV-infected. Zoster: 500 mg PO tid for 7 d. [Generic/Trade: Tabs 125, 250, 500 mg.] ▶K ♀B ▶? $$

VALACYCLOVIR (Valtrex) First-episode genital herpes: 1 g PO bid × 10 d. Recurrent genital herpes: 500 mg PO bid × 3 d; 1 g PO bid × 5–10 d in HIV infection. Chronic suppression of genital herpes: 500–1000 mg PO daily; 500 mg PO bid if HIV infection. Reduction of genital herpes transmission in immunocompetent patients with ≤9 recurrences/yr: 500 mg PO daily by source partner, in conjunction with safer sex practices. Herpes labialis: 2 g PO q12h × 2 doses. Zoster: 1000 mg PO tid × 7 d. [Generic/Trade: Tabs 500,1000 mg.] ▶K ♀B ▶+ $$$$$

NOTE FOR ALL ANTI-HIV DRUGS: *Many serious drug interactions; always check before prescribing. AIDS treatment guidelines available online at www.aidsinfo. nih.gov.*

Antiviral Agents—Anti-HIV—CCR5 Antagonists

MARAVIROC (Selzentry) 150 mg PO bid with strong CYP 3A4 inhibitors (delavirdine, most protease inhibitors, ketoconazole, itraconazole, clarithromycin); 300 mg PO bid with drugs that are not strong CYP 3A4 inducers/inhibitors (NRTIs, tipranavir-ritonavir, nevirapine, enfuvirtide); 600 mg PO bid with strong CYP 3A4 inducers (efavirenz, rifampin, carbamazepine, phenobarbital, phenytoin). Tropism test before treatment; not for dual/mixed or CXCR4-tropic HIV infection. Hepatotoxicity with allergic features. [Trade only: Tabs 150, 300 mg.] ▶LK ♀B ▶- $$$$$

Antiviral Agents—Anti-HIV—Combinations

ATRIPLA (efavirenz + emtricitabine + tenofovir) 1 tab PO once daily on empty stomach, preferably at bedtime. [Trade only: Tabs efavirenz 600 mg + emtricitabine 200 mg + tenofovir 300 mg.] ▶KL ♀D ▶- $$$$$

COMBIVIR (lamivudine + zidovudine) 1 tab PO bid. [Trade only: Tabs lamivudine 150 mg + zidovudine 300 mg.] ▶LK ♀C ▶- $$$$$

EPZICOM (abacavir + lamivudine) 1 tab PO daily. [Trade only: Tabs abacavir 600 mg + lamivudine 300 mg.] ▶LK ♀C ▶- $$$$$

TRIZIVIR (abacavir + lamivudine + zidovudine) 1 tab PO bid. [Trade only: Tabs abacavir 300 mg + lamivudine 150 mg + zidovudine 300 mg.] ▶LK ♀C ▶- $$$$$

TRUVADA (emtricitabine + tenofovir) 1 tab PO daily. [Trade only: Tabs emtricitabine 200 mg + tenofovir 300 mg.] ▶K ♀B ▶- $$$$$

Antiviral Agents—Anti-HIV—Fusion Inhibitors

ENFUVIRTIDE (Fuzeon, T-20) 90 mg SC bid. Peds, ≥6 yo: 2 mg/kg up to 90 mg SC bid. [30-d kit with vials, diluent, syringes, alcohol wipes. Single-dose vials contain 108 mg to provide 90 mg enfuvirtide.] ▶Serum ♀B ▶- $$$$$

Antiviral Agents—Anti-HIV—Integrase Strand Transfer Inhibitor

RALTEGRAVIR (Isentress) 400 mg PO bid. [Trade only: Tabs 400 mg.] ▶Glucuronidation ♀C ▶- $$$$$

Antiviral Agents—Anti-HIV—Non-Nucleoside Reverse Transcriptase Inhibitors

EFAVIRENZ (Sustiva, EFV) Adults & children >40 kg: 600 mg PO qhs. With voriconazole: Use voriconazole 400 mg PO bid & efavirenz 300 mg PO once daily. Peds, ≥3 yo: Give PO qhs 200 mg for 10–15 kg; 250 mg for 15–20 kg; 300 mg for 20 to <25 kg; 350 mg for 25 to <32.5 kg; 400 mg for 32.5 to <40 kg. Do not give with high-fat meal. [Trade only: Caps 50, 100, 200 mg, tabs 600 mg.] ▶L ♀D ▶- $$$$$

ETRAVIRINE (Intelence) Combination therapy for treatment-resistant HIV infection: 200 mg PO bid after meals. [Trade only: Tabs 100 mg.] ▶L ♀B ▶- $$$$$

NEVIRAPINE (Viramune, NVP) 200 mg PO daily × 14 d initially. If tolerated, increase to 200 mg PO bid. Peds. Severe skin reactions & hepatotoxicity. ▶LK ♀C ▶- $$$$$. [Trade only: Tabs 200 mg, susp 50 mg/5 mL (240 mL).]

Antiviral Agents—Anti-HIV—Nucleoside/Nucleotide Reverse Transcriptase Inhibitors

ABACAVIR (Ziagen, ABC) Adult: 300 mg PO bid or 600 mg PO daily. Children ≥3 mo: 8 mg/kg up to 300 mg PO bid. Potentially fatal hypersensitivity. HLA-B*5701 predisposes to hypersensitivity; screen before starting and avoid if positive test. Never rechallenge with abacavir after suspected reaction. [Trade only: Tabs 300 mg, oral soln 20 mg/mL (240 mL).] ▶L ♀C ▶- $$$$$

DIDANOSINE (Videx, Videx EC, ddI) Videx EC, adults: 400 mg PO daily if ≥60 kg, 250 mg PO daily if <60 kg. Dosage reduction of Videx EC with teno-fovir: 250 mg if ≥60 kg, 200 mg if <60 kg. Dosage reduction unclear with tenofovir if CrCl <60 mL/min. Buffered powder, peds: 100 mg/m2 PO bid for age 2 wk-8 mo. 120 mg/m2 PO bid for >8 mo. All formulations usually taken

(cont.)

on empty stomach. [Generic/Trade: Pediatric powder for oral solution 10 mg/mL (buffered with antacid), delayed-release caps 200, 250, 400 mg. Trade only: (Videx EC) delayed-release caps 125 mg, chewable tabs 25, 50, 100, 150, 200 mg.] ▶LK ♀B ▶- $$$$$

EMTRICITABINE (*Emtriva, FTC*)   200 mg cap or 240 mg oral soln PO once daily. Peds, oral soln: 3 mg/kg PO once daily for ≤3 mo, 6 mg/kg up to 240 mg for 3 mo-17 yo. Can give 200 mg cap PO once daily if >33 kg. [Trade only: Caps 200 mg, oral soln 10 mg/mL (170 mL).] ▶K ♀B ▶- $$$$$

LAMIVUDINE (*Epivir, Epivir-HBV, 3TC, ✦Heptovir*)   Epivir for HIV infection. Adults: 150 mg PO bid or 300 mg PO daily. Peds: 4 mg/kg up to 150 mg PO bid. Can use tabs if ≥14 kg. Epivir-HBV for hepatitis B. Adults: 100 mg PO daily. Peds: 3 mg/kg up to 100 mg PO daily. [Trade only: Epivir, 3TC: Tabs 150 (scored), 300 mg, oral soln 10 mg/mL. Epivir-HBV, Heptovir: Tabs 100 mg, oral soln 5 mg/mL.] ▶K ♀C ▶- $$$$$

STAVUDINE (*Zerit, d4T*)   40 mg PO q12h; 30 mg q12h if <60 kg. Peds (<30 kg): 1 mg/ kg PO bid. [Trade only: Caps 15, 20, 30, 40 mg, oral soln 1 mg/mL (200 mL).] ▶LK ♀C ▶- $$$$$

TENOFOVIR (*Viread, TDF*)   300 mg PO daily with a meal. [Trade only: Tab 300 mg.] ▶K ♀B ▶- $$$$$

ZIDOVUDINE (*Retrovir, AZT, ZDV*)   200 mg PO tid or 300 bid. Peds: 160 mg/m2 up to 200 mg PO q8h. [Generic/Trade: Cap 100 mg, tab 300 mg, syrup 50 mg/5 mL (240 mL).] ▶LK ♀C ▶- $$$$$

Antiviral Agents—Anti-HIV—Protease Inhibitors

ATAZANAVIR (*Reyataz, ATV*)   Give atazanavir PO once daily with food. Adults, therapy-naive: 400 mg. With efavirenz or tenofovir, therapy-naïve: Atazanavir 300 mg + ritonavir 100 mg. Therapy-experienced: Atazanavir 300 mg + ritonavir 100 mg. Peds, ≥6 yo: Give with ritonavir 4 mg/kg (max atazanavir 300 mg + ritonavir 100 mg). Therapy-naïve: Atazanavir 8.5 mg/kg for 15-<20 kg, 7 mg/kg for ≥20 kg. Therapy-experienced: Atazanavir 7 mg/kg for ≥25 kg. Therapy-naïve, ritonavir-intolerant, ≥13 yo and ≥39 kg: 400 mg PO once daily. Give atazanavir 2 h before or 1 h after buffered didanosine. [Trade only: Caps 100, 150, 200, 300 mg.] ▶L ♀B ▶- $$$$$

DARUNAVIR (*Prezista*)   Therapy-experienced patients: 600 mg boosted by ritonavir 100 mg PO bid with food. Do not use without ritonavir. [Trade only: Tab 300, 600 mg.] ▶L ♀B ▶- $$$$$

FOSAMPRENAVIR (*Lexiva, 908, ✦Telzir*)   Therapy-naïve adults: 1400 mg PO bid OR 1400 mg + ritonavir 100/200 mg both once daily OR 700 mg + ritonavir 100 mg both bid. Protease inhibitor-experienced adults: 700 mg + ritonavir 100 mg both bid. Peds. Therapy-naïve, 2–5 yo: Susp 30 mg/kg up to 1400 mg PO bid. Therapy-naïve, ≥6 yo: Susp 30 mg/kg up to 1400 mg bid (can use 2 tabs bid if ≥47 kg) OR susp 18 mg/kg up to 700 mg + ritonavir 3 mg/kg up to 100 mg both bid. Therapy-experienced, ≥6 yo: Susp 18 mg/kg up to 700 mg + ritonavir 3 mg/kg up to 100 mg both bid. Take tabs without regard to meals. Adults should take susp without food;

children should take with food. [Trade only: Tabs 700 mg, susp 50 mg/mL.] ▶L ♀C ▶– $$$$$

INDINAVIR (*Crixivan, IDV*) 800 mg PO q8h between meals with water (at least 48 ounces/d to prevent kidney stones). [Trade only: Caps 100, 200, 333, 400 mg.] ▶LK ♀C ▶– $$$$$

LOPINAVIR-RITONAVIR (*Kaletra, LPV/r*) Adults: Therapy-naive patients: 2 tabs PO bid or 4 tabs once daily. 5 mL PO bid or 10 mL once daily of oral soln. Increase oral soln to 6.5 mL PO bid (not once daily) with efavirenz, nevirapine, fosamprenavir, or nelfinavir (dosage increase not needed with tabs). Therapy-experienced patients: No once-daily regimen. 2 tabs or 5 mL oral soln bid. Increase oral soln to 6.5 mL PO bid with efavirenz, nevirapine, or nelfinavir. Consider 3 tabs bid with efavirenz, nevirapine, fosamprenavir without ritonavir, or nelfinavir if reduced lopinavir susceptibility suspected. Peds: Without efavirenz, nevirapine, fosamprenavir, or nelfinavir. Oral soln, 14 d-6 mo: lopinavir 16 mg/kg PO bid. Oral soln, 6 mo-18 yo: 12 mg/kg PO bid for 7-<15 kg, 10 mg/kg PO bid for ≥15 kg-<40 kg. Tabs (100 mg/25 mg), 6 mo-18 yo: Give PO bid 2 tabs for 15–25 kg, 3 tabs for >25–35 kg, 4 tabs for >35 kg. With efavirenz, nevirapine, fosamprenavir, or nelfinavir, 6 mo-18 yo: 13 mg/kg PO bid for 7-<15 kg (oral soln only), 11 mg/kg PO bid for ≥15-<45 kg (oral soln or tabs); use adult dose for >45 kg. Give tabs without regard to meals; give oral soln with food. ▶L ♀C ▶– $$$$$ [Trade only: Caps 133.3/33.3 mg; tabs 200/50 mg, 100/25 mg; oral soln 80/20 mg/mL (160 mL).]

NELFINAVIR (*Viracept, NFV*) 750 mg PO tid or 1250 mg PO bid. Peds: 20–45 mg/kg PO tid. Take with meals. [Trade only: Tab 250, 625 mg, oral powder 50 mg/g (114 g).] ▶L ♀B ▶– $$$$$

RITONAVIR (*Norvir, RTV*) Full-dose regimen (600 mg PO bid) poorly tolerated. Adult doses of 100 mg PO daily to 400 mg PO bid used to boost levels of other protease inhibitors. Peds >1 mo old: Start with 250 mg/m2 and increase q2–3 d by 50 mg/m2 twice daily. Usual dose is 350–400 mg/m2 to max of 600 mg PO bid. If 400 mg/m2 twice daily not tolerated, consider other alternatives. [Trade only: Cap 100 mg, oral soln 80 mg/mL (240 mL).] ▶L ♀B ▶– $$$$$

SAQUINAVIR (*Invirase, SQV*) Take with/after meals. Regimens must contain ritonavir. Saquinavir 1000 mg + ritonavir 100 mg both PO bid within 2 h after meals. Saquinavir 1000 mg PO + Kaletra 400/100 mg both PO bid. [Trade only: Invirase (hard gel) caps 200 mg, tabs 500 mg.] ▶L ♀B ▶– $$$$$

TIPRANAVIR (*Aptivus*) 500 mg boosted by ritonavir 200 mg PO bid with food. Peds: 14 mg/kg with 6 mg/kg ritonavir PO bid; do not exceed adult dose. Hepatotoxicity. [Trade only: Caps 250 mg. Oral soln 100 mg/mL (95 mL in unit-ofuse amber glass bottle).] ▶Feces ♀C ▶– $$$$$

Antiviral Agents—Anti-Influenza

AMANTADINE (*Symmetrel, ✦Endantadine*) CDC no longer recommends for influenza A. Parkinsonism: 100 mg PO bid. Max 300–400 mg/d divided tid-qid. [Generic only: Cap 100 mg. Generic/Trade: Tab 100 mg, syrup 50 mg/5 mL (480 mL).] ▶K ♀C ▶? $$

OSELTAMIVIR (*Tamiflu*) 75 mg PO bid × 5 d starting within 2 d of symptom onset. 75 mg PO daily for prophylaxis. Peds ≥1 yo: Each dose is 30 mg if ≤15 kg, 45 mg if 16–23 kg, 60 mg if 24–40 kg, 75 mg if >40 kg or ≥13 yo. For treatment, give twice daily × 5 d starting within 2 d of symptom onset. For prophylaxis, give once daily × 10 d starting within 2 d of exposure. Take with food to improve tolerability. [Trade only: Caps 30, 45, 75 mg, susp 12 mg/mL (25 mL).] ▶LK ♀C ▶? $$$

Antiviral Agents—Other

ADEFOVIR (*Hepsera*) Chronic hepatitis B: 10 mg PO daily. Nephrotoxic; lactic acidosis and hepatic steatosis; discontinuation may exacerbate hepatitis B; HIV resistance in untreated HIV infection. [Trade only: Tabs 10 mg.] ▶K ♀C ▶- $$$$$

ENTECAVIR (*Baraclude*) Chronic hepatitis B: 0.5 mg PO once daily if treatment naive; 1 mg if lamivudine-resistant or history of viremia despite lamivudine treatment. Give 2h after last meal and 2h before next meal. [Trade only: Tabs 0.5, 1 mg, solution 0.05 mg/mL (210 mL).] ▶K ♀C ▶- $$$$$

INTERFERON ALFA-2B (*Intron A*) Chronic hepatitis B: 5 million units/d or 10 million units 3 times/wk SC/IM × 16 wk if HBeAg +, × 48 wk if HBeAg-. Chronic hepatitis C: 3 million units SC/IM 3 times/wk × 4 mo. Continue for 18–24 mo if ALT normalized. [Trade only: Powder/soln for injection 10, 18, 50 million units/vial. Soln for injection 18, 25 million units/multidose vial. Multidose injection pens 3, 5,10 million units/0.2 mL (1.5 mL), 6 doses/pen.] ▶K ♀C ▶? + $$$$$

INTERFERON ALFACON-1 (*Infergen*) Chronic hepatitis C: 9 mcg SC 3 times/wk × 24 wk. If relapse/no response, increase to 15 mcg SC 3 times/wk. If intolerable adverse effects, reduce to 7.5 mcg SC 3 times/wk. [Trade only: Vials injectable soln 9 mcg/mL (0.3 mL, 0.5 mL).] ▶Plasma ♀C ▶? $$$$

PALIVIZUMAB (*Synagis*) Prevention of respiratory syncytial virus pulmonary disease in high-risk children: 15 mg/kg IM q mo during RSV season. ▶L ♀C ▶? $$$$$

PEGINTERFERON ALFA-2A (*Pegasys*) Chronic hepatitis C: 180 mcg SC in abdomen or thigh once weekly for 48 wk +/− PO ribavirin. Hepatitis B: 180 mcg SC in abdomen or thigh once weekly for 48 wk. May cause or worsen severe autoimmune, neuropsychiatric, ischemic, & infectious diseases. Frequent clinical & lab monitoring. [Trade only: 180 mcg/1 mL solution in single-use vial, 180 mcg/0.5 mL prefilled syringe.] ▶LK ♀C ▶- $$$$$

PEGINTERFERON ALFA-2B (*PEG-Intron*) Chronic hepatitis C: Give SC once weekly for 1 yr. Monotherapy 1 mcg/kg/wk. In combo oral ribavirin: 1.5 mcg/kg/wk. May cause or worsen severe autoimmune, neuropsychiatric, ischemic, & infectious diseases. Frequent clinical & lab monitoring. [Trade only: 50, 80, 120, 150 mcg/0.5 mL single-use vials with diluent, 2 syringes, and alcohol swabs. Disposable single-dose Redipen 50, 80, 120, 150 mcg.] ▶K? ♀C ▶- $$$$$

OVERVIEW OF BACTERIAL PATHOGENS (Selected)

GRAM Positive Aerobic Cocci: *Staph epidermidis* (coagulase negative), *Staph aureus* (coagulase positive), Streptococci: *S pneumoniae* (pneumococcus), *S pyogenes* (Group A), *S agalactiae* (Group B), enterococcus

GRAM Positive Aerobic / Facultatively Anaerobic Bacilli: Bacillus, Corynebacterium diphtheriae, Erysipelothrix rhusiopathiae, Listeria monocytogenes, Nocardia

GRAM Negative Aerobic Diplococci: Moraxella catarrhalis, Neisseria gonorrhoeae, Neisseria meningitidis

GRAM Negative Aerobic Coccobacilli: Haemophilus ducreyi, Haemoph. Influenzae

GRAM Negative Aerobic Bacilli: Acinetobacter, Bartonella species, Bordetella pertussis, Brucella, Burkholderia cepacia, Campylobacter, Francisella tularensis, Helicobacter pylori, Legionella pneumophila, Pseudomonas aeruginosa, Stenotrophomonas maltophilia, Vibrio cholerae, Yersinia

GRAM Neg Facultatively Anaerobic Bacilli: Aeromonas hydrophila, Eikenella corrodens, Pasteurella multocida, Enterobacteriaceae: E coli, Citrobacter, Shigella, Salmonella, Klebsiella, Enterobacter, Hafnia, Serratia, Proteus, Providencia

ANAEROBES: Actinomyces, Bacteroides fragilis, Clostridium botulinum, Clostridium difficile, Clostridium perfringens, Clostridium tetani, Fusobacterium, Lactobacillus, Peptostreptococcus

DEFECTIVE Cell Wall Bacteria: Chlamydia pneumoniae, Chlamydia psittaci, Chlamydia trachomatis, Coxiella burnetii, Mycoplasma pneumoniae, Rickettsia prowazekii, Rickettsia rickettsii, Rickettsia typhi, Ureaplasma urealyticum

SPIROCHETES: Borrelia burgdorferi, Leptospira, Treponema pallidum

MYCOBACTERIA: M avium complex, M kansasii, M leprae, M tuberculosis

RIBAVIRIN—INHALED (*Virazole*) Severe respiratory syncytial virus infection in children: Aerosol 12–18 h/d $\times$ 3–7 d. Beware of sudden pulmonary deterioration; ventilator dysfunction due to drug precipitation. ▶Lung ♀X ▶- $$$$$

RIBAVIRIN—ORAL (*Rebetol, Copegus, Ribasphere*) Hepatitis C. Rebetol: In combo with interferon alfa 2b (Intron A): 600 mg PO bid if >75 kg; 400 mg q am and 600 q pm if ≤75 kg. In combo with peginterferon alfa 2b (PEG-Intron): 400 mg PO bid. Copegus: In combo with peginterferon alfa 2a (Pegasys): For genotype 1/4, 1200 mg/d if ≥75 kg; 1000 mg/d if <75 kg. For genotype 2/3, 800 mg/d PO. For patients coinfected with HIV, Copegus dose is 800 mg/d regardless of genotype. Give bid with food. Decrease ribavirin dose if Hb decreases. [Generic/Trade: Caps 200 mg, Tabs 200, 500 mg. Generic only: Tabs 400, 600 mg. Trade only (Rebetol): Oral soln 40 mg/mL (100 mL).] ▶Cellular, K ♀X ▶- $$$$$

TELBIVUDINE (*Tyzeka*) Chronic hepatitis B: 600 mg PO once daily. [Trade only: Tabs 600 mg.] ▶K ♀B ▶- $$$$$

Carbapenems

DORIPENEM (*Doribax*) 500 mg IV q8h. ▶K ♀B ▶? $$$$$

ERTAPENEM (*Invanz*) 1 g IV/IM q24h. Prophylaxis, colorectal surgery: 1 g IV 1 h before incision. Peds: 15 mg/kg IV/IM q12h (max 1 g/d). Infuse IV over 30 min. ▶K ♀B ▶? $$$$$

IMIPENEM-CILASTATIN (*Primaxin*) 250–1000 mg IV q6–8h. Peds >3 mo: 15–25 mg/kg IV q6h. ▶K ♀C ▶? $$$$$

MEROPENEM (*Merrem IV*) Complicated skin infections 10 mg/kg up to 500 mg IV q8h. Intra-abdominal infections: 20 mg/kg up to 1 g IV q8h. Peds meningitis: 40 mg/kg IV q8h for age ≥3 mo; 2 g IV q8h if >50 kg. ▶K ♀B ▶? $$$$$

Cephalosporins—1st Generation

CEFADROXIL (*Duricef*) 1–2 g/d PO divided once daily-bid. Peds: 30 mg/kg/d divided bid. [Generic/Trade: Tabs 1 g, caps 500 mg, susp 125, 250, & 500 mg/5 mL.] ▶K ♀B ▶+ $$$

CEFAZOLIN (*Ancef*) 0.5–1.5 g IM/IV q6–8h. Peds: 25–50 mg/kg/d divided q6–8h, severe infections 100 mg/kg/d. ▶K ♀B ▶+ $$

CEPHALEXIN (*Keflex, Panixine DisperDose*) 250–500 mg PO qid. Peds 25–50 mg/kg/d. Not for otitis media, sinusitis. [Generic/Trade: Caps 250, 500 mg. Generic only: Tabs 250, 500 mg, susp 125 & 250 mg/5 mL. Panixine DisperDose 125, 250 mg scored tabs for oral susp. Trade only: Caps 333, 750 mg.] ▶K ♀B ▶? $$$

Cephalosporins—2nd Generation

CEFACLOR (*Ceclor, Raniclor*) 250–500 mg PO tid. Peds: 20–40 mg/kg/d PO divided tid. Otitis media: 40 mg/kg/d PO divided bid. Group A streptococcal pharyngitis: 20 mg/kg/d PO divided bid. Extended release: 375–500 mg PO bid. Serum sickness-like reactions with repeated use. [Generic only: Caps 250, 500 mg, susp & chew tabs 125, 187, 250, 375 mg per 5 mL or tab, extended release tabs 375, 500 mg.] ▶K ♀B ▶? $$$$

CEFOXITIN (*Mefoxin*) 1–2 g IM/IV q6–8h. Peds: 80–160 mg/kg/d IV divided q4–8h. ▶K ♀B ▶+ $$$$$

CEFPROZIL (*Cefzil*) 250–500 mg PO bid. Peds otitis media: 15 mg/kg/dose PO bid. Peds group A streptococcal pharyngitis (sec-line to penicillin): 7.5 mg/kg/dose PO bid × 10d. [Generic/Trade: Tabs 250,500 mg, susp 125 & 250 mg/5 mL.] ▶K ♀B ▶+ $$$$

CEFUROXIME (*Zinacef, Ceftin*) 750–1500 mg IM/IV q8h. Peds: 50–100 mg/kg/d IV divided q6–8h, not for meningitis. 250–500 mg PO bid. Peds: 20–30 mg/kg/d susp PO divided bid. [Generic/Trade: Tabs 125, 250, 500 mg, Susp 125 & 250 mg/5 mL.] ▶K ♀B ▶? $$$

Cephalosporins—3rd Generation

CEFDINIR (*Omnicef*) 14 mg/kg/d up to 600 mg/d PO divided once daily or bid. [Generic/Trade: Cap 300 mg. Susp 125 & 250 mg/5 mL.] ▶K ♀B ▶? $$$$

CEFDITOREN (*Spectracef*) 200–400 mg PO bid with food. [Trade only: Tabs 200 mg.] ▶K ♀B ▶? $$$$

CEFIXIME (*Suprax*) 400 mg PO once daily. Gonorrhea: 400 mg PO single-dose. Peds: 8 mg/kg/d divided once daily-bid. [Trade only: Susp 100 & 200 mg/5 mL, Tab 400 mg.] ▶K/Bile ♀B ▶? $$

CEPHALOSPORINS—GENERAL ANTIMICROBIAL SPECTRUM

1st generation: gram positive (including *Staph aureus*); basic gram negative coverage
2nd generation: diminished *Staph aureus*, improved gram negative coverage compared to 1st generation; some with anaerobic coverage
3rd generation: further diminished *Staph aureus*, further improved gram negative coverage compared to 1st & 2nd generation; some with Pseudomonal coverage and diminished gram positive coverage
4th generation: same as 3rd generation plus coverage against *Pseudomonas*

CEFOPERAZONE (*Cefobid*) Usual dose 2–4 g/d IM/IV divided q12h. Max dose: 6–12 g/d IV divided q6–12 h. Possible clotting impairment. ▶Bile/K ♀B ▶? $$$$$

CEFOTAXIME (*Claforan*) Usual dose: 1–2 g IM/IV q6–8h. Peds: 50–180 mg/kg/d IM/IV divided q4–6h. AAP dose for pneumococcal meningitis: 225–300 mg/kg/d IV divided q6–8h. ▶KL ♀B ▶+ $$$$$

CEFPODOXIME (*Vantin*) 100–400 mg PO bid. Peds: 10 mg/kg/d divided bid. [Generic/Trade: Tabs 100, 200 mg. Susp 50 & 100 mL/5 mL.] ▶K ♀B ▶? $$$$

CEFTAZIDIME (*Ceptaz, Fortaz, Tazicef*) 1 g IM/IV or 2 g IV q8–12h. Peds: 30–50 mg/kg IV q8h. ▶K ♀B ▶+ $$$$$

CEFTIBUTEN (*Cedax*) 400 mg PO once daily. Peds: 9 mg/kg up to 400 mg PO once daily. [Trade only: Cap 400 mg, susp 90 mg/5 mL.] ▶K ♀B ▶? $$$$$

CEFTIZOXIME (*Cefizox*) 1–2 g IV q8–12h. Peds: 50 mg/kg/dose IV q6–8h. ▶K ♀B ▶? $$$$$

CEFTRIAXONE (*Rocephin*) 1–2 g IM/IV q24h. Meningitis: 2 g IV q12h. Gonorrhea: single dose 125 mg IM (250 mg if PID). Peds: 50–75 mg/kg/d up to 2 g divided q12–24h. Meningitis: 100 mg/kg/d up to 4 g q12h. Otitis media: 50 mg/kg up to 1 g IM single dose. Dilute in 1% lidocaine for IM. In neonates, fatal lung/kidney precipitation with calcium has been reported. Avoid within 48 h of IV calcium-containing products or solutions, even by separate IV lines. Do not dilute with Ringers/ Hartmann's soln or TPN containing calcium. ▶K/Bile ♀B ▶+ $$$

Cephalosporins—4th Generation

CEFEPIME (*Maxipime*) 0.5–2 g IM/IV q12h. Peds: 50 mg/kg IV q8–12h. ▶K ♀B ▶? $$$$$

Macrolides

AZITHROMYCIN (*Zithromax, Zmax*) 500 mg IV daily. PO: 10 mg/kg up to 500 mg on d 1, then 5 mg/kg up to 250 mg daily to complete 5 d. Group A streptococcal pharyngitis (sec-line to penicillin): 12 mg/kg up to 500 mg PO daily × 5 d. Short regimens for peds otitis media (30 mg/kg PO single dose or 10 mg/kg PO daily × 3 d) and sinusitis (10 mg/kg PO daily × 3 d). Short regimen for adult acute sinusitis or exacerbation of chronic bronchitis:

(cont.)

500 mg PO daily × 3 d. Chlamydia (including pregnancy), chancroid: 1 g PO single dose. Prevention of disseminated Mycobacterium avium complex disease: 1200 mg PO q wk. Acute sinusitis in children: 10 mg/kg PO daily × 3 d. [Generic/Trade: Tab 250, 500, 600 mg, Susp 100 & 200/5 mL. Trade only: Packet 1000 mg. Z-Pak: #6, 250 mg tab. Tri-Pak: #3, 500 mg tab. Zmax extended release oral susp: 2 g in 60 mL single dose bottle.] ▶L ♀B ▶? $$

CLARITHROMYCIN (*Biaxin, Biaxin XL*)   250–500 mg PO bid. Peds: 7.5 mg/kg PO bid. H pylori: See table in GI section. See table for prophylaxis of bacterial endocarditis. Mycobacterium avium complex disease prevention: 7.5 mg/kg up to 500 mg PO bid. Biaxin XL: 1000 mg PO daily with food. [Generic/Trade: Tab 250, 500 mg. Extended release tab 500 mg. Susp 125 & 250 mg/5 mL. Trade only: Biaxin XL-Pak: #14, 500 mg tabs. Generic only: Extended release tab 1000 mg.] ▶KL ♀C ▶? $$$

ERYTHROMYCIN BASE (*Eryc, E-mycin, Ery-Tab, ✦Erybid, Erythromid, P.C.E.*)   250–500 mg PO qid, 333 mg PO tid, or 500 mg PO bid. [Generic/Trade: Tab 250, 333, 500 mg, delayed-release cap 250.] ▶L ♀B ▶+ $

ERYTHROMYCIN ETHYL SUCCINATE (*EES, Eryped*)   400 mg PO qid. Peds: 30–50 mg/kg/d divided qid. [Generic/Trade: Tab 400 tab, susp 200 & 400 mg/5 mL. Trade only (EryPed): Susp 100 mg/2.5 mL (50 mL).] ▶L ♀B ▶+ $

ERYTHROMYCIN LACTOBIONATE, ✦ERYTHROCIN IV 15–20 MG/KG/D (*max 4 g*)   IV divided q6h. Peds: 15–50 mg/kg/d IV divided q6h. ▶L ♀B ▶+ $$$$$

PEDIAZOLE (erythromycin ethyl succinate + sulfisoxazole)   50 mg/kg/d (based on EES dose) PO divided tid-qid. [Generic/Trade: Susp, erythromycin ethyl succinate 200 mg + sulfisoxazole 600 mg/5 mL.] ▶KL ♀C ▶- $$

Penicillins—1st Generation—Natural

BENZATHINE PENICILLIN (*Bicillin L-A, ✦Megacillin*)   1.2 million units IM. Peds <27 kg 0.3–0.6 MU IM, ≥27 kg 0.9 MU IM. Doses last 2–4 wk. [Trade only: for IM use, 600,000 units/mL; 1, 2, and 4 mL syringes.] ▶K ♀B ▶? $$

BICILLIN C-R (procaine penicillin + benzathine penicillin)   For IM use. Not for treatment of syphilis. [Trade only: for IM use 300/300 thousand units/mL procaine/benzathine penicillin; 1, 2, and 4 mL syringes.] ▶K ♀B ▶? $$$

PENICILLIN G Pneumococcal pneumonia & severe infections: 250,000–400,000 units/kg/d (8–12 million units/d in adult)   IV divided q4–6h. Pneumococcal meningitis: 250,000 units/kg/d (24 million units/d in adult) IV divided q2–4h. ▶K ♀B ▶? $$$$

PENICILLIN V (*Veetids, ✦PVF-K, Nadopen-V*)   Adults: 250–500 mg PO qid. Peds: 25–50 mg/kg/d divided bid-qid. AHA doses for pharyngitis: 250 mg (peds) or 500 mg (adults) PO bid-tid × 10 d. [Generic/Trade: Tabs 250, 500 mg, oral soln 125 & 250 mg/5 mL.] ▶K ♀B ▶? $

PROCAINE PENICILLIN (*Wycillin*)   0.6–1.0 million units IM daily (peak 4h, lasts 24h). ▶K ♀B ▶? $$$$$

SEXUALLY TRANSMITTED DISEASES & VAGINITIS

Overview: Treat sexual partners for all except herpes, candida, and bacterial vaginosis. Reference www.cdc.gov/STD/treatment/

Bacterial vaginosis: 1) metronidazole 5 g of 0.75% gel intravaginally daily × 5 d OR 500 mg PO bid × 7 d. 2) clindamycin 5 g of 2% cream intravaginally qhs × 7 d. In pregnancy: 1) metronidazole 500 mg PO bid × 7 d OR 250 mg PO tid × 7 d. 2) clindamycin 300 mg PO bid × 7 d.

Candidal vaginitis: 1) intravaginal clotrimazole, miconazole, terconazole, nystatin, tioconazole, or butoconazole. 2) fluconazole 150 mg PO single dose.

Chancroid: Single dose of: 1) azithromycin 1 g PO or 2) ceftriaxone 250 mg IM.

Chlamydia: First line either azithromycin 1 g PO single dose or doxycycline 100 mg PO bid × 7 d. Second line fluoroquinolones or erythromycin. In pregnancy: 1) azithromycin 1 g PO single dose. 2) amoxicillin 500 mg PO tid × 7 d. Repeat nucleic acid amplification test 3 wk after treatment.

Epididymitis: 1) ceftriaxone 250 mg IM single dose + doxycycline 100 mg PO bid × 10 d. 2) ofloxacin 300 mg PO bid or levofloxacin 500 mg PO daily × 10 d if enteric organisms suspected, or cephalosporin/doxycycline allergic.

Gonorrhea: Single dose: 1) ceftriaxone 125 mg IM. 2) cefixime 400 mg PO. 3) ciprofloxacin 500 mg PO. 4) ofloxacin 400 mg PO. 5) levofloxacin 250 mg PO. Treat chlamydia empirically. Cephalosporin desensitization advised for cephalosporin-allergic patients who cannot take fluoroquinolones (eg, pregnant women). Consider azithromycin 2 g PO single dose for uncomplicated gonorrhea, but no efficacy/safety data for this in pregnant women. Due to high resistance rates, quinolones not recommended if infection acquired in Hawaii or California, recent foreign travel by patient/partner, or in men who have sex with men. See health dept. or www.cdc.gov/std/gisp for current info.

Gonorrhea, disseminated: Initially treat with ceftriaxone 1 g IM/IV q24h until 24–48 h after improvement. Second-line alternatives: 1) ciprofloxacin 400 mg IV q12h. 2) ofloxacin 400 mg IV q12h. 3) levofloxacin 250 mg IV qd. 4) cefotaxime 1 g IV q8h. 5) ceftizoxime 1 g IV q8h. Complete 1 wk of treatment with: 1) cefixime 400 mg PO bid. 2) ciprofloxacin 500 mg PO bid. 3) ofloxacin 400 mg PO bid. 4) levofloxacin 500 mg PO daily. Cephalosporin desensitization advised for cephalosporin-allergic patients who cannot take fluoroquinolones (eg, pregnant women). Due to high resistance rates, quinolones not recommended if infection acquired in Hawaii or California, recent foreign travel by patient/partner, or in men who have sex with men. See health dept. or www.cdc.gov/std/gisp for resistance info.

Gonorrhea, meningitis: ceftriaxone 1–2 g IV q12h for 10–14 d.

Gonorrhea, endocarditis: ceftriaxone 1–2 g IV q12h for at least 4 wk.

Granuloma inguinale: doxycycline 100 mg PO bid × ≥3 wk and until lesions completely healed. Alternative azithromycin 1 g PO once weekly × 3 wk.

Herpes simplex (genital, first episode): 1) acyclovir 400 mg PO tid × 7–10 d. 2) famciclovir 250 PO tid × 7–10 d. 3) valacyclovir 1 g PO bid × 7–10 d.

Herpes simplex (genital, recurrent): 1) acyclovir 400 mg PO tid × 5 d. 2) acyclovir 800 mg PO tid × 2 d or bid × 5 d. 3) famciclovir 125 mg PO bid × 5 d. 4) famciclovir 1000 mg PO bid × 1 d. 5) valacyclovir 500 mg PO bid × 3 d. 6) valacyclovir 1 g PO daily × 5 d.

Herpes simplex (suppressive therapy): 1) acyclovir 400mg PO bid. 2) famciclovir 250 mg PO bid. 3) valacyclovir 500–1000 mg PO daily.

Herpes simplex, recurrent in HIV infection): 1) Acyclovir 400 mg PO tid × 5–10 d. 2) famciclovir 500 mg PO bid × 5–10 d. 3) Valacyclovir 1 g PO bid × 5–10 d.

Herpes simplex (suppressive therapy in HIV infection): 1) Acyclovir 400–800 mg PO bid-tid. 2) Famciclovir 500 mg PO bid. 3) Valacyclovir 500 mg PO bid.

(cont.)

SEXUALLY TRANSMITTED DISEASES & VAGINITIS, continued

Herpes simplex (prevention of transmission in immunocompetent patients with ≤9 *recurrences/yr):* Valacyclovir 500 mg PO daily by source partner, in conjunction with safer sex practices.

Lymphogranuloma venereum: 1) doxycycline 100 mg PO bid × 21 d. Alternative: erythromycin base 500 mg PO bid × 21 d.

Pelvic inflammatory disease (PID), inpatient regimens: 1) cefoxitin 2 g IV q6h + doxycycline 100 mg IV/PO q12h. 2) clindamycin 900 mg IV q8h + gentamicin 2 mg/kg IM/IV loading dose, then 1.5 mg/kg IM/IV q8h (See gentamicin entry for alternative daily dosing). Can switch to PO therapy within 24 h of improvement.

Pelvic inflammatory disease (PID), outpatient treatment: 1) ceftriaxone 250 mg IM single dose + doxycycline 100 mg PO bid +/– metronidazole 500 mg PO bid × 14 d.) ofloxacin 400 mg PO bid/levofloxacin 500 mg PO daily +/– metronidazole 500 mg PO bid × 14 d. Due to high resistance rates, quinolones not recommended if infection acquired in Hawaii or California, recent foreign travel by patient/partner, or in men who have sex with men. See health department or www.cdc.gov/std/gisp for current resistance info.

Proctitis, proctocolitis, enteritis: ceftriaxone 125 mg IM single dose + doxycycline 100 mg PO bid x7d.

Sexual assault prophylaxis: ceftriaxone 125 mg IM single dose + metronidazole 2 g PO single dose + azithromycin 1 g PO single dose/doxycycline 100 mg PO bid × 7 d. Consider giving antiemetic

Syphilis (primary and secondary): 1) benzathine penicillin 2.4 million units IM single dose. 2) doxycycline 100 mg PO bid × 2 weeks if penicillin allergic.

Syphilis (early latent, ie, duration <1 y): 1) benzathine penicillin 2.4 million units IM single dose. 2) doxycycline 100 mg PO bid × 2 weeks if penicillin allergic.

Syphilis (late latent or unknown duration): 1) benzathine penicillin 2.4 million units IM q week × 3 doses.

2) doxycycline 100 mg PO bid × 4 weeks if penicillin allergic.

Syphilis (tertiary): 1) benzathine penicillin 2.4 million units IM q week × 3 doses. 2) doxycycline 100 mg PO bid × 4 weeks if penicillin allergic.

Syphilis (neuro): 1) penicillin G 18–24 million units/d continuous IV infusion or 3–4 million units IV q4h × 10–14 d. 2) procaine penicillin 2.4 million units IM daily + probenecid 500 mg PO qid, both × 10–14 d.

Syphilis in pregnancy: Treat only with penicillin regimen for stage of syphilis as noted above. Use penicillin desensitization protocol if penicillin-allergic.

Trichomonal vaginitis: metronidazole 2 g PO single dose (can use in pregnancy) or tinidazole 2 g PO single dose.

Urethritis, Cervicitis: Test for Chlamydia and gonorrhea with nucleic acid amplification test. Treat based on test results or treat presumptively if high-risk of infection (Chlamydia: age ≤25 y, new/multiple sex partners, or unprotected sex; gonorrhea: population prevalence >5%), esp. if nucleic acid amplification test unavailable or patient unlikely to return for follow-up.

Urethritis (persistent/recurrent): 1) metronidazole/tinidazole 2 g PO single dose + azithromycin 2 g PO single dose (if not used in first episode).

Penicillins—2nd generation—Penicillinase-Resistant

DICLOXACILLIN (*Dynapen*)   250–500 mg PO qid. Peds: 12.5–25 mg/kg/d divided qid. [Generic only: Caps 250, 500 mg.] ▶KL ♀B ▶? $$

NAFCILLIN 1–2 g IM/IV q4h. Peds: 50–200 mg/kg/d divided q4–6h. ▶L ♀B ▶? $$$$$

OXACILLIN (*Bactocill*) 1–2 g IM/IV q4–6h. Peds 150–200 mg/kg/d IM/IV divided q4–6h. ▶KL ♀B ▶? $$$$$

Penicillins—3rd generation—Aminopenicillins

AMOXICILLIN (*Amoxil, DisperMox, Moxatag, Trimox, ✦Novamoxin*) 250–500 mg PO tid, or 500–875 mg PO bid. Acute sinusitis with antibiotic use in past mo &/or drug-resistant S pneumoniae rate >30%: 3–3.5 g/d PO. High-dose for community-acquired pneumonia: 1 g PO tid. Lyme disease: 500 mg PO tid × 14 d for early disease, × 28 d for Lyme arthritis. Chlamydia in pregnancy: 500 mg PO tid × 7 d. Group A streptococcal pharyngitis/ tonsillitis, ≥12 yo: 775 mg ER tab (Moxatag) PO × 10 d. Peds AAP otitis media: 80–90 mg/kg/d divided bid-tid. AAP recommends 5–7 d of therapy for older (≥6 yo) children with non-severe otitis media, and 10 d for younger children and those with severe disease. Peds non-otitis: 40 mg/kg/d PO divided tid or 45 mg/kg/d divided bid. [Generic/Trade: Caps 250, 500 mg, tabs 500, 875 mg, chews 125, 200, 250, 400 mg, susp 125 & 250 mg/5 mL, susp 200 & 400 mg/5 mL. Trade only: Infant drops 50 mg/mL (Amoxil). DisperMox 200, 400, 600 mg tabs for oral susp, Moxatag 775 mg extended-release tab.] ▶K ♀B ▶+ $

AMOXICILLIN-CLAVULANATE (*Augmentin, Augmentin ES-600, Augmentin XR, ✦Clavulin*) 500–875 mg PO bid or 250–500 mg PO tid. Augmentin XR: 2 tabs PO q12h with meals. Peds AAP otitis media: Augmentin ES 90 mg/kg/d divided bid. AAP recommends 5–7 d of therapy for older (≥6 yo) children with non-severe otitis media, and 10 d for younger children and those with severe disease. Peds: 45 mg/kg/d PO divided bid or 40 mg/kg/d divided tid for otitis, sinusitis, pneumonia; 25 mg/kg/d divided bid or 20 mg/kg/d divided tid for less severe infections. [Generic/Trade: (amoxicillin + clavulanate) Tabs 250+125, 500+125, 875+125 mg, chewables and susp 200+28.5, 400+57 mg per tab or 5 mL, (ES) susp 600+42.9 mg/5 mL Trade only: Chewables and susp 125+31.25, 250+62.5 mg per tab or 5 mL. Extended-release tabs (Augmentin XR) 1000+62.5 mg.] ▶K ♀B ▶? $$$$

AMPICILLIN (*Principen, ✦Penbritin*) Usual dose: 1–2 g IV q4–6h. Sepsis, meningitis: 150–200 mg/kg/d IV divided q3–4h. Peds: 50–400 mg/kg/d IM/IV divided q4–6h. [Generic/Trade: Caps 250,500 mg, susp 125 & 250 mg/5 mL.] ▶K ♀B ▶? $ PO $$$$$ IV

AMPICILLIN-SULBACTAM (*Unasyn*) 1.5–3 g IM/IV q6h. Peds: 100–400 mg/kg/d of ampicillin divided q6h. ▶K ♀B ▶? $$$$$

PIVAMPICILLIN (*Pondocillin*) Canada only. Adults: 500–1000 mg PO bid. Infants, 3–12 mo: 40–60 mg/kg/d PO divided bid. Peds, 1–10 yo: 25–35 mg/kg/d PO divided bid up to 525 mg PO bid. [Trade only: Tabs 500 mg (377 mg ampicillin), # 20, oral susp 35 mg/mL (26 mg ampicillin), 100,150,200 mL bottles.] ▶K ♀? ▶? $

Penicillins—4th generation—Extended Spectrum

PIPERACILLIN 3–4 g IM/IV q4–6h. ▶K/BILE ♀B ▶? $$$$$

PIPERACILLIN-TAZOBACTAM (*Zosyn, ✦Tazocin*) 3.375–4.5 g IV q6h. Peds: 300–400 mg/kg/d piperacillin IV divided q6–8h for >6 mo; 150–300 mg/

(cont.)

kg/d IV divided q6–8h for <6 mo. Peds appendicitis/peritonitis: 100 mg/kg piperacillin IV q8h for ≥9 mo; 80 mg/kg IV q8h for 2–9 mo; use adult dose if >40 kg. ▶K ♀B ▶? $$$$$

TICARCILLIN (*Ticar*) 3–4 g IM/IV q4–6h. Peds: 200–300 mg/kg/d divided q4–6h. ▶K ♀B ▶+ $$$$$

TICARCILLIN-CLAVULANATE (*Timentin*) 3.1 g IV q4–6h. Peds: 50 mg/kg up to 3.1 g IV q4–6h. ▶K ♀B ▶? $$$$$

Quinolones—1st Generation

NALIDIXIC ACID (*NegGram*) 1 g PO qid. [Trade only: Tabs 0.25, 0.5, 1 g.] ▶KL ♀C ▶? $$$$

Quinolones—2nd Generation

CIPROFLOXACIN (*Cipro, Cipro XR, ProQuin XR*) 200–400 mg IV q8–12h. 250–750 mg PO bid. Simple UTI: 250 mg bid × 3d or Cipro XR/Proquin XR 500 mg PO daily × 3d. Give Proquin XR with main meal of d. Cipro XR for pyelonephritis or complicated UTI: 1000 mg PO daily × 7–14 d. [Generic/ Trade: Tabs 100, 250, 500, 750 mg. Extended release tabs 500, 1000 mg. Trade only (ProQuin XR) Extended release tabs 500 mg, blister pack 500 mg (#3 tabs).] ▶LK ♀C but teratogenicity unlikely ▶?+ $

LOMEFLOXACIN (*Maxaquin*) 400 mg PO daily. Take at night. Photosensitivity. [Trade only: Tabs 400 mg.] ▶LK ♀C ▶? $$$

NORFLOXACIN (*Noroxin*) Simple UTI: 400 mg PO bid × 3 d. [Trade only: Tabs 400 mg.] ▶LK ♀C ▶? $$$

OFLOXACIN (*Floxin*) 200–400 mg PO bid. [Generic/Trade: Tabs 200, 300, 400 mg.] ▶LK ♀C ▶?+ $$$

Quinolones—3rd Generation

LEVOFLOXACIN (*Levaquin*) 250–750 mg PO/IV daily. [Trade only: Tabs 250, 500, 750 mg, oral soln 25 mg/mL. Leva-Pak: #5, 750 mg tabs.] ▶KL ♀C ▶? $$$$

SBE PROPHYLAXIS

For dental, oral, respiratory tract, or esophageal procedures	
Standard regimen	amoxicillin 2 g PO 1 h before procedure
Unable to take oral meds	ampicillin 2 g IM/IV within 30 min before procedure
Allergic to penicillin	clindamycin 600 mg PO; or cephalexin or cefadroxil 2 g PO; or azithromycin or clarithromycin 500 mg PO 1 h before procedure
Allergic to penicillin and unable to take oral meds	clindamycin 600 mg IV; or cefazolin 1 g IM/IV within 30 min before procedure
Pediatric drug doses	Total pediatric dose should not exceed adult dose. Amoxicillin 50 mg/kg, ampicillin 50 mg/kg, azithromycin 15 mg/kg, cephalexin 50 mg/kg, cefadroxil 50 mg/kg, cefazolin 25 mg/ kg, clarithromycin 15 mg/kg, clindamycin 20 mg/kg.

PENICILLINS—GENERAL ANTIMICROBIAL SPECTRUM

1st generation: Most streptococci; oral anaerobic coverage
2nd generation: Most streptococci; *Staph aureus*
3rd generation: Most streptococci; basic gram negative coverage
4th generation: *Pseudomonas*

Quinolones—4th Generation

GEMIFLOXACIN (*Factive*) 320 mg PO daily × 5–7 d. [Trade only: Tabs 320 mg.] ▶Feces, K ♀C ▶- $$$

MOXIFLOXACIN (*Avelox*) 400 mg PO/IV daily × 5 d (chronic bronchitis exacerbation), 5–14 d (complicated intra-abdominal infection; usually given IV initially), 7 d (uncomplicated skin infections), 10 d (acute sinusitis), 7–14 d (community acquired pneumonia), 7–21 d (complicated skin infections). [Trade only: Tabs 400 mg.] ▶LK ♀C ▶- $$$

Sulfonamides

SULFADIAZINE CNS toxoplasmosis in AIDS. 1000 mg (<60 kg) to 1500 mg (≥60 kg) PO qid for acute treatment; 500–1000 mg PO qid for secondary prevention. Give with pyrimethamine + leucovorin. [Generic only: Tab 500 mg.] ▶K ♀C ▶+ $$$$

TRIMETHOPRIM-SULFAMETHOXAZOLE (*Bactrim, Septra, Sulfatrim, Cotrimoxazole*) One tab PO bid, double strength (DS, 160 mg/800 mg) or single strength (SS, 80 mg/400 mg). Pneumocystis treatment: 15–20 mg/kg/d (based on TMP) IV divided q6–8h or PO divided tid × 21 d total. Pneumocystis prophylaxis: 1 DS tab PO daily. Peds: 5 mL susp/10 kg (up to 20 mL)/dose PO bid. [Generic/Trade: Tabs 80 mg TMP/400 mg SMX (single strength), 160 mg TMP/800 mg SMX (double strength); susp 40 mg TMP/200 mg SMX per 5 mL. 20 mL susp = 2 SS tabs = 1 DS tab.] ▶K ♀C ▶+ $

Tetracyclines

DEMECLOCYCLINE (*Declomycin*) Usual dose: 150 mg PO qid or 300 mg PO bid on empty stomach. SIADH: 600–1200 mg/d PO given in 3–4 divided doses. [Generic/Trade : Tabs 150,300 mg.] ▶K, feces ♀D ▶? + $$$$$

DOXYCYCLINE (*Adoxa, Doryx, Monodox, Oracea, Periostat, Vibramycin, Vibra-Tabs, ✚Doxycin*) 100 mg PO bid on first d, then 50 mg bid or 100 mg daily. 100 mg PO/IV bid for severe infections. Lyme disease: 100 mg PO bid × 14 d for early disease, × 28 d for Lyme arthritis. Periostat for periodontitis: 20 mg PO bid. Oracea for inflammatory rosacea: 40 mg PO every morning on empty stomach. Malaria prophylaxis: 2 mg/kg/d up to 100 mg PO daily starting 1–2 d before exposure until 4 wk after. Avoid in children <8 yo due to teeth staining. [Generic/Trade: Tabs 75,100 mg, caps 20, 50,100 mg. Susp 25 mg/5 mL (60 mL). Trade only: (Vibramycin) Syrup 50 mg/5 mL (480 mL). Delayed Release (Doryx): Tabs 75,100 mg, Caps 40 mg (Oracea). Generic only: Caps 75,150 mg tabs 50,150 mg.] ▶LK ♀D ▶? + $

QUINOLONES- GENERAL ANTIMICROBIAL SPECTRUM

1st generation: gram negative (excluding *Pseudomonas*), urinary tract only, no atypicals

2nd generation: gram negative (including *Pseudomonas*); *Staph aureus* but not *pneumococcus*; some atypicals

3rd generation: gram negative (including *Pseudomonas*); gram positive (including *Staph aureus* and pneumococcus); expanded atypical coverage

4th generation: same as 3rd generation plus enhanced coverage of *pneumococcus*, decreased activity vs. *Pseudomonas*.

MINOCYCLINE (*Minocin, Dynacin, Solodyn, ★Enca*) 200 mg IV/PO initially, then 100 mg q12h. Solodyn for inflammatory acne, ≥12 yo: Give PO once daily at dose of 45 mg for 45–<60 kg, 90 mg for 60–90 kg, 135 mg for 91–136 kg. [Generic/Trade: Caps, tabs 50, 75, 100 mg. Trade only (Solodyn): Extended release tabs 45, 90, 135 mg.] ▶LK ♀D ▷?+ $$$

TETRACYCLINE (*Sumycin*) 250–500 mg PO qid. [Generic/Trade: Caps 250, 500 mg. Trade only: Tabs 250, 500 mg, susp 125 mg/5 mL.] ▶LK ♀D ▷?+ $

Other Antimicrobials

AZTREONAM (*Azactam*) 0.5–2 g IM/IV q6–12h. Peds: 30 mg/kg q6–8h. ▶K ♀B ▷+ $$$$$

CHLORAMPHENICOL (*Chloromycetin*) 50–100 mg/kg/d IV divided q6h. Aplastic anemia. ▶LK ♀C ▷- $$$$$

CLINDAMYCIN (*Cleocin, ★Dalacin C*) 600–900 mg IV q8h. Each IM injection should be ≤600 mg. 150–450 mg PO qid. Peds: 20–40 mg/kg/d IV divided q6–8h or 8–25 mg/kg/d susp PO divided tid-qid. [Generic/Trade: Cap 75, 150, 300 mg. Trade only: Oral soln 75 mg/5 mL.] ▶L ♀B ▷?+ $$$

DAPTOMYCIN (*Cubicin, Cidecin*) Complicated skin infections: 4 mg/kg IV daily × 7–14 d. S aureus bacteremia: 6 mg/kg IV daily × ≥2–6 wk. Infuse over 30 min. ▶K ♀B ▷? $$$$$

DROTRECOGIN (*Xigris*) To reduce mortality in sepsis: 24 mcg/kg/h IV × 96 h. ▶Plasma ♀C ▷? $$$$$

FOSFOMYCIN (*Monurol*) Simple UTI: One 3 g packet PO single-dose. [Trade only: 3 g packet of granules.] ▶K ♀B ▷? $$

LINEZOLID (*Zyvox, ★Zyvoxam*) 400–600 mg IV/PO q12h. Infuse over 30–120 min. Peds ≤11 yo: 10 mg/kg IV/PO q8h. Uncomplicated skin infections: 10 mg/kg PO q8h if <5 yo, q12h if 5–11 yo. Myelosuppression. MAO inhibitor. [Trade only: Tabs 600 mg, susp 100 mg/5 mL.] ▶Oxidation/K ♀C ▷? $$$$$

METRONIDAZOLE (*Flagyl, ★Florazole ER, Trikacide, Nidazol*) Bacterial vaginosis: 500 mg PO bid or Flagyl ER 750 mg PO daily × 7 d. H pylori: See table in GI section. Anaerobic bacterial infections: Load 1 g or 15 mg/kg IV, then 500 mg or 7.5 mg/kg IV/PO q6–8h, each IV dose over 1 h (not to exceed 4 g/d). Peds: 7.5 mg/kg IV q6h. C difficile diarrhea: 500 mg (10–15 mg/kg/dose for peds) PO tid. Trichomoniasis: 2 g PO single dose for patient & sex partners (may be used in pregnancy per CDC). Giardia: 250 mg (5 mg/kg/dose for peds) PO tid × 5–7 d Giardia: 250 mg PO tid × 5–7 d. [Generic/Trade: Tabs 250,500 mg, ER tabs 750 mg, Caps 375 mg.] ▶KL ♀B ▷?- $

NITROFURANTOIN (*Furadantin, Macrodantin, Macrobid*) 50–100 mg PO qid. Peds: 5–7 mg/kg/d divided qid. Macrobid: 100 mg PO bid. [Nitrofurantoin macrocrystals (Macrodantin) generic/trade: Caps 25,50,100 mg. Nitrofurantoin macrocrystals/monohydrate (Macrobid) generic/trade: Caps 100 mg. Furadantin: Susp 25 mg/5 mL. ▶KL ♀B ▶+? $$

RIFAXIMIN (*Xifaxan*) Travelers diarrhea: 200 mg PO tid × 3 d. [Trade only: Tab 200 mg.] ▶Feces, no GI absorption ♀C ▶? $$

SYNERCID (*quinupristin + dalfopristin*) 7.5 mg/kg IV q8–12 h, each dose over 1 h. Not active against E. faecalis. ▶Bile ♀B ▶? $$$$$

TELITHROMYCIN (*Ketek*) 800 mg PO daily × 7–10 d for community-acquired pneumonia. No longer indicated for acute sinusitis or acute exacerbation of chronic bronchitis (risks exceed potential benefit). Contraindicated in myasthenia gravis. [Trade only: 300,400 mg tabs. Ketek Pak: #10, 400 mg tabs.] ▶LK ♀C ▶? $$$

TIGECYCLINE (*Tygacil*) Complicated skin or intra-abdominal infections: 100 mg IV first dose, then 50 mg IV q12h. Infuse over 30–60 min. ▶Bile, K ♀D ▶?+ $$$$$

TRIMETHOPRIM (*Primsol, ♦Proloprim*) 100 mg PO bid or 200 mg PO daily. [Generic only: Tabs 100,200 mg. Primsol: Oral soln 50 mg/5 mL.] ▶K ♀C ▶- $

VANCOMYCIN (*Vancocin*) 1 g IV q12h, each dose over 1h. Peds: 10–15 mg/kg IV q6h. Clostridium difficile diarrhea: 40–50 mg/kg/d up to 500 mg/d PO divided qid × 7–10 d. IV administration ineffective for this indication. [Trade only: Caps 125, 250 mg.] ▶K ♀C ▶? $$$$$

CARDIOVASCULAR

ACE Inhibitors

NOTE: *See also antihypertensive combinations. Hyperkalemia possible, especially if used concomitantly with other drugs that increase K+ (including K+ containing salt substitutes) and in patients with heart failure, diabetes mellitus, or renal impairment. Monitor closely for hypoglycemia during first month of treatment when combined with insulin or oral antidiabetic agents. ACE inhibitors are contraindicated during pregnancy. Contraindicated with a history of angioedema. Renoprotection and decreased cardiovascular morbidity/mortality seen with some ACE inhibitors are most likely a class effect.*

BENAZEPRIL (*Lotensin*) HTN: Start 10 mg PO daily, usual maintenance dose 20–40 mg PO daily or divided bid, max 80 mg/d. [Generic/Trade: Tabs, nonscored 5, 10, 20, 40 mg.] ▶LK ♀- ▶? $$

CAPTOPRIL (*Capoten*) HTN: Start 25 mg PO bid-tid, usual maintenance dose 25–150 mg bid-tid, max 450 mg/d. Heart failure: Start 6.25–12.5 mg PO tid, usual dose 50–100 mg PO tid, max 450 mg/d. Diabetic nephropathy: 25 mg PO tid. [Generic/Trade: Tabs, scored 12.5, 25, 50, 100 mg.] ▶LK ♀- ▶+ $

ACE INHIBITOR DOSING	Hypertension		Heart Failure		
	Initial	Max/d	Initial	Target	Max
benazepril (Lotensin)	10 mg qd*	80 mg	n.r.	n.r.	n.r.
captopril (Capoten)	25 mg bid/tid	450 mg	6.25–12.5 mg tid	50 mg tid	150 mg tid
enalapril (Vasotec)	5 mg qd*	40 mg	2.5 mg bid	10 mg bid	20 mg bid
fosinopril (Monopril)	10 mg qd*	80 mg	10 mg qd	20 mg qd	40 mg qd
lisinopril (Zestril/ Prinivil)	10 mg qd	80 mg	5 mg qd	20 mg qd	40 mg qd
moexipril (Univasc)	7.5 mg qd*	30 mg	n.r.	n.r.	n.r.
perindopril (Aceon)	4 mg qd*	16 mg	n.r.	n.r.	n.r.
quinapril (Accupril)	10–20 mg qd*	80 mg	5 mg bid	10 mg bid	20 mg bid
ramipril (Altace)	2.5 mg qd*	20 mg	2.5 mg bid	5 mg bid	10 mg bid
trandolapril (Mavik)	1–2 mg qd*	8 mg	1 mg qd	4 mg qd	4 mg qd

Data taken from prescribing information. *May require bid dosing for 24-h BP control. n.r. = not recommended

CILAZAPRIL (✦*Inhibace*) (Canada only). HTN: 1.25–10 mg PO daily. [Generic/ Trade: Tabs, scored 1, 2.5, 5 mg.] ▶LK ♀– ▶? $

ENALAPRIL (*enalaprilat, Vasotec*) HTN: Start 5 mg PO daily, usual mainte-nance dose 10–40 mg PO daily or divided bid, max 40 mg/d. If oral therapy not possible, can use enalaprilat 1.25 mg IV q6h over 5 min, and increase up to 5 mg IV q6h if needed. Renal impairment or concomitant diuretic therapy: Start 2.5 mg PO daily. Heart failure: Start 2.5 mg PO bid, usual 10–20 mg PO bid, max 40 mg/d. [Generic/Trade: Tabs, scored 2.5, 5 mg, non-scored 10, 20 mg.] ▶LK ♀– ▶+ $$

FOSINOPRIL (*Monopril*) HTN: Start 10 mg PO daily, usual maintenance dose 20–40 mg PO daily or divided bid, max 80 mg/d. Heart failure: Start 10 mg PO daily, usual dose 20–40 mg PO daily, max 40 mg/d. [Generic/Trade: Tabs, scored 10, non-scored 20, 40 mg.] ▶LK ♀– ▶? $

LISINOPRIL (*Prinivil, Zestril*) HTN: Start 10 mg PO daily, usual maintenance dose 20–40 mg PO daily, max 80 mg/d. Heart failure, acute MI: Start 2.5–5 mg PO daily, usual dose 5–20 mg PO daily, max dose 40 mg. [Generic/Trade: Tabs, non-scored (Zestril) 2.5, 5, 10, 20, 30, 40 mg. Tabs, scored (Prinivil) 10, 20, 40 mg.] ▶K ♀– ▶? $

MOEXIPRIL (*Univasc*) HTN: Start 7.5 mg PO daily, usual maintenance dose 7.5–30 mg PO daily or divided bid, max 30 mg/d. [Generic/Trade: Tabs, scored 7.5, 15 mg.] ▶LK ♀– ▶? $$

PERINDOPRIL (*Aceon,* ✦*Coversyl*) HTN: Start 4 mg PO daily, usual mainte-nance dose 4–8 mg PO daily or divided bid, max 16 mg/d. Reduction of cardio-vascular events in stable coronary artery disease: Start 4 mg PO/d × 2 wk, max 8 mg/d. Elderly (>70 yr): 2 mg PO/d × 1 wk, 4 mg PO/d × 1 wk, max 8 mg/d. [Trade only: Tabs, scored 2, 4, 8 mg.] ▶K ♀– ▶? $$$

QUINAPRIL (*Accupril*) HTN: Start 10–20 mg PO daily (start 10 mg/d if elderly), usual maintenance dose 20–80 mg PO daily or divided bid, max

(cont.)

80 mg/d. Heart failure: Start 5 mg PO bid, usual maintenance dose 10–20 mg bid. [Generic/Trade: Tabs, scored 5, non-scored 10, 20, 40 mg.] ▶LK ♀- ▶? $$

RAMIPRIL (*Altace*) HTN: 2.5 mg PO daily, usual maintenance dose 2.5–20 mg PO daily or divided bid, max 20 mg/d. Heart failure post-MI: Start 2.5 mg PO bid, usual maintenance dose 5 mg PO bid. Reduce risk of MI, stroke, death from cardiovascular causes: 2.5 mg PO daily × 1 wk, then 5 mg daily × 3 wk, increase as tolerated to max 10 mg/d. [Generic/Trade: Caps 1.25, 2.5, 5, 10 mg. Trade only: Tabs 1.25, 2.5, 5, 10 mg.] ▶LK ♀- ▶? $$$

TRANDOLAPRIL (*Mavik*) HTN: Start 1 mg PO daily, usual maintenance dose 2–4 mg PO daily or divided bid, max 8 mg/d. Heart failure/post-MI: Start 0.5–1 mg PO daily, usual maintenance dose 4 mg PO daily. [Generic/Trade: Tabs, 1, 2, 4 mg.] ▶LK ♀- ▶? $$

Aldosterone Antagonists

EPLERENONE (*Inspra*) HTN: Start 50 mg PO daily; max 50 mg bid. Improve survival of stable patients with left ventricular systolic dysfunction (EF ≤40%) and heart failure post-MI: Start 25 mg PO daily; titrate to target dose 50 mg daily within 4 wk, if tolerated. [Trade only: Tabs non-scored 25, 50 mg.] ▶L ♀B ▶? $$$$

SPIRONOLACTONE (*Aldactone*) HTN: 50–100 mg PO daily or divided bid. Edema: 25–200 mg/d. Hypokalemia: 50–100 mg PO daily. Primary hyperaldosteronism, maintenance: 100–400 mg/d PO. Cirrhotic ascites: Start 100 mg once daily or in divided doses. Maintenance 25–200 mg/d. [Generic/Trade: Tabs, non-scored 25; scored 50,100 mg.] ▶LK ♀D ▶+ $

Angiotensin Receptor Blockers (ARBs)

NOTE *See also antihypertensive combinations.*

CANDESARTAN (*Atacand*) HTN: Start 16 mg PO daily, max 32 mg/d. Reduce cardiovascular death and hospitalizations from heart failure (NYHA II-IV and ejection fraction ≤40%): Start 4 mg PO daily, max 32 mg/d; has added effect when used with ACE inhibitor. [Trade only: Tabs, non-scored 4, 8, 16, 32 mg.] ▶K ♀- ▶? $$$

EPROSARTAN (*Teveten*) HTN: Start 600 mg PO daily, max 800 mg/d given daily or divided bid. [Trade only: Tabs non-scored 400, 600 mg.] ▶Fecal excretion ♀- ▶? $$$

IRBESARTAN (*Avapro*) HTN: Start 150 mg PO daily, max 300 mg/d. Type 2 diabetic nephropathy: Start 150 mg PO daily, target dose 300 mg daily. [Trade only: Tabs, non-scored 75, 150, 300 mg.] ▶L ♀- ▶? $$$

LOSARTAN (*Cozaar*) HTN: Start 50 mg PO daily, max 100 mg/d given daily or divided bid. Volume-depleted patients or history of hepatic impairment: Start 25 mg PO daily. Stroke risk reduction in patients with HTN & left ventricular hypertrophy (does not appear to apply to Blacks): Start 50 mg PO daily. If need more BP reduction add HCTZ 12.5 mg PO daily; then increase losartan to

(cont.)

HYPERTENSION THERAPY*

Area of Concern	Blood Pressure Target	Preferred Therapy	Comments
General coronary artery disease prevention	<140/90 mm Hg	ACE inhibitor, angiotensin receptor blocker, calcium channel blocker, thiazide, or combination. Start 2 drugs if systolic BP ≥160 or diastolic BP ≥100	None
High coronary artery disease risk	<130/80 mm Hg	ACE inhibitor, angiotensin receptor blocker, calcium channel blocker, thiazide, or combination. Start 2 drugs if systolic BP ≥160 or diastolic BP ≥100	High coronary artery disease risk is diabetes mellitus, chronic kidney disease, known coronary artery disease or risk equivalent (eg, peripheral artery disease, abdominal aortic aneurysm), 10-year Framingham risk score ≥10%.
Stable angina, unstable angina, MI	<130/80 mm Hg	Beta blocker plus either an ACE inhibitor or an angiotensin receptor blocker	May add dihydropyridine calcium channel blocker or thiazide. Use beta blockers only if hemodynamically stable. If beta-blocker contraindications or intolerable side effects (and no bradycardia or heart failure), may substitute verapamil or diltiazem.
Left heart failure	<120/80 mm Hg	Beta blocker plus either an ACE inhibitor or an angiotensin receptor blocker, plus a loop or thiazide diuretic, plus an aldosterone antagonist (if NYHA class III or IV, or if clinical heart failure and LV ejection fraction <40%).	Avoid verapamil, diltiazem, clonidine, alpha-blockers. For Blacks with New York Heart Association class III or IV heart failure, consider adding hydralazine/isosorbide dinitrate.

*All patients should attempt lifestyle modifications: optimize weight, healthy diet, sodium restriction, exercise, smoking cessation, alcohol moderation. Adapted from *Circulation* 2007;115:2761–2788.

100 mg/d, then increase HCTZ to 25 mg/d. Type 2 diabetic nephropathy: Start 50 mg PO daily, target dose 100 mg daily. [Trade only: Tabs, non-scored 25, 50, 100 mg.] ▶L ♀-▶? $$$

OLMESARTAN (*Benicar*) HTN: Start 20 mg PO daily, max 40 mg/d. [Trade only: Tabs, non-scored 5, 20, 40 mg.] ▶K ♀-▶? $$$

TELMISARTAN (*Micardis*) HTN: Start 40 mg PO daily, max 80 mg/d. [Trade only: Tabs, non-scored 20, 40, 80 mg.] ▶L ♀-▶? $$$

VALSARTAN (*Diovan*) HTN: Start 80–160 mg PO daily, max 320 mg/d. Heart failure: Start 40 mg PO bid, target dose 160 mg bid; there is no evidence of

(cont.)

added benefit when used with adequate dose of ACE inhibitor. Reduce mortality/morbidity post-MI with left ventricular systolic dysfunction/failure: Start 20 mg PO bid, target dose 160 mg bid. [Trade only: Tabs, scored 40 mg, nonscored 80, 160, 320 mg.] ▶L ♀- ▶? $$$

Antiadrenergic Agents

CLONIDINE (*Catapres, Catapres-TTS, ✦Dixarit*) HTN: Start 0.1 mg PO bid, usual maintenance dose 0.2 to 1.2 mg/d divided bid-tid, max 2.4 mg/d. Rebound HTN with abrupt discontinuation, especially at doses ≥0.8 mg/d. Transdermal (Catapres-TTS): Start 0.1 mg/24 h patch q wk, titrate to desired effect, max effective dose 0.6 mg/24 h (two, 0.3 mg/24 h patches). Transdermal Therapeutic System (TTS) is designed for once a week use so that a TTS-1 delivers 0.1 mg/d × 7 d. May supplement first dose of TTS with oral × 2–3 d while therapeutic level is achieved. ADHD (unapproved peds): Start 0.05 mg PO qhs, titrate based on response over 8 wk to max 0.2 mg/d (<45 kg) or 0.4 mg/d (> 45 kg) in 2–4 divided doses. Tourette's syndrome (unapproved peds and adult): 3–5 mcg/kg/d PO divided bid-qid. Opioid withdrawal, adjunct: 0.1–0.3 mg PO tid-qid or 0.1–0.2 mg PO q4h tapering off over d 4–10. Alcohol withdrawal, adjunct: 0.1–0.2 mg PO q4h prn. Smoking cessation: Start 0.1 mg PO bid, increase 0.1 mg/d at weekly intervals to 0.75 mg/d as tolerated; transdermal (Catapres-TTS): 0.1–0.2 mg/24 h patch q wk for 2–3 wk after cessation. Menopausal flushing: 0.1–0.4 mg/d PO divided bid-tid. Transdermal system applied weekly: 0.1 mg/d. [Generic/Trade: Tabs, non-scored 0.1, 0.2, 0.3 mg. Trade only: transdermal weekly patch 0.1 mg/d (TTS-1), 0.2 mg/d (TTS-2), 0.3 mg/d (TTS-3).] ▶LK ♀C ▶? $$

DOXAZOSIN (*Cardura, Cardura XL*) BPH: Immediate release: Start 1 mg PO qhs, max 8 mg/d. Extended release (not approved for HTN): 4 mg PO qam with breakfast, max 8 mg/d. HTN: Start 1 mg PO qhs, max 16 mg/d. Take first dose at bedtime to minimize orthostatic hypotension. [Generic/Trade: Tabs, scored 1, 2, 4, 8 mg. Trade only (Cardura XL): Tabs, extended-release 4, 8 mg.] ▶L ♀C ▶? $$

GUANFACINE (*Tenex*) Start 1 mg PO qhs, increase to 2–3 mg qhs if needed after 3–4 wk, max 3 mg/d. ADHD in children: Start 0.5 mg PO daily, titrate by 0.5 mg q3–4 d as tolerated to 0.5 mg PO tid. [Generic/Trade: Tabs, non-scored 1, 2 mg.] ▶K ♀B ▶? $

METHYLDOPA (*Aldomet*) HTN: Start 250 mg PO bid-tid, max 3000 mg/d. May cause hemolytic anemia. [Generic only: Tabs, non-scored 125, 250, 500 mg.] ▶LK ♀B ▶+ $

PRAZOSIN (*Minipress*) HTN: Start 1 mg PO bid-tid, max 40 mg/d. Take first dose at bedtime to minimize orthostatic hypotension. [Generic/Trade: Caps 1, 2, 5 mg.] ▶L ♀C ▶? $$

TERAZOSIN (*Hytrin*) HTN: Start 1 mg PO qhs, usual effective dose 1–5 mg PO daily or divided bid, max 20 mg/d. Take first dose at bedtime to minimize orthostatic hypotension. BPH: Start 1 mg PO qhs, usual effective dose 10 mg/d, max 20 mg/d. [Generic/Trade: Tabs & Caps 1, 2, 5, 10 mg.] ▶LK ♀C ▶? $$

Anti-Dysrhythmics/Cardiac Arrest

ADENOSINE (*Adenocard*) PSVT conversion (not A-fib): Adult and peds ≥50 kg: 6 mg rapid IV & flush, preferably through a central line. If no response after 1–2 mins then 12 mg. A third dose of 12 mg may be given prn. Peds <50 kg: initial dose 50–100 mcg/kg, subsequent doses 100–200 mcg/kg q1–2 min prn up to a max single dose of 300 mcg/kg or 12 mg whichever is less. Half-life is <10 sec. Give doses by rapid IV push followed by normal saline flush. Need higher dose if on theophylline or caffeine, lower dose if on dipyridamole or carbamazepine. ▶Plasma ♀C ▶? $$$

AMIODARONE (*Cordarone, Pacerone*) Life-threatening ventricular arrhythmia without cardiac arrest: Load 150 mg IV over 10 min, then 1 mg/min × 6h, then 0.5 mg/min × 18h. Mix in D5W. Oral loading dose 800–1600 mg PO daily for 1–3 wk, reduce to 400–800 mg PO daily for 1 mo when arrhythmia is controlled, reduce to lowest effective dose thereafter, usually 200–400 mg PO daily. Photosensitivity with oral therapy. Pulmonary & hepatic toxicity. Hypo or hyperthyroidism possible. Co-administration of fluoroquinolones, macrolides, or azoles may prolong QTc. May increase digoxin levels; discontinue digoxin or decrease dose by 50%. May increase INR with warfarin by up to 100%; decrease warfarin dose by 33–50%. Do not use with grapefruit juice. Do not use with simvastatin >20 mg/d, or lovastatin >40 mg/d; caution with, or atorvastatin; increases risk of myopathy and rhabdomyolysis. Caution with beta blockers and calcium channel blockers. IV therapy may cause hypotension. Contraindicated with marked sinus bradycardia and second or third degree heart block in the absence of a functioning pacemaker. [Trade only: Pacerone: Tabs, 100, 300 mg. Generic/Trade: Tabs, scored 200, 400 mg.] ▶L ♀D ▶- $$$$

ATROPINE (*AtroPen*) Bradyarrhythmia/CPR: 0.5–1.0 mg IV q3–5 min to max 0.04 mg/kg (3 mg). Peds: 0.02 mg/kg/dose; minimum single dose, 0.1 mg; max cumulative dose, 1 mg. AtroPen: Injector pens for insecticide or nerve agent poisoning. [Trade only: Prefilled auto-injector pen: 0.25 mg (yellow), 0.5 mg (blue), 1 mg (dark red), 2 mg (green).] ▶K ♀C ▶- $

BICARBONATE Severe acidosis: 1 mEq/kg IV up to 50–100 mEq/dose. ▶K ♀C ▶? $

DIGOXIN (*Lanoxin, Lanoxicaps, Digitek*) Systolic heart failure/rate control of chronic A-fib: 0.125–0.25 mg PO daily; impaired renal function: 0.0625–0.125 mg PO daily. Rapid A-fib: Load 0.5 mg IV, then 0.25 mg IV q6h × 2 doses, maintenance 0.125–0.375 mg IV/PO daily. [Generic/Trade: Tabs, scored (Lanoxin, Digitek) 0.125, 0.25 mg; elixir 0.05 mg/mL. Trade only: Caps (Lanoxicaps), 0.1, 0.2 mg.] ▶KL ♀C ▶+ $

DIGOXIN IMMUNE FAB (*Digibind, Digifab*) Digoxin toxicity: 2–20 vials IV, one formula is: Number vials = (serum dig level in ng/mL) × (kg)/100. ▶K ♀C ▶? $$$$$

DISOPYRAMIDE (*Norpace, Norpace CR, ✦Rythmodan, Rythmodan-LA*) Rarely indicated, consult cardiologist. Ventricular arrhythmia: 400–800 mg PO daily in divided doses (immediate-release, q6h or extended-release, q12h). Proarrhythmic. [Generic/Trade: Caps, immediate-release 100, 150 mg; extended-release 150 mg. Trade only: Caps, extended-release 100 mg.] ▶KL ♀C ▶+ $$$$

FLECAINIDE (*Tambocor*) Proarrhythmic. Prevention of paroxysmal atrial fib/flutter or PSVT, with symptoms & no structural heart disease: Start 50 mg PO q12h, may increase by 50 mg bid q4 d, max 300 mg/d. Use with AV nodal slowing agent (beta blocker, verapamil, diltiazem) to minimize risk of 1:1 atrial flutter. Life-threatening ventricular arrhythmias without structural heart disease: Start 100 mg PO q12h, may increase by 50 mg bid q 4 d, max 400 mg/d. With severe renal impairment (CrCl<35 mL/min): Start 50 mg PO bid. [Generic/Trade: Tabs, non-scored 50, scored 100, 150 mg.] ▶K ♀C ▶- $$$$

IBUTILIDE (*Corvert*) Recent onset A-fib/flutter: 0.01 mg/kg up to 1 mg IV over 10 mins, may repeat once if no response after 10 additional min. Keep on cardiac monitor ≥4 h. ▶K ♀C ▶? $$$$$

ISOPROTERENOL (*Isuprel*) Refractory bradycardia or third degree AV block: 0.02–0.06 mg IV bolus or infusion 2 mg in 250 mL D5W (8 mcg/mL) at 5 mcg/min. 5 mcg/min = 37 mL/h. Peds: 0.05–2 mcg/kg/min. 10 kg: 0.1 mcg/kg/min = 8 mL/h. ▶LK ♀C ▶? $$$

LIDOCAINE (*Xylocaine, Xylocard*) Ventricular arrhythmia: Load 1 mg/kg IV, then 0.5 mg/kg q8–10 min as needed to max 3 mg/kg. IV infusion: 4 gm in 500 mL D5W (8 mg/mL) at 1–4 mg/min. Peds: 20–50 mcg/kg/min. ▶LK ♀B ▶? $

MEXILETINE (*Mexitil*) Proarrhythmic. Rarely indicated, consult cardiologist. Ventricular arrhythmia: Start 200 mg PO q8h with food or antacid, max dose 1,200 mg/d. [Generic only: Caps, 150, 200, 250 mg.] ▶L ♀C ▶- $$$

SELECTED DRUGS THAT MAY PROLONG THE QT INTERVAL

alfuzosin	erythromycin*†	nicardipine	sertraline
amiodarone*†	felbamate	octreotide	sotalol*†
apomorphine	flecainide*	ofloxacin	sunitinib
arsenic trioxide*	foscarnet	ondansetron	tacrolimus
azithromycin*	fosphenytoin	pentamidine*†	tamoxifen
chloroquine*	gemifloxacin	phenothiazines‡	telithromycin*
chlorpromazine	granisetron	pimozide*†	thioridazine
cisapride*†	haloperidol*‡	polyethylene	tizanidine
clarithromycin*	ibutilide*†	glycol (PEG-salt	tolterodine
clozapine	indapamide*	solution)§	vardenafil
cocaine*	isradipine	procainamide*	venlafaxine
dasatinib	levofloxacin*	quetiapine‡	visicol§
disopyramide*†	lithium	quinidine*†	voriconazole*
dofetilide*	mefloquine	quinine	vorinostat
dolasetron	methadone*†	ranolazine	ziprasidone‡
droperidol*	moexipril/HCTZ	risperidone‡	
epirubicin	moxifloxacin	salmeterol	

Note. This table may not include all drugs that prolong the QT interval or cause torsades. Risk of drug-induced QT prolongation may be increased in women, elderly, hypokalemia, hypomagnesemia, bradycardia, starvation, CHF, & CNS injuries. Hepatorenal dysfunction & drug interactions can increase the concentration of QT interval-prolonging drugs. Coadministration of QT interval-prolonging drugs can have additive effects. Avoid these (and other) drugs in congenital prolonged QT syndrome (www.qtdrugs.org). *Torsades reported in product labeling/case reports. †Increased risk in women. ‡QT prolongation: thioridazine > ziprasidone > risperidone, quetiapine, haloperidol. §May be due to electrolyte imbalance.

PROCAINAMIDE (*Pronestyl*) Ventricular arrhythmia: Load 100 mg IV q10 min or 20 mg/min (150 mL/h) until: 1) QRS widens >50%, 2) dysrhythmia suppressed, 3) hypotension, or 4) total of 17 mg/kg or 1000 mg. Infusion 2 g in 250 mL D5W (8 mg/mL) at 2–6 mg/min (15–45 mL/h). Proarrhythmic. ▶LK ♀C ▶? $

PROPAFENONE (*Rythmol, Rythmol SR*) Proarrhythmic. Prevention of paroxysmal atrial fib/flutter or PSVT, with symptoms & no structural heart disease; or life-threatening ventricular arrhythmias: Start (immediate release) 150 mg PO q8h; may increase after 3–4 d to 225 mg PO q8h; max 900 mg/d. Prolong time to recurrence of symptomatic atrial fib without structural heart disease: 225 mg SR PO q12h, may increase ≥5 d to 325 mg PO q12h, max 425 mg q12h. Consider using with AV nodal slowing agent (beta blocker, verapamil, diltiazem) to minimize risk of 1:1 atrial flutter. [Generic/Trade: Tabs (immediate release), scored 150, 225, 300 mg. Trade only: SR, caps 225, 325, 425 mg.] ▶L ♀C ▶? $$$$

QUINIDINE (*✦Biquin durules*) Arrhythmia: gluconate, extended-release: 324–648 mg PO q8–12h; sulfate, immediate-release: 200–400 mg PO q6–8h; sulfate, extended-release: 300–600 mg PO q8–12h. Proarrhythmic. [Generic gluconate: Tabs, extended-release non-scored 324 mg. Generic sulfate: Tabs, scored immediate-release 200, 300 mg, Tabs, extended-release 300 mg.] ▶LK ♀C ▶+ $$$-gluconate, $-sulfate

SOTALOL (*Betapace, Betapace AF, ✦Rylosol*) Ventricular arrhythmia (Betapace), A-fib/A-flutter (Betapace AF): Start 80 mg PO bid, max 640 mg/d. Proarrhythmic. [Generic/Trade: Tabs, scored 80,120,160,240 mg, Tabs, scored (Betapace AF) 80,120,160 mg.] ▶K ♀B ▶- $$$$

Anti-Hyperlipidemic Agents—Bile Acid Sequestrants

CHOLESTYRAMINE (*Questran, Questran Light, Prevalite, LoCHOLEST, LoCHOLEST Light*) Elevated LDL cholesterol: Powder: Start 4 g PO daily-bid before meals, increase up to max 24 g/d. [Generic/Trade: Powder for oral susp, 4 g cholestyramine resin/9 g powder (Questran, LoCHOLEST), 4 g cholestyramine resin/5 g powder (Questran Light), 4 g cholestyramine resin/5.5 g powder (Prevalite, LoCHOLEST Light). Each available in bulk powder and single dose packets.] ▶Not absorbed ♀C ▶+ $$$

COLESEVELAM (*Welchol*) Glycemic control of type 2 diabetes or reduce elevated LDL cholesterol: 3 tabs PO bid with meals or 6 tabs once daily with a meal, max dose 6 tabs/d. [Trade only: Tabs, non-scored, 625 mg.] ▶Not absorbed ♀B ▶+ $$$$$

COLESTIPOL (*Colestid, Colestid Flavored*) Elevated LDL cholesterol: Tabs: Start 2 g PO daily-bid, max 16 g/d. Granules: Start 5 g PO daily-bid, max 30 g/d. [Generic/Trade: Tab 1 g. Granules for oral susp, 5 g/7.5 g powder.] ▶Not absorbed ♀B ▶+ $$$

Anti-Hyperlipidemic Agents—HMG-CoA Reductase Inhibitors ("Statins") & Combinations

NOTE: *Hepatotoxicity - monitor LFTs initially, approximately 12 weeks after starting/titrating therapy, then annually or more frequently if indicated.*

Evaluate muscle symptoms & creatine kinase before starting therapy. Evaluate muscle symptoms 6-12 weeks after starting/increasing therapy & at each follow-up visit. Obtain creatine kinase when patient complains of muscle soreness, tenderness, weakness, or pain. These factors increase risk of myopathy: advanced age (especially >80, women >men); multisystem disease (eg, chronic renal insufficiency, especially due to diabetes); multiple medications; perioperative periods; alcohol abuse; grapefruit juice (>1 quart/day); specific concomitant medications: fibrates (especially gemfibrozil), nicotinic acid (rare), cyclosporine, erythromycin, clarithromycin, itraconazole, ketoconazole, protease inhibitors, nefazodone, verapamil, amiodarone. Weigh potential risk of combination therapy against potential benefit.

ADVICOR (*lovastatin + niacin*) Hyperlipidemia: 1 tab PO qhs with a low-fat snack. Establish dose using extended-release niacin first, or if already on lovastatin substitute combo product with lowest niacin dose. Aspirin or ibuprofen 30 min prior may decrease niacin flushing reaction. [Trade only: Tabs, non-scored extended release lovastatin/niacin 20/500, 20/750, 20/1000, 40/1000 mg.] ▶LK ♀X ▶- $$$$

ATORVASTATIN (*Lipitor*) Hyperlipidemia/prevention of cardiovascular events, including type 2 DM: Start 10–40 mg PO daily, max 80 mg/d. [Trade only: Tabs, non-scored 10,20,40,80 mg.] ▶L ♀X ▶- $$$

CADUET (*amlodipine + atorvastatin*) Simultaneous treatment of HTN and hypercholesterolemia: Establish dose using component drugs first. Dosing interval: daily [Trade only: Tabs, 2.5/10, 2.5/20, 2.5/40, 5/10, 5/20, 5/40, 5/80, 10/10, 10/20, 10/40, 10/80 mg.] ▶L ♀X ▶- $$$$

FLUVASTATIN (*Lescol, Lescol XL*) Hyperlipidemia: Start 20–80 mg PO qhs, max 80 mg daily (XL) or divided bid. Post percutaneous coronary intervention: 80 mg of extended release PO daily, max 80 mg daily. [Trade only: Caps, 20, 40 mg; tab, extended-release, non-scored 80 mg.] ▶L ♀X ▶- $$$

LOVASTATIN (*Mevacor, Altoprev*) Hyperlipidemia/prevention of cardiovascular events: Start 20 mg PO q pm, max 80 mg/d daily or divided bid. [Generic/Trade: Tabs, non-scored 20,40 mg. Trade only: Tabs, extended-release (Altoprev) 20,40,60 mg.] ▶L ♀X ▶- $

PRAVASTATIN (*Pravachol*) Hyperlipidemia/prevention of cardiovascular events: Start 40 mg PO daily, max 80 mg/d. [Generic/Trade: Tabs, non-scored 10, 20, 40, 80 mg. Generic only: Tabs 30 mg.] ▶L ♀X ▶- $$$

ROSUVASTATIN (*Crestor*) Hyperlipidemia/slow progression of atherosclerosis: Start 10 mg PO daily, max 40 mg/d. [Trade only: Tabs, non-scored 5, 10, 20, 40 mg.] ▶L ♀X ▶- $$$$

SIMCOR (*simvastatin + niacin*) Hyperlipidemia: 1 tab PO qhs with a low-fat snack. If niacin naïve or switching from immediate release niacin, start: 20/500 mg PO q pm. If receiving extended release niacin, do not start with > 40/2000 mg PO q pm. Max 40/2000 mg/d. Aspirin or ibuprofen 30 min prior may decrease niacin flushing reaction. [Trade only: Tabs, non-scored extended release simvastatin/niacin 20/500, 20/750, 20/1000 mg.] ▶LK ♀X ▶- $$$

LIPID REDUCTION BY CLASS/AGENT*

Drug Class/ Agent	Specific Drugs	Low Density Lipoprotein (LDL)	High Density Lipoprotein (HDL)	Triglycer-ides
Bile acid sequestrants	Cholestyramine (4–16 g), colestipol (5–20 g), colesevelam (2.6–3.8 g)	decrease 15–30%	increase 3–5%	No change or increase
Cholesterol absorption inhibitor	Ezetimibe (10 mg). When added to statin therapy, will decrease LDL 25%, increase HDL 3%, decrease TG 14% in addition to statin effects.	decrease 18%	increase 1%	decrease 8%
Fibrates	Fenofibrate (145–200 mg), gemfibrozil (600 mg bid)	decrease 5–20%	increase 10–20%	decrease 20–50%
Lovastatin + extended release niacin	Advicor (20/1000–40/2000 mg)	decrease 30–42%	increase 20–30%	decrease 32–44%
Niacin	Extended release nicotinic acid (Niaspan 1–2 g), immediate release (crystalline) nico-tinic acid (1.5–3 g), sustained release nicotinic acid (Slo-Niacin 1–2 g)	decrease 5–25%	increase 15–35%	decrease 20–50%
Omega 3 fatty acids	Omacor 4 g	No change or increase	increase 9%	decrease 45%
Statins	Atorvastatin (10–80 mg), fluvastatin (20–80 mg), lovastatin (20–80 mg), pravastatin (20–80 mg), rosuvastatin (5–40 mg), simvastatin (20–80 mg)	decrease 18–63%	increase 5–15%	decrease 7–35%
Simvastatin + ezetimibe	Vytorin 10/10–10/80 mg	decrease 45–60%	increase 6–10%	decrease 23–31%

*Adapted from NCEP: JAMA 2001; 285:2486 and prescribing information.

SIMVASTATIN (Zocor) Hyperlipidemia: Start 20–40 mg PO q pm, max 80 mg/d. Reduce cardiovascular mortality/events in high risk for coronary heart disease event: Start 40 mg PO q pm, max 80 mg/d. [Generic/Trade: Tabs, non-scored 5, 10, 20, 40, 80 mg. Generic only: Orally disintegrating tabs 10, 20, 40 ,80 mg.] ▶L ♀X ▶– $$$$

VYTORIN (ezetimibe + simvastatin) Hyperlipidemia: Start 10/20 mg PO q pm, max 10/80 mg/d. Start 10/40 if need >55% LDL reduction. [Trade only: Tabs, non-scored ezetimibe/simvastatin 10/10, 10/20, 10/40, 10/80 mg.] ▶L ♀X ▶– $$$$

Anti-Hyperlipidemic Agents—Other

BEZAFIBRATE (✦Bezalip) Canada only. Hyperlipidemia/hypertriglyceridemia: 200 mg immediate release PO bid-tid, or 400 mg of sustained release PO daily. [Trade only: Immediate release tab: 200 mg. Sustained release tab: 400 mg.] ▶K ♀D ▶– $$$

EZETIMIBE (*Zetia*, *+Ezetrol*) Hyperlipidemia: 10 mg PO daily. [Trade only: Tabs non-scored 10 mg.] ▶L ♀C ▶? $$$$

FENOFIBRATE (*TriCor, Antara, Lipofen, Triglide*, *+Lipidil Micro, Lipidil Supra, Lipidil EZ*) Hypertriglyceridemia: Tricor tabs: 48–145 mg PO daily, max 145 mg daily. Antara: 43–130 mg PO daily; max 130 mg daily. Fenoglide: 40–120 mg PO daily; max 120 mg daily. Lipofen: 50–150 mg PO daily, max 150 mg daily. Lofibra: 54–200 mg PO daily, max 200 mg daily. Triglide: 50–160 mg PO daily, max 160 mg daily. Generic tabs: 54–160 mg, max 160 mg daily. Generic caps: 67–200 mg PO daily; max 200 mg daily. Hypercholesterolemia/mixed dyslipidemia: Tricor tabs: 145 mg PO daily. Antara: 130 mg PO daily. Fenoglide: 120 mg daily. Lipofen: 150 mg daily. Lofibra: 160–200 mg daily, max 200 mg daily. Triglide: 160 mg daily. Generic tabs: 160 mg daily. Generic caps 200 mg PO daily. All formulations, except Antara, Tricor, and Triglide, should be taken with food. [Generic only: Tabs, non-scored 54, 160 mg. Generic caps, 67, 134, 200 mg. Trade only: Tricor tabs, non-scored 48,145 mg. Antara caps 43, 130 mg. Fenoglide non-scored tabs 40, 120 mg. Lipofen non-scored tabs 50,100,150 mg. Lofibra tabs, non-scored 54, 160 mg. Triglide tabs, non-scored 50, 160 mg. Lofibra caps, 67, 134, 200 mg.] ▶LK ♀C ▶- $$$

GEMFIBROZIL (*Lopid*) Hypertriglyceridemia/primary prevention of coronary artery disease: 600 mg PO bid 30 min before meals. [Generic/Trade: Tabs, scored 600 mg.] ▶LK ♀C ▶? $$$

Antihypertensive Combinations

NOTE: *Dosage should first be adjusted by using each drug separately. See component drugs for ♀*

BY TYPE: ACE Inhibitor/Diuretic: *Accuretic, Capozide, Inhibace Plus, Lotensin HCT, Monopril HCT, Prinzide, Uniretic, Vaseretic, Zestoretic.* **ACE Inhibitor/Calcium Channel Blocker:** *Lexxel, Lotrel, Tarka.* **Angiotensin Receptor Blocker/Diuretic:** *Atacand HCT, Avalide, Benicar HCT, Diovan HCT, Hyzaar, Micardis HCT, Teveten HCT.* **Angiotensin Receptor Blocker/Calcium Channel Blocker:** *Exforge.* **Beta-blocker/Diuretic:** *Corzide, Dutoprol, Inderide, Lopressor HCT, Tenoretic, Timolide, Ziac.* **Diuretic combinations:** *Aldactazide, Dyazide, Maxzide, Moduretic, Triazide.* **Diuretic/miscellaneous antihypertensive:** *Aldoril, Apresazide, Clorpres, Minizide.*
BY NAME: ACCURETIC (quinapril + hydrochlorothiazide): Generic/Trade: Tabs, 10/12.5, 20/12.5, 20/25. **Aldactazide** (spironolactone + hydrochlorothiazide): Generic/Trade: Tabs, non-scored 25/25, scored 50/50 mg. **Aldoril** (methyldopa + hydrochlorothiazide): Generic/Trade: Tabs, non-scored, 250/15 (Aldoril-15), 250/25 mg (Aldoril-25). Trade only: Tabs, non-scored, 500/30 (Aldoril D30), 500/50 mg (Aldoril D50). **Apresazide** (hydralazine + hydrochlorothiazide): Generic only: Caps 25/25, 50/50 mg. **Atacand HCT** (candesartan + hydrochlorothiazide, *+Atacand Plus*): Trade only: Tab, non-scored 16/12.5, 32/12.5 mg. **Avalide** (irbesartan + hydrochlorothiazide): Trade only: Tabs, non-scored 150/12.5, 300/12.5, 300/25 mg. **Benicar HCT** (olmesartan + hydrochlorothiazide): Trade only: Tabs, non-scored 20/ 12.5, 40/12.5, 40/25 mg. **Capozide** (captopril + hydrochlorothiazide): Generic/Trade: Tabs, scored 25/15, 25/25, 50/15, 50/25 mg. **Clorpres** (clonidine + chlorthalidone): Trade only: Tabs,

(cont.)

STATINS*		
Minimum Dose for 30–40% LDL Reduction	LDL	LFT Monitoring
atorvastatin 10 mg	–39%	Baseline, 12 wk, semiannually
fluvastatin 40 mg bid	–36%	Baseline, 8 wk
fluvastatin XL 80 mg	–35%	Baseline, 8 wk
lovastatin 40 mg	–31%	Baseline, 6 & 12 wk, semiannually
pravastatin 40mg	–34%	Baseline, prior to dose increase
rosuvastatin 5 mg	–45%	Baseline, 12 wk, semiannually
simvastatin 20 mg	–38%	Get LFTs prior to & 3 mo after dose increase to 80 mg, then semiannually for first yr.

*Adapted from Circulation 2004;110:227–239. Data taken from prescribing information for primary hypercholesterolemia. LDL= low-density lipoprotein, LFT = l iver function tests. Will get ~6% decrease in LDL with every doubling of dose. ACC/AHA/NHLBI schedule for LFT monitoring: baseline, ~12 wk after starting therapy, annually, when clinically indicated. Stop statin therapy if LFTs are >3 times upper limit of normal.

LDL CHOLESTEROL GOALS*			
Definitions			
Risk factors	"Risk factors": Cigarette smoking, HTN (BP ≥140/90 mm Hg or on antihypertensive meds), low HDL (<40 mg/dL), family hx of CHD (1 relative: male <55 yo, female <65 yo), age (male ≥45 yo, female ≥55 yo).		
Lifestyle changes	"Lifestyle changes" refer to dietary modification, weight reduction, exercise.		
Equivalent risk	"Equivalent risk" defined as diabetes, other atherosclerotic disease (peripheral artery disease, abdominal aortic aneurysm, symptomatic carotid artery disease), or multiple risk factors such that 10 yr risk >20%.		
Risk Category	LDL Goal	Lifestyle Changes at LDL	Also Consider Meds at LDL
High risk: CHD or equivalent risk, 10-yr risk >20%	<100 mg/dL; optional <70 with very high risk factors	≥100 mg/dL	≥100 mg/dL (<100: consider Rx options)
Moderately-high risk: 2+ risk factors, 10-yr risk 10–20%	<130 mg/dL	≥130 mg/dL	≥130 mg/dL (100–129: consider Rx options)
Moderate risk: 2+ risk factors, 10-yr risk <10%	<130 mg/dL	≥130 mg/dL	≥160 mg/dL
Lower risk: 0–1 risk factor	<160 mg/dL	≥160 mg/dL	≥190 mg/dL (160–189: Rx optional)

*All 10-yr risks based upon Framingham stratification; calculator available at: http://hin.nhlbi.nih.gov/ atpiii/calculator.asp?usertype=prof. CHD=coronary heart disease. LDL=low density lipoprotein. Adapted from NCEP: JAMA 2001; 285:2486.

scored 0.1/15, 0.2/15, 0.3/15 mg. *Corzide* (nadolol + bendroflumethiazide): Generic/Trade: Tabs 40/5, 80/5 mg. *Diovan HCT* (valsartan + hydrochlorothiazide): Trade only: Tabs, non-scored 80/12.5, 160/12.5, 160/25, 320/12.5, 320/25 mg. *Dutoprol* (metoprolol + hydrochlorothiazide): Trade only: Tabs, non-scored 25/12.5, 50/12.5 mg, scored 100/12.5 mg. *Dyazide* (triamterene + hydrochlorothiazide): Generic/Trade: Caps, (Dyazide) 37.5/25, (generic only) 50/25 mg. *Exforge* (amlodipine + valsartan): Trade only: Tabs, non-scored 5/160, 5/320, 10/160, 10/320 mg. *Hyzaar* (losartan + hydrochlorothiazide): Trade only: Tabs, non-scored 50/12.5, 100/12.5, 100/25 mg. *Inderide* (propranolol + hydrochlorothiazide): Generic/Trade: Tabs, scored 40/25, 80/25. *Inhibace Plus* (cilazapril + hydrochlorothiazide): Trade only: Scored tabs 5 mg cilazapril + 12.5 mg HCTZ. *Lexxel* (enalapril + felodipine): Trade only: Tabs, non-scored 5/2.5, 5/5 mg. *Lopressor HCT* (metoprolol + hydrochlorothiazide): Generic/Trade: Tabs, scored 50/25, 100/25, 100/50 mg. *Lotensin HCT* (benazepril + hydrochlorothiazide): Generic/Trade: Tabs, scored 5/6.25, 10/12.5, 20/12.5, 20/25 mg. *Lotrel* (amlodipine + benazepril): Generic/Trade: Cap, 2.5/10, 5/10, 5/20, 10/20 mg. Trade only: Cap, 5/40, 10/40 mg. *Maxzide* (triamterene + hydrochlorothiazide, ✚*Triazide*): Generic/ Trade: Tabs, scored (Maxzide-25) 37.5/25 (Maxzide) 75/50 mg. *Maxzide-25* (triamterene + hydrochlorothiazide): Generic/ Trade: Tabs, scored (Maxzide-25) 37.5/25 (Maxzide) 75/50 mg. *Micardis HCT* (telmisartan + hydrochlorothiazide, ✚*Micardis Plus*): Trade only: Tabs, non-scored 40/12.5, 80/12.5, 80/25 mg. *Minizide* (prazosin + polythiazide): Trade only: cap, 1/0.5, 2/0.5, 5/0.5 mg. *Moduretic* (amiloride + hydrochlorothiazide, ✚*Moduret*): Generic/Trade: Tabs, scored 5/50 mg. *Monopril HCT* (fosinopril + hydrochlorothiazide): Generic/Trade: Tabs, non-scored 10/12.5, scored 20/12.5 mg. *Prinzide* (lisinopril + hydrochlorothiazide): Generic/Trade: Tabs, non-scored 10/12.5, 20/12.5, 20/25 mg. *Tarka* (trandolapril + verapamil): Trade only: Tabs, non-scored 2/180, 1/240, 2/240, 4/240 mg. *Tenoretic* (atenolol + chlorthalidone): Generic/Trade: Tabs, scored 50/25, non-scored 100/25 mg. *Teveten HCT* (eprosartan + hydrochlorothiazide): Trade only: Tabs, non-scored 600/12.5, 600/25 mg. *Timolide* (timolol + hydrochlorothiazide): Trade only: Tabs, non-scored 10/25 mg. *Uniretic* (moexipril + hydrochlorothiazide): Generic/Trade: Tabs, scored 7.5/12.5, 15/12.5, 15/25 mg. *Vaseretic* (enalapril + hydrochlorothiazide): Generic/ Trade: Tabs, non-scored 5/12.5, 10/25 mg. *Zestoretic* (lisinopril + hydrochloro-thiazide): Generic/Trade: Tabs, non-scored 10/12.5, 20/12.5, 20/25 mg. *Ziac* (biso-prolol + hydrochlorothiazide): Generic/ Trade: Tabs, non-scored 2.5/6.25, 5/6.25, 10/6.25 mg.

Antihypertensives—Other

ALISKIREN (*Tekturna*) HTN: 150 mg PO daily, max 300 mg/d. [Trade only: Tabs, non-scored 150, 300 mg.] ▶LK ♀– ▶? $$$

FENOLDOPAM (*Corlopam*) Severe HTN: 10 mg in 250 mL D5W (40 mcg/mL), start at 0.1 mcg/kg/min titrate q15 min, usual effective dose 0.1–1.6 mcg/kg/min. ▶LK ♀B ▶? $$$

HYDRALAZINE (*Apresoline*) Hypertensive emergency: 10–50 mg IM or 10–20 mg IV, repeat as needed. HTN: Start 10 mg PO bid-qid, max 300 mg/d.

(cont.)

Headaches, peripheral edema, lupus syndrome. [Generic only: Tabs, non-scored 10, 25, 50, 100 mg.] ▶LK ♀C ▶+ $

NITROPRUSSIDE (*Nipride, Nitropress*) Hypertensive emergency: 50 mg in 250 mL D5W (200 mcg/mL), start at 0.3 mcg/kg/min (70 kg adult: 6 mL/h). Max 10 mcg/kg/min. Protect from light. Cyanide toxicity with high doses, hepatic/renal impairment, prolonged infusions; check thiocyanate levels. ▶RBC's ♀C ▶- $

PHENTOLAMINE (*Regitine, Rogitine*) Diagnosis of pheochromocytoma: 5 mg increments IV/IM. Peds 0.05–0.1 mg/kg IV/IM up to 5 mg per dose. Extravasation: 5–10 mg in 10 mL NS local SC injection. ▶Plasma ♀C ▶? $$$

Antiplatelet Drugs

ABCIXIMAB (*ReoPro*) Platelet aggregation inhibition, percutaneous coronary intervention: 0.25 mg/kg IV bolus via separate infusion line before procedure, then 0.125 mcg/kg/min (max 10 mcg/min) IV inf. for 12h. ▶Plasma ♀C ▶? $$$$$

AGGRENOX (*aspirin + dipyridamole*) Prevention of stroke after TIA/stroke: 1 cap PO bid. [Trade only: Caps, 25 mg aspirin/ 200 mg extended-release dipyridamole.] ▶LK ♀D ▶? $$$$

CLOPIDOGREL (*Plavix*) Reduction of thrombotic events: recent AMI/stroke, established peripheral arterial disease: 75 mg PO daily; acute coronary syndrome: non-ST segment elevation: 300 mg loading dose, then 75 mg PO daily in combination with aspirin. ST segment elevation MI: Start with/without 300 mg loading dose, then 75 mg PO daily in combination with aspirin, with/without thrombolytics. [Generic/Trade: Tab, non-scored 75, 300 mg.] ▶LK ♀B ▶? $$$$

DIPYRIDAMOLE (*Persantine*) Antithrombotic: 75–100 mg PO qid. [Generic/Trade: Tabs, non-scored 25, 50, 75 mg.] ▶L ♀B ▶? $$$

EPTIFIBATIDE (*Integrilin*) Acute coronary syndrome: Load 180 mcg/kg IV bolus, then infusion 2 mcg/kg/min up to 72 h. Discontinue prior to CABG. Percutaneous coronary intervention: Load 180 mcg/kg IV bolus just before procedure, followed by infusion 2 mcg/kg/min and a 2nd 180 mcg/kg IV bolus 10 min after the first. Continue for up to 18–24 h (minimum 12 h) post-procedure. Reduce dose with CrCl <50 mL/min; contraindicated in dialysis patients. ▶K ♀B ▶? $$$$$

TICLOPIDINE (*Ticlid*) Due to high incidence of neutropenia and thrombotic thrombocytopenia purpura, other drugs preferred. Platelet aggregation inhibition/reduction of thrombotic stroke: 250 mg PO bid with food. [Generic/Trade: Tab, non-scored 250 mg.] ▶L ♀B ▶? $$$$

TIROFIBAN (*Aggrastat*) Acute coronary syndromes: Start 0.4 mcg/kg/min IV infusion for 30 mins, then decrease to 0.1 mcg/kg/min for 48–108 h or until 12–24 h after coronary intervention. Half dose with CrCl <30 mL/min. Use concurrent heparin to keep PTT twice normal. ▶K ♀B ▶? $$$$$

Beta Blockers

NOTE: *See also antihypertensive combinations. Not first-line for HTN unless to treat angina, post-MI, left ventricular dysfunction. Abrupt discontinuation may precipitate angina, myocardial infarction, arrhythmias, or rebound HTN; discontinue by tapering over 2 weeks. Avoid using nonselective beta-blockers and use agents with beta-1 selectivity cautiously in asthma/COPD. Beta-1 selectivity diminishes at high doses. Avoid in decompensated heart failure, sick sinus syndrome, severe peripheral artery disease.*

ACEBUTOLOL (Sectral, ✦Rhotral) HTN: Start 400 mg PO daily or 200 mg bid, max 1200 mg/d. Beta1 receptor selective. [Generic/Trade: Caps, 200, 400 mg.] ▶LK ♀B ▶- $$

ATENOLOL (Tenormin) Acute MI: 5 mg IV over 5 min, repeat in 10 min. HTN: Start 25–50 mg PO daily or divided bid, max 100 mg/d. Beta1 receptor selective. [Generic/Trade: Tabs, non-scored 25, 100 mg; scored, 50 mg.] ▶K ♀D ▶- $

BETAXOLOL (Kerlone) HTN: Start 5–10 mg PO daily, max 20 mg/d. Beta1 receptor selective. [Generic/Trade: Tabs, scored 10 mg, non-scored 20 mg.] ▶LK ♀C ▶? $$

BISOPROLOL (Zebeta, ✦Monocor) HTN: Start 2.5–5 mg PO daily, max 20 mg/d. Beta1 receptor selective. [Generic/Trade: Tabs, scored 5 mg, non-scored 10 mg.] ▶LK ♀C ▶? $$

CARVEDILOL (Coreg, Coreg CR) Heart failure, immediate release: Start 3.125 mg PO bid, double dose q2 wk as tolerated up to max of 25 mg bid (if <85 kg) or 50 mg bid (if >85 kg). Heart failure, sustained release: Start 10 mg PO daily, double dose q2 wk as tolerated up to max of 80 mg/d. LV dysfunction following acute MI, immediate release: Start 3.125–6.25 mg PO bid, double dose q 3–10 d as tolerated to max of 25 mg bid. LV dysfunction following acute MI, sustained release: Start 10–20 mg PO daily, double dose q 3–10 d as tolerated to max of 80 mg/d. HTN, immediate release: Start 6.25 mg PO bid, double dose q7–14 d as tolerated to max 50 mg/d. HTN, sustained release: Start 20 mg PO daily, double dose q7–14 d as tolerated to max 80 mg/d. Take with food to decrease orthostatic hypotension. Give Coreg CR in the morning. Alpha1, beta1, and beta2 receptor blocker. [Generic/Trade: Tabs, immediate-release non-scored 3.125, 6.25, 12.5, 25 mg. Trade only: Caps, extended-release 10, 20, 40, 80 mg.] ▶L ♀C ▶? $$$$

ESMOLOL (Brevibloc) SVT/HTN emergency: Mix infusion 5 g in 500 mL (10 mg/mL), load with 500 mcg/kg over 1 min (70 kg: 35 mg or 3.5 mL) then infusion 50–200 mcg/kg/min (70 kg: 100 mcg/kg/min = 40 mL/h). Half-life = 9 min. Beta1 receptor selective. ▶K ♀C ▶? $

LABETALOL (Trandate) HTN: Start 100 mg PO bid, max 2400 mg/d. HTN emergency: Start 20 mg IV slow injection, then 40–80 mg IV q10 min prn up to 300 mg or IV infusion 0.5–2 mg/min. Peds: Start 0.3–1 mg/kg/dose (max 20 mg). Alpha1, beta1, and beta2 receptor blocker. [Generic/Trade: Tabs, scored 100, 200, 300 mg.] ▶LK ♀C ▶+ $$$

METOPROLOL (Lopressor, Toprol-XL, ✦Betaloc) Acute MI: 5 mg increments IV q5–15 min up to 15 mg followed by oral therapy. HTN (immediate release): Start 100 mg PO daily or in divided doses, increase as needed up to 450 mg/d; may require multiple daily doses to maintain 24 h BP control. HTN (extended release): Start 25–100 mg PO daily, increase as needed up to 400 mg/d. Heart failure: Start 12.5–25 mg (extended-release) PO daily, double dose every 2 wk as tolerated up to max 200 mg/d. Angina: Start 50 mg PO bid (immediate release) or 100 mg PO daily (extended-release), increase as needed up to 400 mg/d. Beta1 receptor selective. [Generic/Trade: Tabs, scored 50, 100 mg, extended-release 25, 50, 100, 200 mg. Generic only: Tabs, scored 25 mg.] ▶L ♀C ▶? $$

NADOLOL (*Corgard*) HTN: Start 20–40 mg PO daily, max 320 mg/d. Beta1 and beta2 receptor blocker. [Generic/Trade: Tabs, scored 20, 40, 80, 120, 160 mg.] ▶K ♀C ▶- $$

NEBIVOLOL (*Bystolic*) HTN: Start 5 mg PO daily, max 40 mg/d. Beta1 receptor selective at doses of ≤10 mg and in patients who extensively metabolize CYP 2D6; otherwise, inhibits both beta-1 and beta-2 receptors. [Trade only: Tabs, non-scored 2.5, 5, 10 mg.] ▶L ♀C ▶- $$$

OXPRENOLOL (✦*Trasicor Slow-Trasicor*) Canada only. HTN: Regular release: Initially 20 mg PO tid, titrate upwards prn to usual maintenance 120–320 mg/d divided bid-tid. Alternatively, may substitute an equivalent daily dose of sustained release product; do not exceed 480 mg/d. [Trade only: IRegular release tabs: 40, 80 mg. Sustained release tabs: 80, 160 mg.] ▶L ♀D ▶- $$

PINDOLOL (✦*Visken HTN*) Start 5 mg PO bid, max 60 mg/d. Beta1 and beta2 receptor blocker. [Generic only: Tabs, scored 5, 10 mg.] ▶K ♀B ▶? $$$

PROPRANOLOL (*Inderal, Inderal LA, InnoPran XL*) HTN: Start 20–40 mg PO bid or 60–80 mg PO daily, max 640 mg/d; extended-release (Inderal LA) max 640 mg/d; extended-release (InnoPran XL) 80 mg qhs (10 PM), max 120 mg qhs (chronotherapy). Supraventricular tachycardia or rapid atrial fibrillation/flutter: 1 mg IV q2 min. Max of 2 doses in 4 h. Migraine prophylaxis: Start 40 mg PO bid or 80 mg PO daily (extended-release), max 240 mg/d. Beta1 and beta2 receptor blocker. [Generic/Trade: Tabs, scored 40, 60, 80. Caps, extended-release 60, 80, 120, 160 mg. Generic only: Solution 20 & 40 mg/5 mL. Tabs, 10, 20 mg. Trade only: (InnoPran XL qhs) 80, 120 mg.] ▶L ♀C ▶+ $$

Calcium Channel Blockers (CCBs)—Dihydropyridines

NOTE *See also antihypertensive combinations.*

AMLODIPINE (*Norvasc*) HTN: Start 2.5 to 5 mg PO daily, max 10 daily. [Generic/Trade: Tabs, non-scored 2.5, 5, 10 mg. Generic only: Orally disintegrating tabs 2.5, 5, 10 mg.] ▶L ♀C ▶? $$$

FELODIPINE (*Plendil, ✦Renedil*) HTN: Start 2.5–5 mg PO daily, max 10 mg/d. [Generic/Trade: Tabs, extended-release, non-scored 2.5, 5, 10 mg.] ▶L ♀C ▶? $$

ISRADIPINE (*DynaCirc, DynaCirc CR*) HTN: Start 2.5 mg PO bid, max 20 mg/d (max 10 mg/d in elderly). Controlled-release: 5–10 mg PO daily. [Trade only: Tabs, controlled-release 5, 10 mg. Generic only: Immediate release caps 2.5, 5 mg.] ▶L ♀C ▶? $$$$

NICARDIPINE (*Cardene, Cardene SR*) HTN emergency: Begin IV infusion at 5 mg/h, titrate to effect, max 15 mg/h. HTN: Start 20 mg PO tid, max 120 mg/d. Sustained release: Start 30 mg PO bid, max 120 mg/d. [Generic/Trade: Caps, immediate-release 20, 30 mg. Trade only: Caps, sustained-release 30, 45, 60 mg.] ▶L ♀C ▶? $$

NIFEDIPINE (*Procardia, Adalat, Procardia XL, Adalat CC, ✦Adalat XL, Adalat PA*) HTN/angina: Extended-release: 30–60 mg PO daily, max 120 mg/d. Angina: immediate-release: Start 10 mg PO tid, max 120 mg/d. Avoid sublingual administration, may cause excessive hypotension, AMI, stroke. Do not use immediate-release caps for treating HTN. Preterm labor: loading dose: 10 mg PO q20–30

(cont.)

min if contractions persist, up to 40 mg within the first h. Maintenance dose: 10–20 mg PO q4–6h or 60–160 mg extended release PO daily. [Generic/Trade: Caps, 10, 20 mg. Tabs, extended-release 30, 60, 90 mg.] ▶L ♀C ▶+ $$

NISOLDIPINE (*Sular*)   HTN: Start 17 mg PO daily, max 34 mg/d. Take on an empty stomach. [Trade only: Tabs, extended-release 8.5, 17, 25.5, 34 mg. These replace the former 10, 20, 30, 40 mg tabs.] ▶L ♀C ▶? $$$

Calcium Channel Blockers (CCBs)—Other

NOTE *See also antihypertensive combinations.*

DILTIAZEM (*Cardizem, Cardizem LA, Cardizem CD, Cartia XT, Dilacor XR, Diltiazem CD, Diltzac, Diltia XT, Tiazac, Taztia XT*)   Atrial fibrillation/flutter, PSVT: bolus 20 mg (0.25 mg/kg) IV over 2 min. Rebolus 15 min later (if needed) 25 mg (0.35 mg/kg). Infusion 5–15 mg/h. Once daily, extended-release, HTN: Start 120–240 mg PO daily, max 540 mg/d. Once daily, graded extended-release (Cardizem LA), HTN: Start 180–240 mg PO daily, max 540 mg/d. Twice daily, sustained-release, HTN: Start 60–120 mg PO bid, max 360 mg/d. Immediate-release, angina: Start 30 mg PO qid, max 360 mg/d divided tid-qid; extended-release, Start 120–240 mg PO daily, max 540 mg/d. Once daily, graded extended-release (Cardizem LA), angina: Start 180 mg PO daily, doses >360 mg may provide no additional benefit. [Generic/Trade: Tabs, immediate-release, non-scored (Cardizem) 30, scored 60, 90, 120 mg; Caps, extended-release (Cardizem CD, Cartia XT daily) 120, 180, 240, 300, 360 mg, (Diltzac, Taztia XT, Tiazac daily) 120, 180, 240, 300, 360, 420 mg, (Dilacor XR, Diltia XT) 120, 180, 240 mg. Trade only: Tabs, extended-release graded (Cardizem LA daily) 120, 180, 240, 300, 360, 420 mg.] ▶L ♀C ▶+ $$

VERAPAMIL (*Isoptin SR, Calan, Covera-HS, Verelan, Verelan PM, ✦Veramil*)   SVT: 5–10 mg IV over 2 min; peds (1–15 yo): 2–5 mg (0.1–0.3 mg/kg) IV, max dose 5 mg. Angina: immediate-release, start 40–80 mg PO tid-qid, max 480 mg/d; sustained-release, start 120–240 mg PO daily, max 480 mg/d (use bid dosing for doses >240 mg/d with Isoptin SR and Calan SR); (Covera-HS) 180 mg PO qhs, max 480 mg/d. HTN: same as angina, except (Verelan PM) 100–200 mg PO qhs, max 400 mg/d; immediate-release tabs should be avoided in treating HTN. [Generic/Trade: Tabs, immediate-release, scored (Calan) 40, 80, 120 mg; Tabs, sustained-release, non-scored (Isoptin SR) 120, scored 180, 240 mg; Caps, sustained-release (Verelan) 120,180, 240, 360 mg; Caps, extended-release (Verelan PM) 100, 200, 300 mg. Trade only: Tabs, extended-release (Covera HS) 180, 240 mg.] ▶L ♀C ▶+ $$

Diuretics—Carbonic Anhydrase Inhibitors

ACETAZOLAMIDE (*Diamox, Diamox Sequels*)   Glaucoma: 250 mg PO up to qid (immediate release) or 500 mg PO up to bid (sustained release). Max 1 g/d. Acute glaucoma: 250 mg IV q4h or 500 mg IV initially with 125–250 mg q4h, followed by oral therapy. Mountain sickness prophylaxis: 125–250 mg PO bid-tid, beginning 1–2 d prior to ascent and continuing ≥5 d at higher

(cont.)

altitude. Edema: Rarely used, start 250–375 mg IV/PO qam given intermittently (qod or 2 consecutive d followed by none for 1–2 d) to avoid loss of diuretic effect. [Generic only: Tabs, 125, 250 mg. Trade only (Sequels): Caps, extended-release 500 mg.] ▶LK ♀C ▶+ $

Diuretics—Loop

BUMETANIDE (Bumex, ✦Burinex) Edema: 0.5–1 mg IV/IM; 0.5–2 mg PO daily. 1 mg bumetanide is roughly equivalent to 40 mg furosemide. [Generic/Trade: Tabs, scored 0.5, 1, 2 mg.] ▶K ♀C ▶? $

ETHACRYNIC ACID (Edecrin) Rarely used. May be useful in sulfonamide-allergic patients. Edema: 0.5–1.0 mg/kg IV, max 100 mg/dose; 25–100 mg PO daily-bid. [Trade only: Tabs, scored 25 mg.] ▶K ♀B ▶? $$$

FUROSEMIDE (Lasix) Edema: Initial dose 20–80 mg IV/IM/PO, increase dose by 20–40 mg every 6–8h until desired response is achieved, max 600 mg/d. Use lower doses in elderly. [Generic/Trade: Tabs, non-scored 20, scored 40, 80 mg. Generic only: Oral solution 10 mg/mL, 40 mg/5 mL.] ▶K ♀C ▶? $

TORSEMIDE (Demadex) Edema: 5–20 mg IV/PO daily. [Generic/Trade: Tabs, scored 5, 10, 20, 100 mg.] ▶LK ♀B ▶? $

Diuretics—Thiazide Type

NOTE See also antihypertensive combinations.

CHLORTHALIDONE (Thalitone) HTN: 12.5–25 mg PO daily, max 50 mg/d. Edema: 50–100 mg PO daily, max 200 mg/d. Nephrolithiasis (unapproved use): 25–50 mg PO daily. [Trade only: Tabs, non-scored (Thalitone) 15 mg. Generic only: Tabs non-scored 25, 50 mg.] ▶L ♀B, D if used in pregnancy-induced HTN ▶+ $

HYDROCHLOROTHIAZIDE (HCTZ, Esidrix, Oretic, Microzide, HydroDiuril) HTN: 12.5–25 mg PO daily, max 50 mg/d. Edema: 25–100 mg PO daily, max 200 mg/d. [Generic/Trade: Tabs, scored 25, 50 mg; Cap 12.5 mg.] ▶L ♀B, D if used in pregnancy-induced HTN ▶+ $

INDAPAMIDE (Lozol, ✦Lozide) HTN: 1.25–5 mg PO daily, max 5 mg/d. Edema: 2.5–5 mg PO qam. [Generic only: Tabs, non-scored 1.25, 2.5 mg.] ▶L ♀B, D if used in pregnancy-induced HTN ▶? $

METOLAZONE (Zaroxolyn) Edema: 5–10 mg PO daily, max 10 mg/d in heart failure, 20 mg/d in renal disease. If used with loop diuretic, start with 2.5 mg PO daily. [Generic/Trade: Tabs 2.5, 5, 10 mg.] ▶L ♀B, D if used in pregnancy-induced HTN ▶? $$$

Nitrates

ISOSORBIDE DINITRATE (Isordil, Dilatrate-SR, ✦Cedocard SR, Coronex) Angina prophylaxis: 5–40 mg PO tid (7 am, noon, 5 pm), sustained-release: 40–80 mg PO bid (8 am, 2 pm). Acute angina, SL Tabs: 2.5–10 mg SL q5–10 min prn, up to 3 doses in 30 min. [Generic/Trade: Tabs, scored 5, 10, 20, 30 mg. Trade only: Tabs, (Isordil) 40 mg, Cap, extended-release (Dilatrate-SR) 40 mg. Generic only: Tab, sustained-release 40 mg, Tab, sublingual 2.5, 5 mg.] ▶L ♀C ▶? $

ISOSORBIDE MONONITRATE (*ISMO, Monoket, Imdur*) Angina: 20 mg PO bid (8 am and 3 pm). Extended-release: Start 30–60 mg PO daily, max 240 mg/d. [Generic/Trade: Tabs, non-scored (ISMO, bid dosing) 20 mg, scored (Monoket, bid dosing) 10, 20 mg, extended-release, scored (Imdur, daily dosing) 30, 60, non-scored 120 mg.] ▶L ♀C ▶? $$

NITROGLYCERIN INTRAVENOUS INFUSION (*Tridil*) Perioperative HTN, acute MI/Heart failure, acute angina: Mix 50 mg in 250 mL D5W (200 mcg/mL), start at 10–20 mcg/min (3–6 mL/h), then titrate upward by 10–20 mcg/min as needed. [Brand name "Tridil" no longer manufactured, but retained herein for name recognition.] ▶L ♀C ▶? $$

NITROGLYCERIN OINTMENT (*Nitro-BID*) Angina prophylaxis: Start 0.5 inch q8h, maintenance 1–2 inches q8h, max 4 inches q4–6h; 15 mg/inch. Allow for a nitrate-free period of 10–14 h to avoid nitrate tolerance. 1 inch ointment is approximately 15 mg. [Trade only: Ointment, 2%, tubes 1,30,60 g (Nitro-BID).] ▶L ♀C ▶? $

NITROGLYCERIN SPRAY (*Nitrolingual, NitroMist*) Acute angina: 1–2 sprays under the tongue prn, max 3 sprays in 15 min. [Trade only: Nitrolingual solution, 4.9, 12 mL. 0.4 mg/spray (60 or 200 sprays/canister); NitroMist aerosol 0.4 mg/spray (230 sprays/canister) ▶L ♀C ▶? $$$$

NITROGLYCERIN SUBLINGUAL (*Nitrostat, NitroQuick*) Acute angina: 0.4 mg SL under tongue, repeat dose every 5 min as needed up to 3 doses in 15 min. [Generic/Trade: Sublingual tabs, non-scored 0.3, 0.4, 0.6 mg; in bottles of 100 or package of 4 bottles with 25 tabs each.] ▶L ♀C ▶? $

NITROGLYCERIN TRANSDERMAL (*Minitran, Nitro-Dur, ✦Trinipatch*) Angina prophylaxis: 1 patch 12–14 h each d. Allow for a nitrate-free period of 10–14 h each d to avoid nitrate tolerance. [Generic/Trade: Transdermal system 0.1, 0.2, 0.4, 0.6 mg/h. Trade only: (Nitro-Dur) 0.3, 0.8 mg/h.] ▶L ♀C ▶? $$

Pressors/Inotropes

DOBUTAMINE (*Dobutrex*) Inotropic support: 2–20 mcg/kg/min. 70 kg: 5 mcg/kg/min with 1 mg/mL concentration (eg, 250 mg in 250 mL D5W) = 21 mL/h. ▶Plasma ♀D ▶- $

DOPAMINE (*Intropin*) Pressor: Start at 5 mcg/kg/min, increase as needed by 5–10 mcg/kg/min increments at 10 min intervals, max 50 mcg/kg/min. 70 kg: 5 mcg/kg/min with 1600 mcg/mL concentration (eg, 400 mg in 250 mL D5W) = 13 mL/h. Doses in mcg/kg/min: 2–4 = (traditional renal dose, apparently ineffective) dopaminergic receptors; 5–10 = (cardiac dose) dopaminergic and beta1 receptors; >10 = dopaminergic, beta1, and alpha1 receptors. ▶Plasma ♀C ▶- $

EPHEDRINE Pressor 10–25 mg slow IV, repeat q5–10 min prn. [Generic only: Caps, 50 mg.] ▶K ♀C ▶? $

EPINEPHRINE (*EpiPen, EpiPen Jr, Twinject, Adrenalin*) Cardiac arrest: 1 mg IV q3–5 min. Anaphylaxis: 0.1–0.5 mg SC/IM, may repeat SC dose q 10–15 min. Acute asthma & hypersensitivity reactions: Adults: 0.1 to 0.3 mg of 1:1,000 soln SC or IM; Peds: 0.01 mg/kg (up to 0.3 mg) of 1:1,000

(cont.)

CARDIAC PARAMETERS AND FORMULAS	*Normal*
Cardiac output (CO) = heart rate× stroke volume	4–8 L/min
Cardiac index (CI) = CO/BSA	2.8–4.2 L/min/m²
MAP (mean arterial press) = [(SBP – DBP)/3] + DBP	80–100 mm Hg
SVR (systemic vasc resis) = (MAP – CVP) × (80)/CO	800–1200 dyne/sec/cm⁵
PVR (pulm vasc resis) = (PAM – PCWP) × (80)/CO	45–120 dyne/sec/cm⁵
QTc = QT/square root of RR	0.38–0.42
Right atrial pressure (central venous pressure)	0–8 mm Hg
Pulmonary artery systolic pressure (PAS)	20–30 mm Hg
Pulmonary artery diastolic pressure (PAD)	10–15 mm Hg
Pulmonary capillary wedge pressure (PCWP)	8–12 mm Hg (post-MI ~16 mm Hg)

soln SC or IM. [Soln for injection: 1:1,000 (1 mg/mL in 1 mL amps or 10 mL vial). Trade only: EpiPen Auto-injector delivers one 0.3 mg (1:1,000, 0.3 mL) IM dose. EpiPen Jr. Autoinjector delivers one 0.15 mg (1:2,000, 0.3 mL) IM dose. Twinject Auto-injector delivers one 0.15 mg (1:1,000, 0.15 mL) or 0.3 mg (1:1,000, 0.3 mL) IM/SQ dose.] ▶Plasma ♀C ▶? $

INAMRINONE Heart failure: 0.75 mg/kg bolus IV over 2–3 min, then infusion 100 mg in 100 mL NS (1 mg/mL) at 5–10 mcg/kg/min. 70 kg: 5 mcg/kg/ min = 21 mL/h. ▶K ♀C ▶? $$$$$

MIDODRINE (Orvaten, ProAmatine, ◆Amatine) Orthostatic hypotension: 10 mg PO tid while awake. [Generic/Trade: Tabs, scored 2.5, 5, 10 mg.] ▶LK ♀C ▶? $$$$$

MILRINONE (Primacor) Systolic heart failure (NYHA class III,IV): Load 50 mcg/kg IV over 10 min, then begin IV infusion of 0.375–0.75 mcg/kg/min. ▶K ♀C ▶? $$

NOREPINEPHRINE (Levophed) Acute hypotension: 4 mg in 500 mL D5W (8 mcg/mL) start 8–12 mcg/min, adjust to maintain BP, average maintenance rate 2–4 mcg/min, ideally through central line. 3 mcg/min = 22.5 mL/h. ▶Plasma ♀C ▶? $

PHENYLEPHRINE—INTRAVENOUS (Neo-Synephrine) Severe hypotension: 50 mcg boluses IV. Infusion: 20 mg in 250 mL D5W (80 mcg/mL), start 100–180 mcg/min (75–135 mL/min), usual dose once BP is stabilized 40–60 mcg/ min. ▶Plasma ♀C ▶- $

Pulmonary Arterial Hypertension

SILDENAFIL (Revatio) Pulmonary hypertension 20 mg PO tid. Contraindicated with nitrates. [Revatio: Tabs 20 mg.] ▶LK ♀B ▶? $$$$$

Thrombolytics

ALTEPLASE (tpa, t-PA, Activase, Cathflo, ◆Activase rt-PA) Acute MI: 15 mg IV bolus, then 50 mg over 30 min, then 35 mg over the next 60 min; (patient ≤67 kg) 15 mg IV bolus, then 0.75 mg/kg (max 50 mg) over 30 min, then 0.5 mg/kg (max 35 mg) over the next 60 min. Concurrent heparin infusion. Acute ischemic stroke with symptoms ≤3h: 0.9 mg/kg (max 90 mg); give 10% of total dose as an IV bolus, and the remainder IV over 60 min. Multiple exclusion criteria. Acute pulmonary embolism: 100 mg IV over 2h, then restart heparin

THROMBOLYTIC THERAPY FOR ACUTE MI

Indications (if high-volume cath lab unavailable): Clinical history & presentation strongly suggestive of MI within 12 h plus ≥1 of the following: 1 mm ST elevation in ≥2 contiguous leads; new left BBB; or 2 mm ST depression in V1-4 suggestive of true posterior MI.

Absolute contraindications: Previous cerebral hemorrhage, known cerebral aneurysm or arteriovenous malformation, known intracranial neoplasm, recent (<3 mo) ischemic stroke (except acute ischemic stroke <3 h), aortic dissection, active bleeding or bleeding diathesis (excluding menstruation), significant closed head or facial trauma (<3 mo).

Relative contraindications: Severe uncontrolled HTN (>180/110 mm Hg) on presentation or chronic severe HTN; prior ischemic stroke (>3 mo), dementia, other intracranial pathology; traumatic/prolonged (>10 min) cardiopulmonary resuscitation; major surgery (<3 wk); recent (within 2–4 wk) internal bleeding; puncture of non-compressible vessel; pregnancy; active peptic ulcer disease; current use of anticoagulants. For streptokinase/anistreplase: prior exposure (>5 d ago) or prior allergic reaction.

Reference: *Circulation* 2004;110:588–636

when PTT ≤twice normal. Occluded central venous access device: 2 mg/mL in catheter for 2 h. May use second dose if needed. ▶L ♀C ▶? $$$$$
RETEPLASE (*Retavase*) Acute MI: 10 units IV over 2 min; repeat once in 30 min. ▶L ♀C ▶? $$$$$
STREPTOKINASE (*Streptase, Kabikinase*) Acute MI: 1.5 million units IV over 60 min. ▶L ♀C ▶? $$$$$
TENECTEPLASE (*TNKase*) Acute MI: Single IV bolus dose over 5 sec based on body weight; <60 kg, 30 mg; 60–69 kg, 35 mg; 70–79 kg, 40 mg; 80–89 kg, 45 mg; ≥90kg, 50 mg. ▶L ♀C ▶? $$$$$
UROKINASE (*Kinlytic*) PE: 4400 units/kg IV loading dose over 10 min, followed by IV infusion 4400 units/kg/h for 12 h. Occluded IV catheter: 5000 units instilled into catheter, remove solution after 5 min. ▶L ♀B ▶? $$$$$

Volume Expanders

ALBUMIN (*Albuminar, Buminate, Albumarc, ✦Plasbumin*) Shock, burns: 500 mL of 5% solution IV infusion as rapidly as tolerated, repeat in 30 min if needed. ▶L ♀C ▶? $$$$$
DEXTRAN (*Rheomacrodex, Gentran, Macrodex*) Shock/hypovolemia: 20 mL/kg up to 500 mL IV. ▶K ♀C ▶? $$
HETASTARCH (*Hespan, Hextend*) Shock/hypovolemia: 500–1000 mL IV 6% solution. ▶K ♀C ▶? $$
PLASMA PROTEIN FRACTION (*Plasmanate, Protenate, Plasmatein*) Shock/hypovolemia: 5% soln 250–500 mL IV prn. ▶L ♀C ▶? $$$

Other

BIDIL (*hydralazine + isosorbide dinitrate*) Heart failure (adjunct to standard therapy in black patients): Start 1 tab PO tid, increase as tolerated to max 2 tabs bid. May decrease to ½ tab tid with intolerable side effects; try to increase dose when side effects subside. [Trade only: Tabs, scored 37.5/20 mg.] ▶LK ♀C ▶? $$$$$

CILOSTAZOL (*Pletal*) Intermittent claudication: 100 mg PO bid on empty stomach. 50 mg PO bid with cytochrome P450 3A4 inhibitors (eg, ketoconazole, itraconazole, erythromycin, diltiazem) or cytochrome P450 2C19 inhibitors (eg, omeprazole). Avoid grapefruit juice. [Generic/Trade: Tabs 50, 100 mg.] ▶L ♀C ▶? $$$$

NESIRITIDE (*Natrecor*) Hospitalized patients with decompensated heart failure with dyspnea at rest: 2 mcg/kg IV bolus over 60 sec, then 0.01 mcg/kg/min IV infusion for up to 48 h. Do not initiate at higher doses. Limited experience with increased doses. 1.5 mg vial in 250 mL D5W (6 mcg/mL). 70 kg: 2 mcg/kg bolus = 23.3 mL, 0.01 mcg/kg/min infusion = 7 mL/h. Symptomatic hypotension. May increase mortality. Not indicated for outpatient infusion, for scheduled repetitive use, to improve renal function, or to enhance diuresis. ▶K, plasma ♀C ▶? $$$$$

PENTOXIFYLLINE (*Trental*) 400 mg PO tid with meals. [Generic/Trade: Tabs 400 mg.] ▶L ♀C ▶? $$$

RANOLAZINE (*Ranexa*) Chronic angina: 500 mg PO bid, max 2000 mg daily. Reserve for angina not controlled with other antianginal drugs. Get baseline and follow-up EKGs; evaluate effects on QT interval. Contraindicated with pre-existing QT prolongation, hepatic impairment, QT prolonging drugs. Many drug interactions. [Trade only: Tabs, extended release 500, 1000 mg.] ▶LK ♀C ▶? $$$$$

CONTRAST MEDIA

MRI Contrast—Gadolinium-based (all non-iodinated)

NOTE *Avoid gadolinium-based contrast agents if severe renal insufficiency (GFR <30 mL/min/1.73 m2) due to risk of nephrogenic systemic fibrosis / nephrogenic fibrosing dermopathy. Similarly avoid in acute renal insufficiency of any severity due to hepatorenal syndrome or during the perioperative phase of liver transplant.*

GADOBENATE (*MultiHance*) Non-ionic IV contrast for MRI. ▶K ♀C ▶? $$$$
GADODIAMIDE (*Omniscan*) Non-ionic IV contrast for MRI. ▶K ♀C ▶? $$$$
GADOPENTETATE (*Magnevist*) IV contrast for MRI. ▶K ♀C ▶? $$$
GADOTERIDOL (*Prohance*) Non-ionic IV contrast for MRI. ▶K ♀C ▶? $$$$
GADOVERSETAMIDE (*OptiMARK*) IV contrast for MRI. ▶K ♀C ▶- $$$$

MRI Contrast—Other (all non-iodinated)

FERUMOXIDES (*Feridex*) Non-ionic, iron-based IV contrast for hepatic MRI. ▶L ♀C ▶? $$$$
FERUMOXSIL (*GastroMARK*) Non-ionic, iron-based, oral GI contrast for MRI. ▶L ♀B ▶? $$$$
MANGAFODIPIR (*Teslascan*) Manganese-based IV contrast for MRI. ▶L ♀- ▶- $$$$

Radiography Contrast

NOTE *Beware of allergic or anaphylactoid reactions. Avoid IV contrast in renal insufficiency or dehydration. Hold metformin (Glucophage) prior to or at the time of iodinated contrast dye use and for 48 h after procedure. Restart after procedure only if renal function is normal.*

BARIUM SULFATE NON-IODINATED GI (eg, oral, rectal) contrast. ▶Not absorbed ♀? ▶+ $

DIATRIZOATE (*Cystografin, Gastrografin, Hypaque, MD-Gastroview, RenoCal, Reno-DIP, Reno-60, Renografin*) Iodinated, ionic, high osmolality IV or GI contrast. ▶K ♀C ▶? $

IODIXANOL (*Visipaque*) Iodinated, non-ionic, iso-osmolar IV contrast. ▶K ♀B ▶? $$$

IOHEXOL (*Omnipaque*) Iodinated, non-ionic, low osmolality IV and oral/body cavity contrast. ▶K ♀B ▶? $$$

IOPAMIDOL (*Isovue*) Iodinated, non-ionic, low osmolality IV contrast. ▶K ♀? ▶? $$

IOPROMIDE (*Ultravist*) Iodinated, non-ionic, low osmolality IV contrast. ▶K ♀B ▶? $$$

IOTHALAMATE (*Conray, ✦Vascoray*) Iodinated, ionic, high osmolality IV contrast. ▶K ♀B ▶- $

IOVERSOL (*Optiray*) Iodinated, non-ionic, low osmolality IV contrast. ▶K ♀B ▶? $$

IOXAGLATE (*Hexabrix*) Iodinated, ionic, low osmolality IV contrast. ▶K ♀B ▶- $$$

IOXILAN (*Oxilan*) Iodinated, non-ionic, low osmolality IV contrast. ▶K ♀B ▶- $$$

DERMATOLOGY

Acne Preparations

ADAPALENE (*Differin*) Apply qhs. [Trade only: gel 0.1% & 0.3% (15,45 g) cream 0.1% (15,45 g), soln 0.1% pad (30 mL).] ▶Bile ♀C ▶? $$

AZELAIC ACID (*Azelex, Finacea, Finevin*) Apply bid. [Trade only: cream 20%, 30 g, 50 g (Azelex, Finevin), gel 15% 30, 50 g (Finacea).] ▶K ♀B ▶? $$$

BENZACLIN (*clindamycin + benzoyl peroxide*) Apply bid. [Trade only: gel clindamycin 1% + benzoyl peroxide 5%; 25, 50 g, gel pump clindamycin 1% + benzoyl peroxide 5%; 50 g.] ▶K ♀C ▶+ $$$

BENZAMYCIN (*erythromycin base + benzoyl peroxide*) Apply bid. [Generic/Trade: gel erythromycin 3% + benzoyl peroxide 5%; 23.3, 46.6 g.] ▶LK ♀C ▶? $$$

BENZOYL PEROXIDE (*Benzac, Benzagel 10%, Desquam, Clearasil, ✦Solugel, Benoxyl*) Apply daily; increase to bid-tid if needed. [OTC and Rx generic: liquid 2.5,5,10%, bar 5,10%, mask 5%, lotion 5,5.5,10%, cream 5,10%, cleanser 10%, gel 2.5,4,5, 6,10,20%.] ▶LK ♀C ▶? $

CLENIA (*sulfacetamide + sulfur*) Apply 1–3 times daily. [Generic only: lotion (sodium sulfacetamide 10% & sulfur 5%) 25 g. Trade only (sodium sulfacetamide 10% & sulfur 5%): cream 28 g, foaming wash 170,340 g.] ▶K ♀C ▶? $$

CLINDAMYCIN—TOPICAL (*Cleocin T, Clindagel, ClindaMax, Evoclin, ✦Dalacin T*) Apply daily (Evoclin) or bid (Cleocin T). [Generic/Trade: gel 1% 7.5, 30 g, lotion 1% 60 mL, solution 1% 30, 60 mL. Trade only: foam 1% 50, 100 g (Evoclin), gel 1% 40, 75 mL (Clindagel).] ▶L ♀B ▶- $$

DIANE-35 (*cyproterone + ethinyl estradiol*) Canada only. 1 tab PO daily for 21 consecutive d, stop for 7 d, repeat cycle. [Rx trade only: blister pack of 21 tabs 2 mg/0.035 mg cyproterone acetate/ethinyl estradiol.] ▶L ♀X ▶- $$

DUAC (*clindamycin + benzoyl peroxide*) (*✦Clindoxyl*) Apply qhs. [Trade only: gel clindamycin 1% + benzoyl peroxide 5%; 45 g.] ▶K ♀C ▶+ $$$$

ERYTHROMYCIN—TOPICAL (*Eryderm, Erycette, Erygel, A/T/S, ✦Sans-Acne, Erysol*) apply bid. [Generic only: solution 1.5% 60 mL, 2% 60,120 mL, pads 2%, gel 2% 30,60 g, ointment 2% 25 g.] ▶L ♀B ▶? $$

ISOTRETINOIN (*Accutane, Amnesteem, Claravis, Sotret, ✦Clarus*) 0.5–2 mg/kg/d PO divided bid for 15–20 wk. Typical target dose is 1 mg/kg/d. Can only be prescribed by healthcare professionals who are registered with the iPledge program. Potent teratogen; use extreme caution. May cause depression. Not for long-term use. [Generic/Trade: caps 10, 20, 40 mg. Generic only (Sotret & Claravis): caps 30 mg.] ▶LK ♀X ▶- $$$$$

ROSULA (*sulfacetamide + sulfur*) Apply 1–3 times daily. [Trade only: gel (sodium sulfacetamide 10% & sulfur 5%) 45 mL, aqueous cleanser (sodium sulfacetamide 10% & sulfur 5%) 355 mL, soap (sodium sulfacetamide 10% & sulfur 4%) 473 mL.] ▶K ♀C ▶? $$$$

SALICYLIC ACID (*Akurza, Clearasil Cleanser, Stridex Pads*) Apply/wash area up to three times daily. [Generic/Trade: OTC: pads, foam, mask scrub, 0.5%, 1%, 2%. Rx/Trade: cream 6%, 12 oz. (Akurza), lotion 6%, 12 oz. (Akurza).] ▶Not absorbed ♀? ▶? $

SULFACETAMIDE—TOPICAL (*Klaron, Rosula NS*) Apply bid. [Generic/Trade: lotion 10% 59, 118 mL. Trade only (Rosula NS): Single-use pads 10%.] ▶K ♀C ▶? $$

SULFACET-R (*sulfacetamide + sulfur*) Apply 1–3 times daily. [Trade (Sulfacet-R) and generic: lotion (sodium sulfacetamide 10% & sulfur 5%) 25 g.] ▶K ♀C ▶? $$

TAZAROTENE (*Tazorac, Avage*) Acne (Tazorac): Apply 0.1% cream qhs. Psoriasis: apply 0.05% cream qhs, increase to 0.1% prn. [Trade only (Tazorac): Cream 0.05% and 0.1% - 30, 60 g, Gel 0.05% and 0.1% - 30, 100 g. Trade only (Avage): Cream 0.1% 15, 30 g.] ▶L ♀X ▶? $$$$

TRETINOIN—TOPICAL (*Retin-A, Retin-A Micro, Renova, Retisol-A, ✦Stieva-A, Rejuva-A, Vitamin A Acid Cream*) Apply qhs. [Generic/Trade: cream 0.025% 20,45 g, 0.05% 20,45 g, 0.1% 20,45 g, gel 0.025% 15,45 g, 0.1% 15,45 g, liquid 0.05% 28 mL. Trade only: Renova cream 0.02% & 0.05% 40,60 g, Retin-A Micro gel 0.04%, 0.1% 20,45 g.] ▶LK ♀C ▶? $$

ZIANA (*clindamycin + tretinoin*) Apply qhs. [Trade only: gel clindamycin 1.2% + tretinoin 0.025% 30, 60 g.] ▶LK ♀C ▶? $$$$

Actinic Keratosis Preparations

DICLOFENAC—TOPICAL (*Solaraze, Voltaren*) Solaraze: Actinic/solar keratoses: apply bid to lesions × 60–90 d. Voltaren: Osteoarthritis of areas amenable to topical therapy: 2 g (upper extremities) to 4 g (lower extremities) 4 times daily. [Trade only: gel 3% 50 (Solaraze), 100 g (Solaraze, Voltaren).] ▶L ♀B ▶? $$$$$

FLUOROURACIL—TOPICAL (*5-FU, Carac, Efudex, Fluoroplex*) Actinic keratoses: apply bid × 2–6 wk. Superficial basal cell carcinomas: apply 5% cream/solution bid. [Trade only: Cream 0.5% 30 g (Carac), 5% 25 g (Efudex), 1% 30 g (Fluoroplex). Generic/Trade: Solution 2% & 5% 10 mL (Efudex), Cream 5% 40 g.] ▶L ♀X ▶- $$$$$

METHYLAMINOLEVULINATE (*Metvix, Metvixia*) Apply cream to non-hyperkeratotic actinic keratoses lesion and surrounding area on face or scalp; cover with dressing for 3 h; remove dressing and cream and perform illumination therapy. Repeat in 7 d. [Trade only: cream: 16%, 2 g tube.] ▶Not absorbed ♀C ▶? ?

Antibacterials (Topical)

BACITRACIN (*♣Baciguent*) Apply daily-tid. [OTC Generic/Trade: ointment 500 units/g 1,15,30 g.] ▶Not absorbed ♀C ▶? $

FUSIDIC ACID—TOPICAL (*♣Fucidin*) Canada only Apply tid-qid. [Canada trade only: cream 2% fusidic acid 5,15,30 g, ointment 2% sodium fusidate 5,15,30 g.] ▶L ♀? ▶? $

GENTAMICIN—TOPICAL (*Garamycin*) Apply tid-qid. [Generic/Trade: ointment 0.1% 15,30 g, cream 0.1% 15,30 g.] ▶K ♀D ▶? $

MAFENIDE (*Sulfamylon*) Apply daily-bid. [Trade only: cream 37, 114, 411 g, 5% topical solution 50 g packets.] ▶LK ♀C ▶? $$$

METRONIDAZOLE—TOPICAL (*Noritate, MetroCream, MetroGel, MetroLotion, ♣Rosasol*) Rosacea: Apply daily (1%) or bid (0.75%). [Trade only: Gel (MetroGel) 1% 45,60 g, Cream (Noritate) 1% 30,60 g. Generic/Trade: Gel 0.75% 29 g. Cream 0.75% 45 g. Lotion (MetroLotion) 0.75% 59 mL.] ▶KL ♀B(- in 1st trimester) ▶- $$$

MUPIROCIN (*Bactroban, Centany*) Impetigo/infected wounds: Apply tid. Nasal methicillin-resistant Staph aureus eradication: 0.5 g in each nostril bid × 5 d. [Generic/Trade: Cream 2% 15, 30 g, ointment 2% 22 g, 2% nasal ointment 1 g single-use tubes (for MRSA eradication).] ▶Not absorbed ♀B ▶? $$$

NEOSPORIN CREAM (*neomycin + polymyxin*) Apply daily-tid. [OTC Trade only: neomycin 3.5 mg/g + polymyxin 10,000 units/g 15 g and unit dose 0.94 g.] ▶K ♀C ▶? $

NEOSPORIN OINTMENT (*bacitracin + neomycin + polymyxin*) Apply daily-tid. [OTC Generic/Trade: bacitracin 400 units/g + neomycin 3.5 mg/g + polymyxin 5,000 units/g 2,4,9.6,14.2,15, 30 g and unit dose 0.94 g.] ▶K ♀C ▶? $

POLYSPORIN (*bacitracin + polymyxin, ♣Polytopic*) apply ointment/aerosol/powder daily-tid. [OTC Trade only: ointment 15,30 g and unit dose 0.9 g, powder 10 g, aerosol 90 g.] ▶K ♀C ▶? $

RETAPAMULIN (*Altabax*) Impetigo: Apply bid for 5 d. [Trade only: ointment 1% 5, 10, 15 g.] ▶Not absorbed ♀B ▶? $$$

SILVER SULFADIAZINE (*Silvadene*, *✦Dermazin, Flamazine, SSD*) Apply daily-bid. [Generic/Trade: cream 1% 20,50,85,400,1000 g.] ▶LK ♀B ▶- $

Antifungals (Topical)

BUTENAFINE (*Lotrimin Ultra, Mentax*) Apply daily-bid. [Trade only. Rx: cream 1% 15,30 g (Mentax). OTC: cream 1% 12, 24 g (Lotrimin Ultra).] ▶L ♀B ▶? $

CICLOPIROX (*Loprox, Penlac, ✦Stieprox shampoo*) Cream, lotion: Apply bid. Nail solution: apply daily to affected nails; apply over previous coat; remove with alcohol every 7 d. Seborrheic dermatitis (Loprox shampoo): shampoo twice/wk × 4 wk. [Trade only: gel (Loprox) 0.77% 30, 45, 100 g, shampoo (Loprox) 1% 120 mL. Generic/Trade: nail solution (Penlac) 8% 6.6 mL, cream (Loprox) 0.77% 15, 30, 90 g, lotion (Loprox TS) 0.77% 30, 60 mL.] ▶K ♀B ▶? $$$$

CLOTRIMAZOLE—TOPICAL (*Lotrimin, Mycelex, ✦Canesten, Clotrimaderm*) Apply bid. [Note that Lotrimin brand cream, lotion, solution are clotrimazole, while Lotrimin powders and liquid spray are miconazole. OTC & Rx generic/Trade: cream 1% 15, 30, 45, 90 g, solution 1% 10,30 mL. Trade only: lotion 1% 30 mL.] ▶L ♀B ▶? $

ECONAZOLE Tinea pedis, cruris, corporis, tinea versicolor: apply daily. Cutaneous candidiasis: apply bid. [Generic only: cream 1% 15, 30, 85 g.] ▶Not absorbed ♀C ▶? $$

KETOCONAZOLE—TOPICAL (*Extina, Nizoral, Xolegel, ✦Ketoderm*) Tinea/candidal infections: Apply daily. Seborrheic dermatitis: apply cream daily-bid for 4 wk or gel daily for 2 wk or foam bid for 4 wk. Dandruff: apply 1% shampoo twice a wk. Tinea versicolor: apply shampoo to affected area, leave on for 5 min, rinse. [Generic/Trade: cream 2% 15, 30, 60 g, shampoo 2% (120 mL). Trade only: shampoo 1% (OTC), gel 2%, 15 g (Rx, Xolegel) foam 2%, 50, 100 g (Rx, Extina).] ▶L ♀C ▶? $$

MICONAZOLE—TOPICAL (*Monistat-Derm, Micatin, Lotrimin*) Tinea, candida: Apply bid. [Note that Lotrimin brand cream, lotion, solution are clotrimazole, while Lotrimin powders and liquid spray are miconazole. OTC generic: ointment 2% 29 g, spray 2% 105 mL, solution 2% 7.39, 30 mL. Generic/Trade: cream 2% 15,30,90 g, powder 2% 90 g, spray powder 2% 90,100 g, spray liquid 2% 105,113 mL.] ▶L ♀+ ▶? $

NAFTIFINE (*Naftin*) Tinea: Apply daily (cream) or bid (gel). [Trade only: cream 1% 15, 30, 60, 90 g, gel 1% 20, 40, 60, 90 g.] ▶LK ♀B ▶? $$$

NYSTATIN—TOPICAL (*Mycostatin, ✦Nilstat, Nyaderm, Candistatin*) Candidiasis: Apply bid-tid. [Generic/Trade: cream 100,000 units/g 15, 30, 240 g, ointment 100,000 units/g 15, 30 g, powder 100,000 units/g 15 g.] ▶Not absorbed ♀C ▶? $

OXICONAZOLE (*Oxistat, Oxizole*) Tinea pedis, cruris, and corporis: Apply daily-bid. Tinea versicolor (cream only): apply daily. [Trade only: cream 1% 15, 30, 60 g, lotion 1% 30 mL.] ▶? ♀B ▶? $$$

SERTACONAZOLE (*Ertaczo*) Tinea pedis: Apply bid. [Trade only: cream 2% 15, 30, 60 g.] ▶Not absorbed ♀C ▶? $$

TERBINAFINE—TOPICAL (*Lamisil, Lamisil AT*) Tinea: Apply daily-bid. [Trade only: cream 1% 15,30 g, gel 1% 5,15,30 g OTC Trade only (Lamisil AT): cream 1% 12,24 g, spray pump solution 1% 30 mL.] ▶L ♀B ▶? $$$

TOLNAFTATE (*Tinactin, ✦ZeaSorb AF*) Apply bid. [OTC Generic/Trade: cream 1% 15,30 g, solution 1% 10,15 mL, powder 1% 45,90 g, spray powder 1% 100,105,150 g, spray liquid 1% 60,120 mL. Trade only: gel 1% 15 g.] ▶? ♀? ▶? $

Antiparasitics (Topical)

A-200 (*pyrethrins + piperonyl butoxide*) (✦R&C) Lice: Apply shampoo, wash after 10 min. Reapply in 5–7 d. [OTC Generic/Trade: shampoo (0.33% pyrethrins, 4% piperonyl butoxide) 60,120,240 mL.] ▶L ♀C ▶? $

CROTAMITON (*Eurax*) Scabies: Apply cream/lotion topically from chin to feet, repeat in 24 h, bathe 48 h later. Pruritus: massage prn. [Trade only: cream 10% 60 g, lotion 10% 60,480 mL.] ▶? ♀C ▶? $$

LINDANE (✦Hexit) Other drugs preferred. Scabies: Apply 30–60 mL of lotion, wash after 8–12 h. Lice: 30–60 mL of shampoo, wash off after 4 min. Can cause seizures in epileptics or if overused/misused in children. Not for infants. [Generic only: lotion 1% 60, 480 mL, shampoo 1% 60, 480 mL.] ▶L ♀B ▶? $

MALATHION (*Ovide*) Apply to dry hair, let dry naturally, wash off in 8–12 h. [Trade only: lotion 0.5% 59 mL.] ▶? ♀B ▶? $$

PERMETHRIN (*Elimite, Acticin, Nix, ✦Kwellada-P*) Scabies: Apply cream from head (avoid mouth/ nose/eyes) to soles of feet & wash after 8–14 h. 30 g is typical adult dose. Lice: Saturate hair and scalp with 1% rinse, wash after 10 min. Do not use in children <2 mo old. May repeat therapy in 7 d, as necessary. [Trade only: cream (Elimite, Acticin) 5% 60 g. OTC Generic/Trade: liquid creme rinse (Nix) 1% 60 mL.] ▶L ♀B ▶? $$

RID (*pyrethrins + piperonyl butoxide*) Lice: Apply shampoo/mousse, wash after 10 min. Reapply in 5–10 d. [OTC Generic/Trade: shampoo 60,120,240 mL. Trade only: mousse 5.5 oz.] ▶L ♀C ▶? $

Antipsoriatics

ACITRETIN (*Soriatane*) 25–50 mg PO daily. Avoid pregnancy during therapy and for 3 yr after discontinuation. [Trade only: cap 10, 25 mg.] ▶L ♀X ▶- $$$$$

ALEFACEPT (*Amevive*) 7.5 mg IV or 15 mg IM once weekly × 12 doses. May repeat with 1 additional 12-wk course after 12 wk have elapsed since last dose. ▶? ♀B ▶? $$$$$

ANTHRALIN (*Anthra-Derm, Drithocreme, ✦Anthrascalp, Anthranol, Anthraforte, Dithranol*) Apply daily. Short contact periods (ie, 15–20 min) followed by removal may be preferred. [Trade only: ointment 0.1% 42.5 g, 0.25% 42.5 g, 0.4% 60 g, 0.5% 42.5 g, 1% 42.5 g, cream 0.1% 50 g, 0.2% 50 g, 0.25% 50 g, 0.5% 50 g. Generic/Trade: cream 1% 50 g.] ▶? ♀C ▶- $$

CALCIPOTRIENE (*Dovonex*) Apply bid. [Trade only: ointment 0.005% 30, 60, 100 g, cream 0.005% 30, 60, 100 g. Generic/Trade: Scalp solution 0.005% 60 mL.] ▶L ♀C ▶? $$$

EFALIZUMAB (*Raptiva*)   0.7 mg/kg SC × 1 then 1 mg/kg SC q wk. [Trade only: single use vials, 125 mg.] ▶L ♀C ▶? $$$$$

TACLONEX (*calcipotriene + betamethasone*)   Apply daily for up to 4 wk. [Trade only: (calcipotriene 0.005% + betamethasone dipropionate 0.064%) ointment 15, 30, 60, 100 g, Topical susp 15, 30, 60 g.] ▶L ♀C ▶? $$$$$

Antivirals (Topical)

ACYCLOVIR—TOPICAL (*Zovirax*)   Herpes genitalis: apply oint q3h (6 times/d) × 7 d. Recurrent herpes labialis: apply cream 5 times/d for 4 d. [Trade only: ointment 5% 15 g, cream 5% (2 & 5 g).] ▶K ♀C ▶? $$$$$

DOCOSANOL (*Abreva*)   Oral-facial herpes (cold sores): apply 5x/d until healed. [OTC: Trade only: cream 10% 2 g.] ▶Not absorbed ♀B ▶? $

IMIQUIMOD (*Aldara*)   Genital/perianal warts: apply 3 times weekly during sleeping h for up to 16 wk. Wash off after 8 h. Nonhyperkeratotic, nonhypertrophic actinic keratoses on face/scalp in immunocompetent adults: apply 2 times weekly during sleeping h for 16 wk. Wash off after 8 h. Primary superficial basal cell carcinoma: apply 5 times weekly for 6 wk. Wash off after 8 h. [Trade only: cream 5% 250 mg single use packets.] ▶Not absorbed ♀C ▶? $$$$$

PENCICLOVIR (*Denavir*)   Herpes labialis (cold sores): apply cream q2h while awake × 4 d. [Trade only: cream 1% tubes 1.5 g.] ▶Not absorbed ♀B ▶? $$

PODOFILOX (*Condylox, ✦Condyline, Wartec*)   External genital warts (gel and solution) and perianal warts (gel only): apply bid for 3 consecutive d of a wk and repeat for up to 4 wk. [Generic/Trade: Solution 0.5% 3.5 mL. Trade only: Gel 0.5% 3.5 g.] ▶? ♀C ▶? $$$

PODOPHYLLIN (*Podocon-25, Podofin, Podofilm*)   Warts: apply by physician. Not to be dispensed to patients. [Not to be dispensed to patients. For hospital/clinic use; not intended for outpatient prescribing. Trade only: Liquid 25% 15 mL.] ▶? ♀- $$$

SINECATECHINS (*Veregen*)   Apply tid to external genital warts for up to 16 wk. [Trade only: ointment 15% 15 g.] ▶Unknown ♀C ▶? $$$$$

Atopic Dermatitis Preparations

PIMECROLIMUS (*Elidel*)   Atopic dermatitis: Apply bid. [Trade only: cream 1% 30, 60, 100 g.] ▶L ♀C ▶? $$$$

TACROLIMUS—TOPICAL (*Protopic*)   Atopic dermatitis: Apply bid. [Trade only: ointment 0.03% & 0.1% 30, 60, 100 g ▶Minimal absorption ♀C ▶? $$$$

Corticosteroid / Antimicrobial Combinations

CORTISPORIN (*neomycin + polymyxin + hydrocortisone*)   Apply bid-qid. [Trade only: Cream 7.5 g, Ointment 15 g.] ▶LK ♀C ▶? $$$

FUCIDIN H (*fusidic acid + hydrocortisone*)   Canada only. Apply tid. [Canada trade only: cream 2% fusidic acid, 1% hydrocortisone acetate 30 g.] ▶L ♀? ▶? $$

LOTRISONE (*clotrimazole + betamethasone*) (*✚Lotriderm*) Apply bid. Do not use for diaper rash. [Generic/Trade: cream (clotrimazole 1% + betamethasone 0.05%) 15 g, lotion (clotrimazole 1% + betamethasone 0.05%) 30 mL.] ▶L ♀C ▶? $$$

MYCOLOG II (*nystatin + triamcinolone*) Apply bid. [Generic/Trade: cream 15,30,60,120 g, ointment 15,30,60,120 g.] ▶L ♀C ▶? $

Hemorrhoid Care

DIBUCAINE (*Nupercainal*) Apply cream/ointment tid-qid prn. [OTC Generic/Trade: ointment 1% 30 g.] ▶L ♀? ▶? $

PRAMOXINE (*Anusol Hemorrhoidal Ointment, Fleet Pain Relief, Proctofoam NS*) Ointment/pads/foam up to 5 times/d prn. [OTC Trade only: ointment (Anusol Hemorrhoidal Ointment), pads (Fleet Pain Relief), aerosol foam (ProctoFoam NS).] ▶Not absorbed ♀+ ▶+ $

STARCH (*Anusol Suppositories*) 1 Supp up to 6 times/d prn. [OTC Trade only: suppositories (51% topical starch; soy bean oil, tocopheryl acetate).] ▶Not absorbed ♀+ ▶+ $

WITCH HAZEL (*Tucks*) Apply to anus/perineum up to 6 times/d prn. [OTC Generic/Trade: pads, gel.] ▶? ♀+ ▶+ $

Other Dermatologic Agents

ALITRETINOIN (*Panretin*) Apply bid-qid to cutaneous Kaposi's lesions [Trade only: gel 0.1%, 60 g.] ▶Not absorbed ♀D ▶- $$$$$

ALUMINUM CHLORIDE (*Drysol, Certain Dri*) Apply qhs. [Rx: Generic/Trade: solution 20%: 37.5 mL bottle, 35, 60 mL bottle with applicator. OTC: Trade only (Certain Dri): solution 12.5%: 36 mL bottle.] ▶K ♀? ▶? $

BECAPLERMIN (*Regranex*) Diabetic ulcers: Apply gel daily. [Trade only: gel 0.01%, 2 & 15 g.] ▶Minimal absorption ♀C ▶? $$$$$

CALAMINE apply lotion tid-qid prn for poison ivy/oak or insect bite itching. [OTC Generic only: lotion 120, 240, 480 mL.] ▶? ♀? ▶? $

CAPSAICIN (*Zostrix, Zostrix-HP*) Arthritis, post-herpetic or diabetic neuralgia: apply cream up to tid-qid. [OTC Generic/Trade: cream 0.025% 45,60 g, 0.075% 30,60 g, lotion 0.025% 59 mL, 0.075% 59 mL, gel 0.025% 15,30 g, 0.05% 43 g, roll-on 0.075% 60 mL.] ▶? ♀? ▶? $

COAL TAR (*Polytar, Tegrin, Cutar, Tarsum*) Apply shampoo at least twice a wk, or for psoriasis apply daily-qid. [OTC Generic/Trade: shampoo, conditioner, cream, ointment, gel, lotion, soap, oil.] ▶? ♀? ▶? $

DOXEPIN—TOPICAL (*Zonalon*) Pruritus: Apply qid for up to 8 d. [Trade only: cream 5% 30,45 g.] ▶L ♀B ▶- $

EFLORNITHINE (*Vaniqa*) Reduction of facial hair: Apply to face bid. [Trade only: cream 13.9% 30 g.] ▶K ♀C ▶? $$$

EMLA (*prilocaine + lidocaine—topical*) Topical anesthesia: Apply 2.5 g cream or 1 disc to region at least 1 h before procedure. Cover cream with an occlusive dressing. [Trade only: cream (2.5% lidocaine + 2.5% prilocaine) 5 g, disc 1 g. Generic/Trade: cream (2.5% lidocaine + 2.5% prilocaine) 30 g.] ▶LK ♀B ▶? $$

CORTICOSTEROIDS—TOPICAL

Potency*	Generic	Trade Name	Forms	Frequency
Low	alclometasone dipropionate	Aclovate	0.05% C/O	bid-tid
Low	clocortolone pivalate	Cloderm	0.1% C	tid
Low	desonide	DesOwen, Tridesilon	0.05% C/L/O	bid-tid
Low	hydrocortisone	Hytone, others	0.5% C/L/O; 1% C/L/O; 2.5% C/L/O	bid-qid
Low	hydrocortisone acetate	Cortaid, Corticaine	0.5% C/O, 1% C/O/Sp	bid-qid
Medium	betamethasone valerate	Luxiq	0.1% C/L/O; 0.12% F (Luxiq)	qd-bid
Medium	desoximetasone‡	Topicort	0.05% C	bid
Medium	fluocinolone	Synalar	0.01% C/S; 0.025% C/O	bid-qid
Medium	flurandrenolide	Cordran	0.025% C/O; 0.05% C/L/O/T	bid-qid
Medium	fluticasone propionate	Cutivate	0.005% O; 0.05% C/L	qd-bid
Medium	hydrocortisone butyrate	Locoid	0.1% C/O/S	bid-tid
Medium	hydrocortisone valerate	Westcort	0.2% C/O	bid-tid
Medium	mometasone furoate	Elocon	0.1% C/L/O	qd
Medium	triamcinolone‡	Aristocort, Kenalog	0.025% C/L/O; 0.1% C/L/O/S	bid-tid
High	amcinonide	Cyclocort	0.1% C/L/O	bid-tid
High	betamethasone dipropionate‡	Maxivate, others	0.05% C/L/O (non-Diprolene)	qd-bid
High	desoximetasone‡	Topicort	0.05% G; 0.25% C/O	bid
High	diflorasone diacetate‡	Maxiflor	0.05% C/O	bid
High	fluocinonide	Lidex	0.05% C/G/O/S	bid-qid
High	halcinonide	Halog	0.1% C/O/S	bid-tid
High	triamcinolone‡	Aristocort, Kenalog	0.5% C/O	bid-tid
Very high	betamethasone dipropionate‡	Diprolene, Diprolene AF	0.05% C/G/L/O	qd-bid
Very high	clobetasol	Temovate, Cormax, Olux	0.05% C/G/O/L/S/Sp/F (Olux)	bid
Very high	diflorasone diacetate‡	Psorcon	0.05% C/O	qd-tid
Very high	halobetasol propionate	Ultravate	0.05% C/O	qd-bid

*Potency based on vasoconstrictive assays, which may not correlate with efficacy. Not all available products are listed, including those lacking potency ratings. ‡These drugs have formulations in more than once potency category. C, cream; O, ointment; L, lotion; T, tape; F, foam; S, solution; G, gel; Sp, spray.

HYALURONIC ACID (*Bionect, Restylane*) Moderate to severe facial wrinkles: Inject into wrinkle/fold (Restylane). Protection of dermal ulcers: apply gel/cream/spray to wound bid or tid (Bionect). [Rx: Injection 0.4 mL and 0.7 mL syringe. Cream 0.2% 25 g. Gel 0.2% 30 g. Spray 20 mL.] ▶? ♀? ▶? $$$$$

HYDROQUINONE (*Eldopaque, Eldoquin, Eldoquin Forte, EpiQuin Micro, Esoterica, Glyquin, Lustra, Melanex, Solaquin, Claripel, ✦Ultraquin*) Hyperpigmentation: Apply to area bid. [OTC Generic/Trade: cream 1.5%, lotion 2%. Rx Generic/Trade: solution 3%, gel 4%, cream 4%.] ▶? ♀C ▶? $$$

LACTIC ACID (*Lac-Hydrin, Amlactin, ✦Dermalac*) Apply lotion/cream bid. [Trade only: lotion 12% 150, 360 mL. Generic/OTC: cream 12% 140, 385 g. AmLactin AP is lactic acid (12%) with pramoxine (1%).] ▶? ♀? ▶? $$

LIDOCAINE—TOPICAL (*Xylocaine, Lidoderm, Numby Stuff, LMX, Zingo, ✦Maxilene*) Apply prn. Dose varies with anesthetic procedure, degree of anesthesia required and individual patient response. Postherpetic neuralgia: apply up to 3 patches to affected area at once for up to 12 h within a 24 h period. Apply 30 min prior to painful procedure (ELA-Max 4%). Discomfort with anorectal disorders: apply prn (ELA-Max 5%). Intradermal powder injection for venipuncture / IV cannulation, 3–18 yo (Zingo): 0.5 mg to site 1–10 min prior. [For membranes of mouth and pharynx: spray 10%, ointment 5%, liquid 5%, solution 2,4%, dental patch. For urethral use: jelly 2%. Patch (Lidoderm) 5%. Intradermal powder injection system: 0.5 mg (Zingo). OTC: Trade only: liposomal lidocaine 4% (ELA-Max).] ▶LK ♀B ▶+ $$

MINOXIDIL—TOPICAL (*Rogaine, Rogaine Forte, Rogaine Extra Strength, Minoxidil for Men, Theroxidil Extra Strength, ✦Minox, Apo-Gain*) Androgenetic alopecia in men or women: 1 mL to dry scalp bid. [OTC Trade only: solution 2%, 60 mL, 5%, 60 mL, 5% (Rogaine Extra Strength, Theroxidil Extra Strength - for men only) 60 mL, foam 5% 60 g.] ▶K ♀C ▶- $$

MONOBENZONE (*Benoquin*) Extensive vitiligo: Apply bid-tid. [Trade only: cream 20% 35.4 g.] ▶Minimal absorption ♀C ▶? $$

OATMEAL (*Aveeno*) Pruritus from poison ivy/oak, varicella: Apply lotion qid prn. Also bath packets for tub. [OTC Generic/Trade: lotion, packets.] ▶Not absorbed ♀? ▶? $

PANAFIL (*papain + urea + chlorophyllin copper complex*) Debridement of acute or chronic lesions: Apply to clean wound and cover daily-bid. [Trade only: Ointment: 6, 30 g, spray 33 mL.] ▶? ♀? ▶? $$$

PLIAGIS (*tetracaine + lidocaine—topical*) Apply 20–30 min prior to superficial dermatological procedure (60 min for tattoo removal). [Trade only: cream lidocaine 7% + tetracaine 7%.] ▶Minimal absorption ♀B ▶? $$

PRAMOSONE (*pramoxine + hydrocortisone*) (*✦Pramox HC*) Inflammatory and pruritic manifestations of corticosteroid-responsive dermatoses: Apply tid-qid. [Trade only: 1% pramoxine/1% hydrocortisone acetate: cream 30, 60 g, oint 30 g, lotion 60, 120, 240 mL. 1% pramoxine/2.5% hydrocortisone acetate: cream 30, 60 g, oint 30 g, lotion 60, 120 mL.] ▶Not absorbed ♀C ▶? $$$

SELENIUM SULFIDE (*Selsun, Exsel, Versel*) Dandruff, seborrheic dermatitis: Apply 5–10 mL lotion/shampoo twice weekly × 2 wk then less frequently, thereafter. Tinea versicolor: Apply 2.5% lotion/shampoo to affected area daily ×

(cont.)

7 d. [OTC Generic/Trade: lotion/shampoo 1% 120,210,240, 330 mL, 2.5% 120 mL. Rx Generic/Trade: lotion/shampoo 2.5% 120 mL.] ▶? ♀C ▶? $

SOLAG (*mequinol + tretinoin*) (*◆Solage*) Apply to solar lentigines bid. [Trade only: soln 30 mL (mequinol 2% + tretinoin 0.01%).] ▶Not absorbed ♀X ▶? $$$$

SYNERA (*tetracaine + lidocaine—topical*) Apply 20–30 min prior to superficial dermatological procedure. [Trade only: patch lidocaine 70 mg + tetracaine 70 mg.] ▶Minimal absorption ♀B ▶? $$

TRI-LUMA (*fluocinolone + hydroquinone + tretinoin*) Melasma of the face: apply qhs × 4–8 wk. [Trade only: soln 30 g (fluocinolone 0.01% + hydroquinone 4% + tretinoin 0.05%).] ▶Minimal absorption ♀C ▶? $$$$

VUSION (*miconazole—topical + zinc oxide + white petrolatum*) Apply to affected diaper area with each change for 7 d. [Trade only: ointment 50 g.] ▶Minimal absorption ♀C ▶? $$$$$

ENDOCRINE & METABOLIC

Androgens/Anabolic Steroids

NOTE *See OB/GYN section for other hormones.*

METHYLTESTOSTERONE (*Android, Methitest, Testred, Virilon*) Advancing inoperable breast cancer in women who are 1–5 yr postmenopausal: 50–200 mg/d PO in divided doses. Hypogonadism in men: 10–50 mg PO daily. [Generic only: Caps 10 mg,Tabs 10, 25 mg.] ▶L ♀X ▶? ©III $$$

NANDROLONE (*Deca-Durabolin*) Anemia of renal disease: women 50–100 mg IM q wk, men 100–200 mg IM q wk. [Generic only: Injection 50, 100 & 200 mg/mL.] ▶L ♀X ▶– ©III $$

OXANDROLONE (*Oxandrin*) Weight gain: 2.5 mg PO bid-qid for 2–4 wk. [Generic/Trade: Tabs 2.5, 10 mg.] ▶L ♀X ▶? ©III $$$$$

TESTOSTERONE (*Androderm, AndroGel, Delatestryl, Depo-Testosterone, Striant, Testim, Testopel, Testro AQ, ◆Andriol*) Injectable enanthate or cypionate: 50–400 mg IM q2–4 wk. Transdermal - Androderm: 5 mg patch to nonscrotal skin qhs. AndroGel 1%: Apply 5 g from gel pack or 4 pumps (5 g) from dispenser daily to shoulders/upper arms/abdomen. Testim: One tube (5 g) daily to shoulders/upper arms. Pellet - Testopel: 2–6 (150–450 mg testosterone) pellets SC q 3–6 mo. Buccal- Striant: 30 mg q 12 h on upper gum above the incisor tooth; alternate sides for each application. [Trade only: Patch 2.5 & 5 mg/24 h (Androderm). Gel 1% 2.5, 5 g packet & 75 g multidose pump (AndroGel). Gel 1%, 5 g tube (Testim). Pellet 75 mg (Testopel). Buccal: blister packs - 30 mg (Striant). Generic/Trade: Injection 100, 200 mg/mL (cypionate), 200 mg/mL (ethanate).] ▶L ♀X ▶– ©III $$$$$

Bisphosphonates

ALENDRONATE (*Fosamax, Fosamax Plus D, ◆Fosavance*) Postmenopausal osteoporosis prevention (5 mg PO daily or 35 mg PO weekly) & treatment (10

(cont.)

mg daily, 70 mg PO weekly or 70 mg/vit D3 2800 IU PO weekly). Treatment of glucocorticoid-induced osteoporosis in men & women: 5 mg PO daily or 10 mg PO daily (postmenopausal women not taking estrogen). Treatment of osteoporosis in men: 10 mg PO daily, 70 mg PO weekly, or 70 mg/vit D3 2800 IU PO weekly. Paget's disease in men & women: 40 mg PO daily × 6 mon. May cause severe esophagitis. [Generic/Trade (Fosamax): Tabs 5, 10, 35, 40, 70 mg. Trade only: Oral soln 70 mg/75 mL (single dose bottle). Fosamax Plus D: 70 mg + either 2800 or 5600 units of vitamin D3.] ▶K ♀C ▶- $$

CLODRONATE (✦*Ostac, Bonefos*) Canada only. IV single dose - 1500 mg slow infusion over ≥4 h. IV multiple dose - 300 mg slow infusion daily over 2–6 h up to 10 d. Oral - following IV therapy, maintenance 1600–2400 mg/d in single or divided doses. Max PO dose 3200 mg/d; duration of therapy is usually 6 mon. [Generic/Trade: Caps 400 mg.] ▶K ♀D- $$$$$

ETIDRONATE (*Didronel*) Paget's disease: 5–10 mg/kg PO daily × 6 mo or 11–20 mg/kg daily × 3 mo. [Generic/Trade: Tabs 200, 400 mg.] ▶K ♀C ▶? $$$$

IBANDRONATE (*Boniva*) Treatment/prevention of postmenopausal osteoporosis. Oral: 2.5 mg PO daily or 150 mg PO q mo. IV: 3 mg IV every 3 mo. [Trade only: 2.5, 150 mg tabs.] ▶K ♀C ▶? $$$$

PAMIDRONATE (*Aredia*) Hypercalcemia of malignancy: 60–90 mg IV over 2–24 h. Wait ≥7 d before considering retreatment. ▶K ♀D ▶? $$$$$

RISEDRONATE (*Actonel, Actonel Plus Calcium*) Prevention & treatment of postmenopausal osteoporosis: 5 mg PO daily, 35 mg PO weekly, 75 mg PO on two consecutive d each mo, or 150 mg once monthly. Treatment of osteoporosis in men: 35 mg PO weekly. Prevention & treatment of glucocorticoid-induced osteoporosis: 5 mg PO daily. Paget's disease: 30 mg PO daily × 2 mo. May cause esophagitis. [Generic/Trade: Tabs 5, 30, 35 mg. Trade only: 75, 150 mg; 35/1250 mg (calcium).] ▶K ♀C ▶? $$$

ZOLEDRONIC ACID (*Reclast, Zometa, ✦Aclasta*) Treatment of osteoporosis: 5 mg (Reclast) once yrly IV infusion over ≥15 min. Hypercalcemia (Zometa): 4 mg IV infusion over ≥15 min. Wait ≥7 d before considering retreatment. Paget's Disease (Reclast): 5 mg IV single dose. Multiple myeloma and metastatic bone lesions from solid tumors (Zometa): 4 mg IV infusion over ≥15 min q3–4 wk. ▶K ♀D ▶? $$$$$

Corticosteroids

NOTE *See also dermatology, ophthalmology.*

BETAMETHASONE (*Celestone, Celestone Soluspan, ✦Betaject*) Anti-inflammatory/Immunosuppressive: 0.6–7.2 mg/d PO divided bid-qid; up to 9 mg/d IM. Fetal lung maturation, maternal antepartum: 12 mg IM q24h × 2 doses. [Trade only: Syrup 0.6 mg/5 mL.] ▶L ♀C ▶- $$$$$

CORTISONE (*Cortone*) 25–300 mg PO daily. [Generic only: Tabs 5, 10, 25 mg.] ▶L ♀D ▶- $

DEXAMETHASONE (*Decadron, Dexpak, ✦Dexasone*) Anti-inflammatory/immunosuppressive: 0.5–9 mg/d PO/IV/IM, divided bid-qid. Cerebral edema: 10–20 mg IV load, then 4 mg IM q6h (off-label IV use common) or 1–3 mg PO tid. Bronchopulmonary dysplasia in preterm infants: 0.5 mg/kg PO/IV divided q12h ×

3 d, then taper. Croup: 0.6 mg/kg PO or IM × 1. Acute asthma: >2 yo: 0.6 mg/kg to max 16 mg PO daily × 2 d. Fetal lung maturation, maternal antepartum: 6 mg IM q12h × 4 doses. Antiemetic, prophylaxis: 8 mg IV or 12 mg PO prior to chemotherapy; 8 mg PO daily × 2–4 d. Antiemetic, treatment: 10–20 mg PO/IV q4–6h. [Generic/Trade: Tabs 0.5, 0.75. Generic only: Tabs 0.25, 1.0, 1.5, 2, 4, 6 mg; elixir 0.5 mg/5 mL; solution 0.5 mg/5 mL, 1 mg/1 mL (concentrate). Trade only: Dexpak (51 total 1.5 mg tabs for a 13 d taper).] ▶L ♀C ▶– $

FLUDROCORTISONE (Florinef) Mineralocorticoid activity: 0.1 mg PO 3 times weekly to 0.2 mg PO daily. [Generic only: Tabs 0.1 mg.] ▶L ♀C ▶? $

HYDROCORTISONE (Cortef, Cortenema, Solu-Cortef) 100–500 mg IV/IM q2–6h prn (sodium succinate). 20–240 mg/d PO divided tid- qid. Ulcerative colitis: 100 mg retention enema qhs (laying on side for ≥1 h) for 21 d. [Generic/Trade: Tabs 5, 10, 20 mg, Enema 100 mg/60 mL.] ▶L ♀C ▶– $

METHYLPREDNISOLONE (Solu-Medrol, Medrol, Depo-Medrol) Oral (Medrol): dose varies, 4–48 mg PO daily. Medrol Dosepak tapers 24 to 0 mg PO over 7 d. IM/Joints (Depo-Medrol): dose varies, 4–120 mg IM q1–2 wk. Parenteral (Solu-Medrol): dose varies, 10–250 mg IV/IM. Acute spinal cord injury: 30 mg/kg IV over 15 min, followed in 45 min by a 5.4 mg/kg IV infusion × 23–47h. Peds: 0.5–1.7 mg/kg PO/IV/IM divided q6–12h. [Trade only: Tabs 2, 16, 32 mg. Generic/Trade: Medrol Dosepak (4 mg-21 tabs).] ▶L ♀C ▶– $

PREDNISOLONE (Flo-Pred, Prelone, Pediapred, Orapred, Orapred ODT) 5–60 mg PO daily. [Generic/Trade: Syrup 15 mg/5 mL (Prelone; wild cherry flavor). Solution 5 mg/5 mL (Pediapred, raspberry flavor), 15 mg/5 mL (Orapred; grape flavor). Trade only: Orally disintegrating tablets 10, 15, 30 mg (Orapred ODT). Susp 5 mg/5 mL, 15 mg/5 mL (Flo-Pred; cherry flavor). Generic only: Tabs 5 mg. Syrup 5 mg/5 mL.] ▶L ♀C ▶+ $$

PREDNISONE (Deltasone, Sterapred, ✦Winpred) 1–2 mg/kg or 5–60 mg PO daily. [Trade only: Sterapred (5 mg tabs): tapers 30 to 5 mg PO over 6d or 30 to 10 mg over 12d), Sterapred DS (10 mg tabs: tapers 60 to 10 mg over 6d, or 60 to 20 mg PO over 12d) taper packs. Generic only: Tabs 1, 2.5, 5, 10, 20, 50 mg. Solution 5 mg/5 mL & 5 mg/mL (Prednisone Intensol).] ▶L ♀C ▶+ $

TRIAMCINOLONE (Aristospan, Kenalog, Trivaris) 4–48 mg PO/IM daily. Intraarticular 2.5–40 mg (Kenalog, Trivaris), 2–20 mg (Aristospan). [Trade only: Injection 10 mg/mL & 40 mg/mL (Kenalog), 5 mg/mL & 20 mg/mL (Aristospan), 8 mg (80 mg/mL) syringe (Trivaris).] ▶L ♀C ▶– $

Diabetes-Related—Alphaglucosidase Inhibitors

ACARBOSE (Precose, ✦Glucobay) Start 25 mg PO tid with meals, and gradually increase as tolerated to maintenance 50–100 mg tid. [Generic/Trade: Tabs 25, 50, 100 mg.] ▶Gut/K ♀B ▶– $$$

MIGLITOL (Glyset) Start 25 mg PO tid with meals, maintenance 50–100 tid. [Trade only: Tabs 25, 50, 100 mg.] ▶K ♀B ▶– $$$

Diabetes-Related—Combinations

ACTOPLUS MET (pioglitazone + metformin) 1 tab PO daily-bid. If inadequate control with metformin monotherapy, start 15/500 or 15/850 PO daily-bid. If inadequate control with pioglitazone monotherapy, start 15/500 bid or

(cont.)

CORTICOSTER-OIDS	Approximate Equivalent Dose (mg)	Relative Anti-inflammatory Potency	Relative Mineralocorti-coid Potency	Biological Half-life (h)
betamethasone	0.6–0.75	20–30	0	36–54
cortisone	25	0.8	2	8–12
dexamethasone	0.75	20–30	0	36–54
fludrocortisone	n.a.	10	125	18–36
hydrocortisone	20	1	2	8–12
methylprednis-olone	4	5	0	18–36
prednisolone	5	4	1	18–36
prednisone	5	4	1	18–36
triamcinolone	4	5	0	12–36

n.a., not available.

15/850 daily. Max 45/2550 mg/d. Obtain LFTs before therapy & periodically thereafter. [Trade only: Tabs 15/500, 15/850 mg.] ▶KL ♀C ▶? $$$$

AVANDAMET (*rosiglitazone + metformin*) Initial therapy (drug naive): Start 2/500 mg PO daily or bid. If inadequate control with metformin alone, select tab strength based on adding 4 mg/d rosiglitazone to existing metformin dose. If inadequate control with rosiglitazone alone, select tab strength based on adding 1000 mg/d metformin to existing rosiglitazone dose. Max 8/2000 mg/d. Obtain LFTs before therapy & periodically thereafter. [Trade only: Tabs 2/500, 4/500, 2/1000, 4/1000 mg.] ▶KL ♀C ▶? $$$$$

AVANDARYL (*rosiglitazone + glimepiride*) Initial therapy (drug naive): Start 4/1 mg PO daily. If switching from monotherapy with a sulfonylurea or glita-zone, consider 4/2 mg PO daily. Max 8/4 mg per d. Obtain LFTs before therapy & periodically thereafter. [Trade only: Tabs 4/1, 4/2, 4/4, 8/2, 8/4 mg rosigli-tazone/glimepiride.] ▶LK ♀C ▶? $$$$

DUETACT (*pioglitazone + glimepiride*) Start 30/2 mg PO daily. May start up to 30/4 mg PO daily if prior glimepiride therapy, or up to 30/2 mg PO daily if prior pioglitazone therapy; max 30/4 mg per d. Obtain LFTs before therapy & periodically thereafter. [Trade only: Tabs 30/2, 30/4 mg pioglitazone/glimepiride.] ▶LK ♀C ▶- $$$$

GLUCOVANCE (*glyburide + metformin*) Initial therapy (drug naive): Start 1.25/250 mg PO daily or bid with meals; max 10/2000 mg daily. Inadequate control with a sulfonylurea or metformin alone: Start 2.5/500 or 5/500 mg PO bid with meals; max 20/2000 mg daily. [Generic/Trade: Tabs 1.25/250, 2.5/500, 5/500 mg.] ▶KL ♀B ▶? $$$

JANUMET (*sitagliptin + metformin*) 1 tab PO bid. Individualize based on patient's current therapy. If inadequate control with metformin monotherapy, start 50/500 or 50/1000 bid based on current metformin dose. If inadequate control on sitagliptin, start 50/500 bid. Max 100/2000 mg/d. Give with meals. [Trade only: Tabs 50/500, 50/1000 mg sitagliptin/metformin.] ▶K ♀B ▶? $$$$

METAGLIP (*glipizide + metformin*) Initial therapy (drug naive): Start 2.5/250 mg PO daily to 2.5/500 mg PO bid with meals; max 10/2000 mg daily. Inadequate control with a sulfonylurea or metformin alone: Start 2.5/500 or 5/500 mg PO bid with meals; max 20/2000 mg daily. [Generic/Trade: Tabs 2.5/250, 2.5/500, 5/500 mg.] ▶KL ♀C ▷? \$\$\$

Diabetes-Related—"Glitazones" (Thiazolidinediones)

PIOGLITAZONE (*Actos*) Start 15–30 mg PO daily, max 45 mg/d. Monitor LFTs. [Trade only: Tabs 15, 30, 45 mg.] ▶L ♀C ▷- \$\$\$\$
ROSIGLITAZONE (*Avandia*) Diabetes monotherapy or in combination with metformin or sulfonylurea: Start 4 mg PO daily or divided bid, max 8 mg/d. Obtain LFTs before therapy & periodically thereafter. [Trade only: Tabs 2, 4, 8 mg.] ▶L ♀C ▷- \$\$\$\$

Diabetes-Related—Insulins

INSULIN—INJECTABLE COMBINATIONS (*Humalog Mix 75/25, Humalog Mix 50/50, Humulin 70/30, Humulin 50/50, Novolin 70/30, Novolog Mix 70/30*) Diabetes: Doses vary, but typically total insulin 0.3–1 unit/kg/d SC in divided doses (Type 1), and 0.5–1.5 unit/kg/d SC in divided doses (Type 2). Administer rapid-acting insulin mixtures (Humalog, NovoLog) within 15 min before. Administer regular insulin mixtures 30 min before meals. [Trade only: Insulin lispro protamine susp / insulin lispro (Humalog Mix 75/25,

DIABETES NUMBERS*

Criteria for diagnosis:	Self-monitoring glucose goals	
Pre-diabetes: Fasting glucose 100–125 mg/dL		
Diabetes:† Fasting glucose ≥126 mg/dL,		
random glucose with symptoms: ≥200 mg/dL,	Prandial	90–130 mg/dL
or ≥200 mg/dL 2 h after 75 g oral glucose load	Postprandial	<180 mg/dL
Estimated average glucose (eAG): eAG (mg/dL) =		
(28.7 × A1C) − 46.7	A1C General goal <7%;	
	Normal <6%	

Complications prevention & management: Aspirin‡ (75–162 mg/d) in Type 1 & 2 adults for primary prevention (those with an increased cardiovascular risk, including >40 yo or additional risk factors) and secondary prevention (those with vascular disease); statin therapy to achieve 30–40% LDL reduction regardless of baseline LDL (for those with vascular disease, those >40 yo and additional risk factor, or those <40 yo but LDL >100 mg/dL); ACE inhibitor or ARB if hypertensive or micro-/macro-albuminuria; pneumococcal vaccine (revaccinate one time if age >65 and previously received vaccine at age <65 and >5 yr ago). Every visit: Measure weight & BP (goal <130/80 mm Hg); visual foot exam; review self-monitoring glucose record; review/adjust meds; review self-mgmt skills, dietary needs, and physical activity; smoking cessation counseling. Twice a year: A1C in those meeting treatment goals with stable glycemia (quarterly if not); dental exam. Annually: Fasting lipid profile [goal LDL <100 mg/dL, consider LDL <70mg/dL, HDL >40 mg/dL (>50 mg/dL in women), TG <150 mg/dL], q2 yr with low-risk lipid values; creatinine; albumin to creatinine ratio spot collection; dilated eye exam; flu vaccine; foot exam.

*See recommendations at: care.diabetesjournals.org. Reference: Diabetes Care 2008;30 (Suppl 1):S12-S54. Glucose values are plasma. †Confirm diagnosis with glucose testing on subsequent day. ‡Avoid aspirin if <21 yo due to Reye's Syndrome risk; use if <30 yo has not been studied. LDL is primary target of therapy.

Humalog Mix 50/50). Insulin aspart protamine/insulin aspart (Novolog Mix 70/30). NPH and regular mixtures (Humulin 70/30, Novolin 70/30 or Humulin 50/50). Insulin available in pen form: Novolin 70/30 InnoLet, Novolog Mix 70/30 FlexPen, Humulin 70/30, Humalog Mix 75/25 KwikPen, Humalog Mix 50/50 KwikPen.] ▶LK ♀B/C ▶+ $$$$

INSULIN—INJECTABLE INTERMEDIATE/LONG-ACTING (*Novolin N, Humulin N, Lantus, Levemir*) Diabetes: Doses vary, but typically total insulin 0.3–0.5 unit/kg/d SC in divided doses (Type 1), and 1–1.5 unit/kg/d SC in divided doses (Type 2). Generally, 50–70% of insulin requirements are provided by rapid or short-acting insulin and the remainder from intermediate- or long-acting insulin. Lantus: Start 10 units SC daily (same time everyday) in insulin naive patients. Levemir: Type 2 DM (inadequately controlled on oral meds): Start 0.1–0.2 units/kg once daily in evening or 10 units SC daily or BID. [Trade only: Injection NPH (Novolin N, Humulin N). Insulin glargine (Lantus). Insulin detemir (Levemir). Insulin available in pen form: Novolin N InnoLet, Humulin N Pen, Lantus OptiClik (reusable), Lantus SoloStar (prefilled-disposable), Levemir InnoLet, Levemir FlexPen. Premixed preparations of NPH and regular insulin also available.] ▶LK ♀B/C ▶+ $$$$

INSULIN—INJECTABLE SHORT/RAPID-ACTING (*Apidra, Novolin R, NovoLog, Humulin R, Humalog, ◆NovoRapid*) Diabetes: Doses vary, but typically total insulin 0.3–0.5 unit/kg/d SC in divided doses (Type 1), 1–1.5 unit/kg/d SC in divided doses (Type 2). Generally, 50–70% of insulin requirements provided by rapid or short-acting insulin and remainder from intermediate- or long-acting insulin. Administer rapid-acting insulin (Humalog, NovoLog, Apidra) within 15 min before/immediately after meal. Administer regular insulin 30 min before meals. Severe hyperkalemia: 5–10 units regular insulin plus concurrent dextrose IV. Profound hyperglycemia (eg, DKA): 0.1 unit regular/kg IV bolus, then initial infusion 100 units regular in 100 mL NS (1 unit/mL), at 0.1 units/kg/h. 70 kg: 7 units/h (7 mL/h). [Trade only: Injection regular (Novolin R, Humulin R). Insulin glulisine (Apidra). Insulin lispro (Humalog). Insulin aspart (NovoLog). Insulin available in pen form: Novolin R InnoLet, Humulin R, Apidra OptiClik, Humalog KwikPen, Novolog FlexPen.] ▶LK ♀B/C ▶+ $$$

Diabetes-Related—Meglitinides

NATEGLINIDE (*Starlix*) 120 mg PO tid ≤30 min before meals; use 60 mg PO tid in patients who are near goal A1C. [Trade only: Tabs 60, 120 mg.] ▶L ♀C ▶? $$$$

REPAGLINIDE (*Prandin, ◆Gluconorm*) Start 0.5– 2 mg PO tid before meals, maintenance 0.5–4 mg tid-qid, max 16 mg/d. [Trade only: Tabs 0.5, 1, 2 mg.] ▶L ♀C ▶? $$$$

Diabetes-Related—Sulfonylureas—2nd Generation

GLICLAZIDE (◆*Diamicron, Diamicron MR*) Canada only. Immediate release: Start 80–160 mg PO daily, max 320 mg PO daily (≥160 mg in divided doses). Modified release: Start 30 mg PO daily, max 120 mg PO daily. [Generic/Trade: Tab 80 mg (Diamicron). Trade only: Tabs, modified release 30 mg (Diamicron MR).] ▶KL ♀C ▶? $

INJECTABLE INSULINS*		Onset (h)	Peak (h)	Duration (h)
Rapid/short-acting:	Insulin aspart (NovoLog)	<0.2	1–3	3–5
	Insulin glulisine (Apidra)	0.30–0.4	1	4–5
	Insulin lispro (Humalog)	0.25–0.5	0.5–2.5	≤5
	Regular (Novolin R, Humulin R)	0.5–1	2–3	3–6
Intermediate/long-acting:	NPH (Novolin N, Humulin N)	2–4	4–10	10–16
	Insulin detemir (Levemir)	n.a.	flat action profile	up to 23†
	Insulin glargine (Lantus)	2–4	peakless	24
Mixtures:	Insulin aspart protamine suspension/aspart (NovoLog Mix 70/30, NovoLog Mix 50/50)	0.25	1–4 (biphasic)	up to 24
	Insulin lispro protamine suspension/insulin lispro (HumaLog Mix 75/25, HumaLog Mix 50/50)	<0.25	1–3 (biphasic)	10–20
	NPH/Reg (Humulin 70/30, Humulin 50/50, Novolin 70/30)	0.5–1	2–10 (biphasic)	10–20

*These are general guidelines, as onset, peak, and duration of activity are affected by the site of injection, physical activity, body temperature, and blood supply. † Dose dependent duration of action, range from 6 to 23 h. n.a., not available.

GLIMEPIRIDE (*Amaryl*) Start 1–2 mg PO daily, usual 1–4 mg/d, max 8 mg/d. [Generic/Trade: Tabs 1, 2, 4 mg. Generic only: Tabs 8 mg.] ▶LK ♀C ▶– $$
GLIPIZIDE (*Glucotrol, Glucotrol XL*) Start 5 mg PO daily, usual 10–20 mg/d, max 40 mg/d (divide bid if >15 mg/d). Extended release: Start 5 mg PO daily, usual 5–10 mg/d, max 20 mg/d. [Generic/Trade: Tabs 5, 10 mg; Extended release tabs 2.5, 5, 10 mg.] ▶LK ♀C ▶? $
GLYBURIDE (*Micronase, DiaBeta, Glynase PresTab, ✦Euglucon*) Start 1.25–5 mg PO daily, usual 1.25–20 mg daily or divided bid, max 20 mg/d. Micronized tabs: Start 1.5–3 mg PO daily, usual 0.75–12 mg/d divided bid, max 12 mg/d. [Generic/Trade: Tabs (scored) 1.25, 2.5, 5 mg. micronized Tabs (scored) 1.5, 3, 4.5, 6 mg.] ▶LK ♀B ▶? $

Diabetes-Related—Other

A1C HOME TESTING (*Metrika A1CNow*) For home A1C testing [Fingerstick blood ▶None ♀+ ▶+ $
DEXTROSE (*Glutose, B-D Glucose, Insta-Glucose, Dex-4*) Hypoglycemia: 0.5–1 g/kg (1–2 mL/kg) up to 25 g (50 mL) of 50% soln IV. Dilute to 25% for pediatric administration. [OTC Generic/Trade: Chewable tabs 4 g (Dex-4), 5 g (Glutose). Trade only: Oral gel 40%.] ▶L ♀C ▶? $
EXENATIDE (*Byetta*) Type 2 DM adjunctive therapy when inadequate control on metformin, a sulfonylurea, or a glitazone (alone or in combination): 5 mcg SC bid (within 1 h before the morning and evening meals, or 1 h before the two main meals of the d ≥6h apart). May increase to 10 mcg SC bid after 1 mo.

(cont.)

[Trade only: prefilled pen (60 doses each) 5 mcg/dose, 1.2 mL; 10 mcg/dose, 2.4 mL.] ▶K ♀C ▶? $$$$$

GLUCAGON (*GlucaGen*) Hypoglycemia: 1 mg IV/IM/SC, onset 5–20 min. Diagnostic aid: 1 mg IV/IM/SC. [Trade only: injection 1 mg.] ▶LK ♀B ▶? $$$

GLUCOSE HOME TESTING (*Accu-Chek Active, Accu-Check Advantage, Accu-Check Aviva, Accu-Check Compact, Accu-Check Compact Plus, Accu-Check Complete, Accu-Check Voicemate, FreeStyle Flash, FreeStyle Freedom, FreeStyle Freedom Lite, FreeStyle Lite, OneTouch Ultra, OneTouch UltraMini, OneTouch UltraSmart, Precision Xtra, ReliOn, Sidekick, True Track Smart System, Clinistix, Clinitest, Diastix, Tes-Tape*) Use for home glucose monitoring. [Plasma: Accu-Check meters, FreeStyle meters, OneTouch meters, Precision Xtra, ReliOn, Sidekick, True Track. Urine: Clinistix, Clinitest, Diastix, Tes-Tape.] ▶None ♀+ ▶+ $$

METFORMIN (*Glucophage, Glucophage XR, Glumetza, Fortamet, Riomet*) Diabetes: Immediate release: Start 500 mg PO daily-bid or 850 mg PO daily with meals, may gradually increase to max 2550 mg/d. Extended release: Glucophage XR: 500 mg PO daily with evening meal; increase by 500 mg q wk to max 2000 mg/d (may divide bid). Glumetza: 1000 mg PO daily with evening meal; increase by 500 mg q wk to max 2000 mg/d (may divide bid). Fortamet: 500–1000 mg daily with evening meal; increase by 500 mg q wk to max 2500 mg/d. Polycystic ovary syndrome (unapproved, immediate release): 500 mg PO tid. [Generic/Trade: Tabs 500, 850,1000 mg, extended release 500, 750 mg. Trade only, extended release: Fortamet 500, 1000 mg; Glumetza 500, 1000 mg. Trade only: oral soln 500 mg/5 mL (Riomet).] ▶K ♀B ▶? $

PRAMLINTIDE (*Symlin, Symlinpen*) Type 1 DM with mealtime insulin therapy: Initiate 15 mcg SC immediately before major meals & titrate by 15 mcg increments (if significant nausea has not occurred for ≥3 d) to maintenance 30–60 mcg as tolerated. Type 2 DM with mealtime insulin therapy: Initiate 60 mcg SC immediately before major meals and increase to 120 mcg as tolerated (if significant nausea has not occurred for 3–7 d). [Trade only: 600 mcg/mL in 5 mL vials, 1000 mcg/mL pen injector (Symlinpen) 1.5 & 2.7 mL.] ▶K ♀C ▶? $$$$

SITAGLIPTIN (*Januvia*) Type 2 DM: 100 mg PO daily. [Trade only: Tabs 25, 50, 100 mg.] ▶K ♀B ▶? $$$$

Diagnostic Agents

COSYNTROPIN (*Cortrosyn, ✦Synacthen*) Rapid screen for adrenocortical insufficiency: 0.25 mg (0.125 mg if <2 yo) IM/ IV over 2 min; measure serum cortisol before and 30–60 min after. ▶L ♀C ▶? $

Gout-Related

ALLOPURINOL (*Aloprim, Zyloprim*) Mild gout or recurrent calcium oxalate stones: 200–300 mg PO daily-bid, max 800 mg/d. [Generic/Trade: Tabs 100, 300 mg.] ▶K ♀C ▶+ $

COLBENEMID (*colchicine + probenecid*) 1 tab PO daily × 1 wk, then 1 tab PO bid. [Generic only: Tabs 0.5 mg colchicine + 500 mg probenecid.] ▶KL ♀C ▶? $$$

COLCHICINE Rapid treatment of acute gouty arthritis: 0.6 mg PO q1h for up to 3h (max 3 tabs). Gout prophylaxis: 0.6 mg PO bid if CrCl ≥50 mL/min, 0.6 mg PO daily if CrCl 35–49 mL/min, 0.6 mg PO q2–3 d if CrCl 10–34 mL/min. [Generic only: Tabs 0.6 mg.] ▶L ♀C ▶? $

PROBENECID (✦*Benuryl*) Gout: 250 mg PO bid × 7 d, then 500 bid. Adjunct to penicillin injection: 1–2 g PO. [Generic only: Tabs 500 mg.] ▶KL ♀B ▶? $

Minerals

CALCIUM ACETATE (*PhosLo*) Hyperphosphatemia: Initially 2 tabs/caps PO with each meal. [Generic/Trade: Gel caps 667 mg (169 mg elem Ca).] ▶K ♀+ ▶? $$$

CALCIUM CARBONATE (*Caltrate, Mylanta Children's, Os-Cal, Oyst-Cal, Tums, Surpass, Viactiv, ✦Calsan*) Supplement: 1–2 g elem Ca/d or more PO with meals divided bid-qid. Antacid: 1000–3000 mg PO q2h prn or 1–2 pieces gum chewed prn, max 7000 mg/d. [OTC Generic/Trade: tab 500, 650, 750, 1000, 1250, 1500 mg, chew tab 400, 500, 750,850, 1000, 1177, 1250 mg, cap 1250 mg, gum 300, 450 mg, susp 1250 mg/5 mL. Calcium carbonate is 40% elem Ca and contains 20 mEq of elem Ca/g calcium carbonate. Not more than 500 mg elem Ca/dose. Available in combination with sodium fluoride, vitamin D and/or vitamin K. Trade examples: Caltrate 600 + D = 600 mg elemental Ca/200 units vit D, Os-Cal 500 + D = 500 mg elemental Ca/200 units vit D, Os-Cal Extra D = 500 mg elemental Ca/400 units vit D, Tums (regular strength) = 200 mg elemental Ca, Tums (ultra) = 400 mg elemental Ca, Viactiv (chew) 500 mg elemental Ca+ 100 units vit D + 40 mcg vit K.] ▶K ♀+ (? 1st trimester) ▶? $

CALCIUM CHLORIDE 500–1000 mg slow IV q1–3 d. [Generic only: injectable 10% (1000 mg/10 mL) 10 mL ampules, vials, syringes.] ▶K ♀+ ▶+ $

CALCIUM CITRATE (*Citracal*) 1–2 g elem Ca/d or more PO with meals divided bid-qid. [OTC: Trade only (mg elem Ca): 200 & 250 mg with 200 units vitamin D and 250 mg with 125 units vitamin D and 80 mg of magnesium. Chew tabs 500 mg with 200 units vitamin D. OTC: Generic/Trade: Tabs 200 mg, 315 mg with 200 units vitamin D.] ▶K ♀+ ▶+ $

CALCIUM GLUCONATE 2.25–14 mEq slow IV. 500–2000 mg PO bid-qid. [Generic only: Injectable 10% (1000 mg/10 mL, 4.65 mEq/10 mL) 1, 10, 50, 100, 200 mL. OTC Generic only: Tab 50, 500, 650, 975,1000 mg. Chew tab 650 mg.] ▶K ♀+ ▶+ $

FERRIC GLUCONATE COMPLEX (*Ferrlecit*) 125 mg elem iron IV over 10 min or diluted in 100 mL NS IV over 1 h. Peds ≥6 yo: 1.5 mg/kg (max 125 mg) elem iron diluted in 25 mL NS & administered IV over 1h. ▶KL ♀B ▶? $$$$$

FERROUS GLUCONATE (*Fergon*) 800–1600 mg ferrous gluconate PO divided tid. [OTC Generic/Trade: Tab (ferrous gluconate) 240. Generic only: Tab 27, 300, 324, 325 mg.] ▶K ♀+ ▶+ $

FERROUS SULFATE (*Fer-in-Sol, Feosol, ✦Ferodan, Slow-Fe*) 500–1000 mg ferrous sulfate (100–200 mg elem iron) PO divided tid. Liquid: Adults 5–10 mL tid, non-infant children 2.5–5 mL tid. Many other available formulations. [OTC Generic/Trade (mg ferrous sulfate): Tabs, extended-release 160 mg; tabs 324 & 325 mg; drops 75 mg/0.6 mL. OTC Generic only: Tabs, extended-release 50 mg; elixir 220 mg/5 mL.] ▶K ♀+ ▶+ $

FLUORIDE (*Luride*, ✦*Fluor-A-Day*, *Fluotic*)   Adult dose: 10 mL topical rinse swish & spit daily. Peds daily dose based on fluoride content of drinking water (table). [Generic only: chew tab 0.5,1 mg, tab 1 mg, drops 0.125 mg, 0.25 mg, and 0.5 mg/dropperful, lozenges 1 mg, sol. 0.2 mg/mL, gel 0.1%, 0.5%, 1.23%, rinse (sodium fluoride) 0.05,0.1,0.2%).] ▶K ♀? ▶? $

IRON DEXTRAN (*InFed, DexFerrum*, ✦*Dexiron, Infufer*)   25–100 mg IM daily prn. Equations used to calculate IV dose (weight & Hb). ▶KL ♀– ▶? $$$$

IRON POLYSACCHARIDE (*Niferex, Niferex-150, Nu-Iron 150*)   50–200 mg PO divided daily-tid. [OTC Trade only: Cap 60 mg (Niferex). OTC Generic/Trade: Cap 150 mg (Niferex-150, Nu-Iron 150), liquid 100 mg/5 mL (Niferex). 1 mg iron polysaccharide = 1 mg elemental iron.] ▶K ♀+ ▶+ $$

IRON SUCROSE (*Venofer*)   Iron deficiency with hemodialysis: 5 mL (100 mg elem iron) IV over 5 min or diluted in 100 mL NS IV over ≥15 min. Iron deficiency in non-dialysis chronic kidney disease: 10 mL (200 mg elem iron) IV over 5 min. ▶KL ♀B ▶? $$$$$

MAGNESIUM CHLORIDE (*Slow-Mag*)   2 tabs PO daily. [OTC Trade only: enteric coated tab 64 mg. 64 mg tab Slow-Mag = 64 mg elem magnesium.] ▶K ♀A ▶+ $

MAGNESIUM GLUCONATE (*Almora, Magtrate, Maganate*, ✦*Maglucate*)   500–1000 mg PO divided tid. [OTC Generic only: tab 500 mg, liquid 54 mg elem Mg/5 mL.] ▶K ♀A ▶+ $

MAGNESIUM OXIDE (*Mag-200, Mag-Ox 400*)   400–800 mg PO daily. [OTC Generic/Trade: cap 140,250,400,420,500 mg.] ▶K ♀A ▶+ $

MAGNESIUM SULFATE   Hypomagnesemia: 1 g of 20% soln IM q6h × 4 doses, or 2 g IV over 1 h (monitor for hypotension). Peds: 25–50 mg/kg IV/IM q4–6h

(cont.)

FLUORIDE SUPPLEMENTATION

Age	<0.3 ppm in drinking water	0.3–0.6 ppm in drinking water	>0.6 ppm in drinking water
0–0.5 yo	—*	—	—
0.5–3 yo	0.25 mg PO qd	—	—
3–6 yo	0.5 mg PO qd	0.25 mg PO qd	—
6–16 yo	1 mg PO qd	0.5 mg PO qd	—

* No supplementation necessary

INTRAVENOUS SOLUTIONS

Solution	Dextrose	Calories/ Liter	Na*	K*	Ca*	Cl*	Lactate*	Osm*
0.9 NS	0 g/L	0	154	0	0	154	0	310
LR	0 g/L	9	130	4	3	109	28	273
D5 W	50 g/L	170	0	0	0	0	0	253
D5 0.2 NS	50 g/L	170	34	0	0	34	0	320
D5 0.45 NS	50 g/L	170	77	0	0	77	0	405
D5 0.9 NS	50 g/L	170	154	0	0	154	0	560
D5 LR	50 g/L	179	130	4	2.7	109	28	527

* All given in mEq/L

for 3–4 doses, max single dose 2 g. Eclampsia: 4–6 g IV over 30 min, then 1–2 g/h. Drip: 5 g in 250 mL D5W (20 mg/mL), 2 g/h = 100 mL/h. Preterm labor: 6 g IV over 20 min, then 1–3 g/h titrated to decrease contractions. Monitor respirations & reflexes. If needed, may reverse toxic effects with calcium gluconate 1 g IV. Torsades de pointes: 1–2 g IV in D5W over 5–60 min. ▶K ♀A ▶+ $

PHOSPHORUS (*Neutra-Phos, K-Phos*) 1 cap/packet PO qid. 1–2 tabs PO qid. Severe hypophosphatemia (eg, <1 mg/dl): 0.08–0.16 mmol/kg IV over 6h. [OTC: Trade only: (Neutra-Phos, Neutra-Phos K) tab/cap/packet 250 mg (8 mmol) phosphorus. Rx: Trade only: (K-Phos) tab 250 mg (8 mmol) phosphorus.] ▶K ♀C ▶? $

POTASSIUM (*Cena-K, Effer-K, K+8, K+10, Kaochlor, Kaon, Kaon Cl, Kay Ciel, Kaylixir, K+Care, K+Care ET, K-Dur, K-G Elixir, K-Lease, K-Lor, Klor-con, Klorvess, Klorvess Effervescent, Klotrix, K-Lyte, K-Lyte Cl, K-Norm, Kolyum, K-Tab, K-vescent, Micro-K, Micro-K LS, Slow-K, Ten-K, Tri-K*) IV infusion 10 mEq/h (diluted). 20–40 mEq PO daily-bid. [Injectable, many different products in a variety of salt forms (ie, chloride, bicarbonate, citrate, acetate, gluconate), available in tabs, caps, liquids, effervescent tabs, packets. Potassium gluconate is available OTC.] ▶K ♀C ▶? $

ZINC ACETATE (*Galzin*) Dietary supplement: 8–12 mg (elemental) daily. Zinc deficiency: 25–50 mg (elemental) daily. Wilson's disease: 25–50 mg (elemental) tid. [Trade: cap 25, 50 mg elemental zinc.] ▶Minimal absorption ♀A ▶- $

ZINC SULFATE (*Orazinc, Zincate*) Dietary supplement: 8–12 mg (elemental) daily. Zinc deficiency: 25–50 mg (elemental) daily. [OTC Generic/Trade: tab 66, 110, 200 mg; Rx: cap 220 mg.] ▶Minimal absorption ♀A ▶- $

Nutritionals

BANANA BAG Alcoholic malnutrition (one formula): Add thiamine 100 mg + folic acid 1 mg + IV multivitamins to 1 liter NS and infuse over 4h. Magnesium sulfate 2 g may be added. "Banana bag" is jargon and not a valid drug order; also known as "rally pack"; specify individual components. ▶KL ♀+ ▶+ $

FAT EMULSION (*Intralipid, Liposyn*) Dosage varies. ▶L ♀C ▶? $$$$$

FORMULAS—INFANT (*Enfamil, Similac, Isomil, Nursoy, Prosobee, Soyalac, Alsoy, Nutramigen Lipil*) Infant meals. [OTC: Milk-based (Enfamil, Similac, SMA) or soy-based (Isomil, Nursoy, ProSobee, Soyalac, Alsoy).] ▶L ♀+ ▶+ $

LEVOCARNITINE (*Carnitor*) 10–20 mg/kg IV at each dialysis session. [Generic/Trade: Tabs 330 mg, Oral solution 1 g /10 mL ▶KL ♀B ▶? $$$$$

OMEGA-3 FATTY ACID (*fish oil, Lovaza, Promega, Cardio-Omega 3, Sea-Omega, Marine Lipid Concentrate, MAX EPA, SuperEPA 1200*) Hypertriglyceridemia: Lovaza: 4 caps PO daily or divided bid; 2–4 g EPA+DHA content daily. Lovaza is only FDA approved fish oil, previously known as Omacor. Marine Lipid Concentrate, Super EPA 1200 mg cap contains EPA 360 mg + DHA 240 mg, daily dose = 4–8 caps. [Trade: (Lovaza) 1 g cap (total 840 mg EPA+DHA). Generic/Trade: cap, shown as EPA+DHA mg content, 240 (Promega Pearls), 300 (Cardi-Omega 3, Max EPA), 320 (Sea-Omega), 400 (Promega), 500 (Sea-Omega), 600 (Marine Lipid Concentrate, SuperEPA 1200), 875 mg (SuperEPA 2000).] ▶L ♀C ▶? $$

POTASSIUM (oral forms)

Effervescent Granules: 20 mEq: Klorvess Effervescent, K-vescent
Effervescent Tablets: 25 mEq: Effer-K, K+Care ET, K-Lyte, K-Lyte/Cl, Klor-Con/EF 50 mEq: K-Lyte DS, K-Lyte/Cl 50
Liquids: 20 mEq/15 mL: Cena-K, Kaochlor S-F, K-G Elixir, Kaochlor 10%, Kay Ciel, Kaon, Kaylixir, Klorvess, Kolyum, Potasalan, Twin-K 30 mEq/15 mL: Rum-K 40 mEq/15 mL: Cena-K, Kaon-Cl 20% 45 mEq/15 mL: Tri-K
Powders: 15 mEq/pack: K+Care 20 mEq/pack: Gen-K, K+Care, Kay Ciel, K-Lor, Klor-Con 25 mEq/pack: K+Care, Klor-Con 25
Tablets/Capsules: 8 mEq: K+8, Klor-Con 8, Slow-K, Micro-K 10 mEq: K+10, K-Norm, Kaon-Cl 10, Klor-Con 10, Klotrix, K-Tab, K-Dur 10, Micro-K 10 20 mEq: Klor-Con M20, K-Dur 20

RALLY PACK Alcoholic malnutrition (one formula): Add thiamine 100 mg + folic acid 1 mg + IV multivitamins to 1 liter NS and infuse over 4h. Magnesium sulfate 2 g may be added. "Rally pack" is jargon and not a valid drug order; also known as "Banana Bag"; specify individual components. ▶KL ♀C ▶- $

Phosphate Binders

LANTHANUM CARBONATE (*Fosrenol*) Hyperphosphatemia in end stage renal disease: Start 750–1500 mg/d PO in divided doses with meals. Titrate dose q2–3 wk in increments of 750 mg/d until acceptable serum phosphate is reached. Most will require 1500–3000 mg/d to reduce phosphate <6.0 mg/dL. [Trade only: chewable tabs 250, 500, 750, 1000 mg.] ▶Not absorbed ♀C ▶? $$$$$

SEVELAMER (*Renagel, Renvela*) Hyperphosphatemia: 800–1600 mg PO tid with meals. [Trade only: sevelamer hydrochloride (Renagel): Tabs 400, 800 mg; sevelamer carbonate (Renvela): Tab 800 mg.] ▶Not absorbed ♀C ▶? $$$$$

Thyroid Agents

LEVOTHYROXINE (*L-Thyroxine, Levolet, Levo-T, Levothroid, ✦Levoxyl, Novothyrox, Synthroid, Thyro-Tabs, Tirosint, Unithroid, T4, ✦Eltroxin, Euthyrox*) Start 100–200 mcg PO daily (healthy adults) or 12.5–50 mcg PO daily (elderly or CV disease), increase by 12.5–25 mcg/d at 3–8 wk intervals. Usual maintenance dose 100–200 mcg/d, max 300 mcg/d. [Generic/Trade: Tabs 25, 50, 75, 88, 100, 112, 125, 137, 150, 175, 200, 300 mcg. Trade only: Caps: 25, 50, 75, 100, 125, 150 mcg in 7 d blister packs, Tabs: 13 mcg (Tirosint).] ▶L ♀A ▶+ $

LIOTHYRONINE (*T3, Cytomel, Triostat*) Start 25 mcg PO daily, max 100 mcg/d. [Trade only: Tabs 5, 25, 50 mcg.] ▶L ♀A ▶? $$

METHIMAZOLE (*Tapazole*) Start 5–20 mg PO tid or 10–30 mg PO daily, then adjust. [Generic/Trade: Tabs 5, 10. Generic only: Tabs 15, 20 mg.] ▶L ♀D ▶+ $$$

PROPYLTHIOURACIL (*PTU, ✦Propyl Thyracil*) Start 100 mg PO tid, then adjust. Thyroid storm: 200–300 mg PO qid, then adjust. [Generic only: Tabs 50 mg.] ▶L ♀D (but preferred over methimazole) ▶+ $

PEDIATRIC REHYDRATION SOLUTIONS

Brand	Glucose	Calories/ Liter	Na*	K*	Cl*	Citrate*	Phos*	Ca*	Mg*
CeraLyte 50 (premeasured powder packet)	0 g/L	160	50	20	40	30	0	0	0
CeraLyte 70 (premeasured powder packet)	0 g/L	160	70	20	60	30	0	0	0
CeraLyte 90 (premeasured powder packet)	0 g/L	160	90	20	80	30	0	0	0
Infalyte	30 g/L	140	50	25	45	34	0	0	0
Kao Lectrolyte (premeasured powder packet)	20 g/L	90	50	20	40	30	0	0	0
Lytren (Canada)	20 g/L	80	50	25	45	30	0	0	0
Naturalyte	25 g/L	100	45	20	35	48	0	0	0
Pedialyte and Pedialyte Freezer Pops	25 g/L	100	45	20	35	30	0	0	0
Rehydralyte	25 g/L	100	75	20	65	30	0	0	0
Resol	20 g/L	80	50	20	50	34	5	4	4

* All given in mEq/L

SODIUM IODIDE I-131 (*Hicon, Iodotope, Sodium Iodide I-131 Therapeutic*) Specialized dosing for hyperthyroidism and thyroid carcinoma. [Generic/Trade: Caps & oral solution: radioactivity range varies at the time of calibration. Hicon is a kit containing caps and a concentrated oral solution for dilution and cap preparation.] ▶K ♀X ▶– $$$$$

Vitamins

ASCORBIC ACID (*vitamin C, ✦Redoxon*) 70–1000 mg PO daily. [OTC: Generic only: tab 25,50,100,250,500,1000 mg, chew tab 100,250,500 mg, time-released tab 500 mg, 1000,1500 mg, time-released cap 500 mg, lozenge 60 mg, liquid 35 mg/0.6 mL, oral solution 100 mg/mL, syrup 500 mg/5 mL.] ▶K ♀C ▶? $

CALCITRIOL (*Rocaltrol, Calcijex*) 0.25–2 mcg PO daily. [Generic/Trade: Cap 0.25, 0.5 mcg. Oral soln 1 mcg/mL. Injection 1,2 mcg/mL.] ▶L ♀C ▶? $$

CYANOCOBALAMIN (*vitamin B12, CaloMist, Nascobal*) Deficiency states: 100–200 mcg IM q mo or 1000–2000 mcg PO daily for 1–2 wk followed by 1000 mcg PO daily, 500 mcg intranasal weekly (Nascobal: 1 spray one nostril once weekly), or 50–100 mcg intranasal daily (CaloMist: 1–2 sprays each

(cont.)

nostril daily). [OTC Generic only: tab 100, 500, 1000, 5000 mcg; lozenges 100, 250, 500 mcg. Rx Trade only: nasal spray 500 mcg/spray (Nascobal 2.3 mL), 25 mcg/spray (CaloMist, 18 mL).] ▶K ♀C ▶+ $

DIATX (*folic acid + niacinamide + cobalamin + pantothenic acid + pyridoxine + d-biotin + thiamine + ascorbic acid + riboflavin*)   1 tab PO daily. [Trade only: Each tab contains folic acid 5 mg + niacinamide 20 mg + cobalamin 1 mg + pantothenic acid 10 mg + pyridoxine 50 mg + d-biotin 300 mcg + thiamine 1.5 mg + vitamin C 60 mg + riboflavin 1.5 mg. Diatreatment Fe: adds 100 mg ferrous fumarate per tab. Diatreatment Zn adds 25 mg of zinc oxide per tab.] ▶LK ♀? ▶? $$$

DOXERCALCIFEROL (*Hectorol*)   Secondary hyperparathyroidism on dialysis: Oral: 10 mcg PO 3x/wk. May increase q8 wk by 2.5 mcg/dose; max 60 mcg/wk. IV: 4 mcg IV 3x/wk. May increase dose q8 wk by 1–2 mcg/dose; max 18 mcg/wk. Secondary hyperparathyroidism not on dialysis: Start 1 mcg PO daily, may increase by 0.5 mcg/dose q 2 wk. Max 3.5 mcg/d. [Trade only: Caps 0.5, 2.5 mcg.] ▶L ♀B ▶? $$$$$

FOLGARD (*folic acid + cyanocobalamin + pyridoxine*)   1 tab PO daily. [Trade only: folic acid 0.8 mg + cyanocobalamin 0.115 mg + pyridoxine 10 mg tab.] ▶K ♀? ▶? $

FOLIC ACID (*folate, Folvite*)   0.4–1 mg IV/IM/PO/SC daily. [OTC Generic only: Tab 0.4,0.8 mg. Rx Generic 1 mg.] ▶K ♀A ▶+ $

FOLTX (*folic acid + cyanocobalamin + pyridoxine*)   1 tab PO daily. [Trade only: folic acid 2.5 mg/ cyanocobalamin 2 mg/ pyridoxine 25 mg tab.] ▶K ♀A ▶+ $

MULTIVITAMINS (*MVI*)   Dose varies with product. Tabs come with and without iron. [OTC & Rx: Many different brands and forms available with and without iron (tab, cap, chew tab, drops, liquid).] ▶LK ♀+ ▶+ $

NEPHROCAP (*ascorbic acid + folic acid + niacin + thiamine + riboflavin + pyridoxine + pantothenic acid + biotin + cyanocobalamin*)   1 cap PO daily. If on dialysis, take after treatment. [Generic/Trade: vitamin C 100 mg/folic acid 1 mg/ niacin 20 mg/ thiamine 1.5 mg/ riboflavin 1.7 mg/ pyridoxine 10 mg/ pantothenic acid 5 mg/ biotin 150 mcg/ cyanocobalamin 6 mcg.] ▶K ♀? ▶? $

NEPHROVITE (*ascorbic acid + folic acid + niacin + thiamine + riboflavin + pyridoxine + pantothenic acid + biotin + cyanocobalamin*)   1 tab PO daily. If on dialysis, take after treatment. [Generic/Trade: vitamin C 60 mg/folic acid 1 mg/ niacin 20 mg/ thiamine 1.5 mg/ riboflavin 1.7 mg/ pyridoxine 10 mg/ pantothenic acid 10 mg/ biotin 300 mcg/ cyanocobalamin 6 mcg.] ▶K ♀? ▶? $

NIACIN (*vitamin B3, nicotinic acid, Niacor, Nicolar, Slo-Niacin, Niaspan*)   Niacin deficiency: 10–500 mg PO daily. Hyperlipidemia: Start 50–100 mg PO bid-tid with meals, increase slowly, usual maintenance range 1.5–3 g/d, max 6 g/d. Extended-release (Niaspan): Start 500 mg qhs, increase monthly as needed up to max 2000 mg. Extended-release formulations not listed here may have greater hepatotoxicity. Titrate slowly and use aspirin or NSAID 30 min before niacin doses to decrease flushing reaction. [OTC: Generic only: tab 50,100,250,500 mg, timed-release cap 125,250,400 mg, timed-release tab 250,500 mg, liquid 50 mg/5 mL. Trade only: 250,500,

(cont.)

750 mg (Slo-Niacin). Rx: Trade only: tab 500 mg (Niacor), timed-release cap 500 mg, timed-release tab 500,750,1000 mg (Niaspan, $$$$).] ▶K ♀C ▷? $

PARICALCITOL (*Zemplar*) Prevention/treatment of secondary hyperparathyroidism with renal insufficiency: 1–2 mcg PO daily or 2–4 mcg PO 3 times/wk; increase dose by 1 mcg/d or 2 mcg/wk until desired PTH level is achieved. Prevention/treatment of secondary hyperparathyroidism with renal failure (CrCl<15 mL/min): 0.04–0.1 mcg/kg (2.8–7 mcg) IV 3 times/wk at dialysis; increase dose by 2–4 mcg q 2–4 wk until desired PTH level is achieved. Max dose 0.24 mcg/kg (16.8 mcg). [Trade only: Caps 1, 2, 4 mcg.] ▶L ♀C ▷? $$$$$

PHYTONADIONE (*vitamin K, Mephyton, AquaMephyton*) Single dose of 0.5–1 mg IM within 1h after birth. Excessive oral anticoagulation: Dose varies based on INR. INR 5–9: 1–2.5 mg PO (≤5 mg PO may be given if rapid reversal necessary); INR >9 with no bleeding: 5–10 mg PO; Serious bleeding & elevated INR: 10 mg slow IV infusion. Adequate daily intake 120 mcg (males) and 90 mcg (females). [Trade only: Tab 5 mg.] ▶L ♀C ▷ + $

PYRIDOXINE (*vitamin B6*) 10–200 mg PO daily. INH overdose: 1 g IV/IM q 30 min, total dose of 1 g for each gram of INH ingested. [OTC Generic only: Tab 25,50,100 mg, timed-release tab 100 mg.] ▶K ♀A ▷+ $

RIBOFLAVIN (*vitamin B2*) 5–25 mg PO daily. [OTC Generic only: tab 25,50,100 mg.] ▶K ♀A ▷+ $

THIAMINE (*vitamin B1*) 10–100 mg IV/IM/PO daily. [OTC Generic only: tab 50,100,250,500 mg, enteric coated tab 20 mg.] ▶K ♀A ▷+ $

TOCOPHEROL (*vitamin E, ✦Aquasol E*) RDA is 22 units (natural, d-alpha-tocopherol) or 33 units (synthetic, d,l-alpha-tocopherol) or 15 mg (alpha-tocopherol). Max recommended 1000 mg (alpha-tocopherol). Antioxidant: 400–800 units PO daily. [OTC Generic only: tab 200,400 units, cap 73.5, 100, 147, 165, 200, 330, 400, 500, 600, 1000 units, drops 50 mg/mL.] ▶L ♀A ▷? $

VITAMIN A RDA: 900 MCG RE (*retinol equivalents*) (males), 700 mcg RE (females). Treatment of deficiency states: 100,000 units IM daily × 3 d, then 50,000 units IM daily for 2 wk. 1 RE = 1 mcg retinol or 6 mcg beta-carotene. Max recommended daily dose 3000 mcg. [OTC: Generic only: cap 10,000, 15,000 units. Trade only: tab 5,000 units. Rx: Generic: 25,000 units. Trade only: soln 50,000 units/mL.] ▶L ♀A (C if exceed RDA, × in high doses) ▷+ $

VITAMIN D (*vitamin D2, ergocalciferol, Calciferol, Drisdol, ✦Osteoforte*) Familial hypophosphatemia (Vitamin D Resistant Rickets): 12,000–500,000 units PO daily. Hypoparathyroidism: 50,000–200,000 units PO daily. Adequate daily intake adults: 19–50 yo: 5 mcg (200 units) ergocalciferol; 51–70 yo: 10 mcg (400 units); >70 yo: 15 mcg (600 units). [OTC: Generic: 200, 400, 800 units, 1000 units, 2000 units (cap/tab).Trade only: soln 8000 units/mL. Rx: Trade only: cap 50,000 units, inj 500,000 units/mL.] ▶L ♀A (C if exceed RDA) ▷+ $

Other

BROMOCRIPTINE (*Parlodel*) Hyperprolactinemia: Start 1.25–2.5 mg PO qhs, then increase q3–7 d to usual effective dose of 2.5–15 mg/d, max 40 mg/d. Acromegaly: Usual effective dose is 20–30 mg/d, max 100 mg/d. Doses >20

(cont.)

mg/d can be divided bid. Also approved for Parkinson's Disease, but rarely used. Take with food to minimize dizziness and nausea. [Generic/Trade: Tabs 2.5 mg. Caps 5 mg.] ▶L ♀B ▶- $$$$$

CABERGOLINE (*Dostinex*) Hyperprolactinemia: 0.25–1 mg PO twice/wk. [Generic/Trade: Tabs 0.5 mg.] ▶L ♀B ▶- $$$$$

CALCITONIN (*Miacalcin, Fortical, ✦Calcimar, Caltine*) Skin test before using injectable product: 1 unit intradermally and observe for local reaction. Osteoporosis: 100 units SC/IM or 200 units (1 spray) intranasal daily (alternate nostrils). Paget's disease: 50–100 units SC/IM daily. Hypercalcemia: 4 units/kg SC/IM q12h. May increase after 2 d to max of 8 units/kg q6h. [Trade only: nasal spray 200 units/activation in 3.7 mL bottle (minimum of 30 doses/bottle).] ▶Plasma ♀C ▶? $$$$

DESMOPRESSIN (*DDAVP, Stimate, ✦Minirin, Octostim*) Diabetes insipidus: 10–40 mcg intranasally daily or divided bid-tid, 0.05–1.2 mg/d PO or divided bid-tid, or 0.5–1 mL/d SC/IV in 2 divided doses. Hemophilia A, von Willebrand's disease: 0.3 mcg/kg IV over 15–30 min, or 150–300 mcg intranasally. Enuresis: 0.2–0.6 mg PO qhs. Not for children <6 yo. [Trade only: Stimate nasal spray 150 mcg/0.1 mL (1 spray), 2.5 mL bottle (25 sprays). Generic/Trade (DDAVP nasal spray): 10 mcg/0.1 mL (1 spray), 5 mL bottle (50 sprays). Note difference in concentration of nasal solutions. Rhinal Tube: 2.5 mL bottle with 2 flexible plastic tube applicators with graduation marks for dosing. Generic only: Tabs 0.1, 0.2 mg.] ▶LK ♀B ▶? $$$$

SODIUM POLYSTYRENE SULFONATE (*Kayexalate*) Hyperkalemia: 1 g/kg up to 15–60 g PO or 30–50 g retention enema (in sorbitol) q6h prn. Irrigate with tap water after enema to prevent necrosis. [Generic only: Susp 15 g/60 mL. Powdered resin.] ▶Fecal excretion ♀C ▶? $$$$

SOMATROPIN (*human growth hormone, Genotropin, Humatrope, Norditropin, Norditropin NordiFlex, Nutropin, Nutropin AQ, Nutropin Depot, Omnitrope, Protropin, Serostim, Serostim LQ, Saizen, Tev-Tropin, Valtropin, Zorbtive*) Dosages vary by indication and product. [Single dose vials (powder for injection with diluent). Tev-Tropin: 5 mg vial (powder for injection with diluent, stable for 14 d when refrigerated). Genotropin: 1.5, 5.8, 13.8 mg cartridges. Humatrope: 6, 12, 24 mg pen cartridges, 5 mg vial (powder for injection with diluent, stable for 14 d when refrigerated). Nutropin AQ: 10 mg multiple dose vial & 5, 10, 20 mg/pen cartridges. Norditropin: 5,10,15 mg pen cartridges. Norditropin NordiFlex: 5, 10, 15 mg prefilled pens. Omnitrope: 1.5, 5.8 mg vial (powder for injection with diluent). Saizen: pre-assembled reconstitution device with autoinjector pen. Serostim: 4, 5, 6 mg single dose vials, 4 & 8.8 mg multidose vials and 8.8 mg cartridges for autoinjector. Valtropin: 5 mg single dose vial, 5 mg prefilled syringe. Zorbtive: 8.8 mg vial (powder for injection with diluent, stable for 14 d when refrigerated).] ▶LK ♀B/C ▶? $$$$$

TERIPARATIDE (*Forteo*) Treatment of postmenopausal women or men with primary or hypogonadal osteoporosis and high risk for fracture: 20 mcg SC daily in thigh or abdomen for ≤2 yr. [Trade only: 28-dose pen injector (20 mcg/dose).] ▶LK ♀C ▶- $$$$$

VASOPRESSIN (*Pitressin, ADH, ✦Pressyn AR*)   Diabetes insipidus: 5–10 units IM/SC bid-qid prn. Cardiac arrest: 40 units IV; may repeat if no response after 3 min. Septic shock: 0.01–0.1 units/min IV infusion, usual dose <0.04 units/min. Variceal bleeding: 0.2–0.4 units/min initially (max 0.9 units/min).] ▶LK ♀C ▶? $$$$$

ENT

Antihistamines—Nonsedating

DESLORATADINE (*Clarinex, ✦Aerius*)   Adults & children ≥12 yo: 5 mg PO daily. 6–11 yo: 1 teaspoonful (2.5 mg) PO daily. 12 mo - 5 yo: ½ teaspoonful (1.25 mg) PO daily. 6–11 mo: 2 mL (1 mg) PO daily. [Trade only: Tabs 5 mg. Fast-dissolve RediTabs 2.5 & 5 mg. Syrup 0.5 mg/mL.] ▶LK ♀C ▶+ $$$
FEXOFENADINE (*Allegra*)   60 mg PO bid or 180 mg daily. 6–12 yo: 30 mg PO bid. [Generic/Trade: Tabs 30, 60, 180 mg, Caps 60 mg. Trade only: Susp 30 mg/5 mL, orally disintegrating tab 30 mg.] ▶LK ♀C ▶+ $$$
LORATADINE (*Claritin, Claritin Hives Relief, Claritin RediTabs, Alavert, Tavist ND*)   Adults & children ≥6 yo: 10 mg PO daily. 2–5 yo: 5 mg PO daily. [OTC: Generic/Trade: Tabs 10 mg. Fast-dissolve tabs (Alavert, Claritin RediTabs) 5, 10 mg. Syrup 1 mg/mL. Rx: Trade only: Chew tab 5 mg (Claritin).] ▶LK ♀B ▶+ $

Antihistamines—Other

CETIRIZINE (*Zyrtec, ✦Reactine, Aller-Relief*)   Adults & children ≥6 yo: 5–10 mg PO daily. 2–5 yo: 2.5 mg PO daily-bid. 6–23 mo: 2.5 mg PO daily. [OTC: Generic/Trade: Tabs 5, 10 mg. Syrup 5 mg/5 mL. Chewable tabs, grape-flavored 5, 10 mg.] ▶LK ♀B ▶-$$$
CHLORPHENIRAMINE (*Chlor-Trimeton, Aller-Chlor*)   4 mg PO q4–6h. Max 24 mg/d. [OTC: Trade only: Tabs, extended-release 12 mg. Generic/Trade: Tabs 4 mg. Syrup 2 mg/5 mL. Tabs, extended release 8 mg.] ▶LK ♀B ▶- $
CLEMASTINE (*Tavist-1*)   1.34 mg PO bid. Max 8.04 mg/d. [OTC: Generic/Trade: Tabs 1.34 mg. Rx: Generic/Trade: Tabs 2.68 mg, Syrup 0.67 mg/5 mL. Rx: Generic only: Syrup 0.5 mg/5 mL.] ▶LK ♀B ▶- $
CYPROHEPTADINE (*Periactin*)   Start 4 mg PO tid. Max 32 mg/d. [Generic only: Tabs 4 mg. Syrup 2 mg/5 mL.] ▶LK ♀B ▶- $
DEXCHLORPHENIRAMINE (*Polaramine*)   2 mg PO q4–6h. Timed release tabs: 4 or 6 mg PO at qhs or q8–10h. [Generic only: Tabs, immediate release 2 mg, timed release 4, 6 mg. Syrup 2 mg/5 mL.] ▶LK ♀? ▶- $$
DIPHENHYDRAMINE (*Benadryl, Banophen, Allermax, Diphen, Diphenhist, Dytan, Siladryl, Sominex, ✦Allerdryl, Nytol*)   Allergic rhinitis, urticaria, hypersensitivity reactions: 25–50 mg IV/IM/PO q4–6h. Peds: 5 mg/kg/d divided q4–6h. EPS: 25–50 mg PO tid-qid or 10–50 mg IV/IM tid-qid. Insomnia: 25–50 mg PO qhs. Peds ≥12 yo: 50 mg PO qhs. [OTC: Trade only: Tabs 25, 50 mg, Chew tabs 12.5 mg. OTC & Rx: Generic only: Caps 25, 50 mg,

(cont.)

softgel cap 25 mg. OTC: Generic/Trade: Solution 6.25 or 12.5 mg per 5 mL. Rx: Trade only: (Dytan) Susp 25 mg/mL, Chew tabs 25 mg.] ▶LK ♀B ▶- $

HYDROXYZINE (*Atarax, Vistaril*)   25–100 mg IM/PO daily-qid or prn. [Generic only: Tabs 10, 25, 50, 100 mg, Caps 100 mg, Syrup 10 mg/5 mL. Generic/Trade: Caps 25, 50 mg, Susp 25 mg/5 mL (Vistaril). (Caps = Vistaril, Tabs = Atarax) ▶L ♀C ▶- $$

LEVOCETIRIZINE (*Xyzal*)   Adults & children ≥12 yo: 5 mg PO daily. 6–11 yo: 2.5 mg PO daily. [Trade only: Tabs 5 mg, scored, oral soln 2.5 mg/5 mL.] ▶K ♀B ▶- $$$

MECLIZINE (*Antivert, Bonine, Medivert, Meclicot, Meni-D, ✦Bonamine*)   Motion sickness: 25–50 mg PO 1 h prior to travel, then 25–50 mg PO daily. Vertigo: 25 mg PO q6h prn. [Rx/OTC/Generic/Trade: tabs 12.5, 25 mg. Chew tabs 25 mg. Rx/Trade only: tabs 50 mg.] ▶L ♀B ▶? $

Antitussives / Expectorants

BENZONATATE (*Tessalon, Tessalon Perles*)   100–200 mg PO tid. Swallow whole. Do not chew. Numbs mouth; possible choking hazard. [Generic/Trade: Softgel caps: 100, 200 mg.] ▶L ♀C ▶? $$

DEXTROMETHORPHAN (*Benylin, Delsym, Dexalone, Robitussin Cough, Vick's 44 Cough*)   10–20 mg PO q4h or 30 mg PO q6–8h. Sustained action liquid 60 mg PO q12h. [OTC: Trade only: Caps 15 mg (Robitussin) & 30 mg (DexAlone), Susp, extended release 30 mg/5 mL (Delsym). Generic/Trade: Syrup 5, 7.5, 10, 15 mg/5 mL. Generic only: Lozenges 5, 10 mg.] ▶L ♀+ ▶+ $

GUAIFENESIN (*Robitussin, Hytuss, Guiatuss, Mucinex*)   100–400 mg PO q4h. 600–1200 mg PO q12h (extended release). 100–200 mg/dose if 6–11 yo. 50–100 mg/dose if 2–5 yo. [Rx-Generic/Trade: Extended release tabs 600, 1200 mg. OTC-Generic/Trade: Liquid & Syrup 100 mg/5 mL. OTC-Trade only: Caps 200 mg (Hytuss), Extended release tabs 600 mg (Mucinex). OTC-Generic only: Tabs 100, 200, 400 mg.] ▶L ♀C ▶+ $

Decongestants

NOTE See ENT - Nasal Preparations for nasal spray decongestants.

PHENYLEPHRINE (*Sudafed PE*)   10 mg PO q4h. [OTC: Trade only: Tabs 10 mg.] ▶L ♀C ▶+ $

PSEUDOEPHEDRINE (*Sudafed, Sudafed 12 Hour, Efidac/24, Dimetapp Decongestant Infant Drops, PediaCare Infants' Decongestant Drops, Triaminic Oral Infant Drops, ✦Pseudofrin*)   Adult: 60 mg PO q4–6h. Peds: 30 mg/dose if 6–12 yo, 15 mg/dose if 2–5 yo. Extended release tabs: 120 mg PO bid or 240 mg PO daily. Dimetapp, PediaCare, & Triaminic Infant Drops: (7.5 mg/0.8 mL): Give PO q4–6h. Max 4 doses/d. 2–3 yo: 1.6 mL. 12–23 mo: 1.2 mL. 4–11 mo: 0.8 mL. 0–3 mo: 0.4 mL. [OTC: Generic/Trade: Tabs 30, 60 mg, Tabs, extended release 120 mg (12 h), Infant drops 7.5 mg/0.8 mL, Solution 15 & 30 mg/5 mL. Trade only: Chew tabs 15 mg, Tabs, extended release 240 mg (24 h).] ▶L ♀C ▶+ $

ENT COMBINATIONS (selected)	Decon-gestant	Antihis-tamine	Anti-tussive	Typical Adult Doses
OTC				
Actifed Cold & Allergy	PE	CH	-	1 tab q4-6h
Actifed Cold & Sinus‡	PS	CH	-	2 tabs q 6h
Allerfrim, Aprodine	PS	TR	-	1 tab or 10 mL q4-6h
Benadryl Allergy/Cold‡	PE	DPH	-	2 tabs q 4h
Benadryl-D Allergy/Sinus Tablets	PE	DPH	-	1 tab q 4 h
Claritin-D 12 hour, Alavert D-12	PS	LO	-	1 tab q12h
Claritin-D 24 hour	PS	LO	-	1 tab daily
Dimetapp Cold & Allergy Elixir	PE	BR	-	20mL q 4h
Dimetapp DM Cold & Cough	PE	BR	DM	20mL q 4h
Drixoral Cold & Allergy	PS	DBR	-	1 tab q12h
Mucinex-DM Extended-Release	-	-	GU,DM	1-2 tab q12h
Robitussin CF	PE	-	GU, DM	10 mL q4h*
Robitussin DM, Mytussin DM	-	-	GU, DM	10 mL q4h*
Robitussin PE, Guiatuss PE	PE	-	GU	10 mL q4h*
Triaminic Cold & Allergy	PE	CH	-	10 mL q4h
Rx Only				
Allegra-D 12- hour	PS	FE	-	1 tab q12h
Allegra-D 24- hour	PS	FE	-	1 tab daily
Bromfenex	PS	BR	-	1 cap q12h
Clarinex-D24-hour	PS	DL	-	1 tab daily
Deconamine	PS	CH	-	1 tab or 10 mL tid-qid
Deconamine SR, Chlordrine SR	PS	CH	-	1 tab q12h
Deconsal II	PE	-	GU	1-2 tabs q12h
Dimetane-DX	PS	BR	DM	10 mL PO q4h
Duratuss	PE	-	GU	1 tab q12h
Duratuss HD©III	PE	-	GU, HY	5-10mL q4-6h
Entex PSE, Guaifenex PSE 120	PS	-	GU	1 tab q12h
Histussin D ©III	PS	-	HY	5 mL qid
Histussin HC ©III	PE	CH	HY	10 mL q4h
Humibid DM	-	-	GU, DM	1 tab q12h
Hycotuss ©III	-	-	GU, HY	5mL pc & qhs
Phenergan/Dextromethorphan	-	PR	DM	5 mL q4-6h
Phenergan VC	PE	PR	-	5 mL q4-6h
Phenergan VC w/codeine©V	PE	PR	CO	5 mL q4-6h
Robitussin AC ©V (generic only)	-	-	GU, CO	10 mL q4h*
Robitussin DAC ©V (generic only)	PS	-	GU, CO	10 mL q4h*
Rondec Syrup	PE	CH	-	5 mL qid†
Rondec DM Syrup	PE	CH	DM	5 mL qid†
Rondec Oral Drops	PE	CH	-	0.75 to 1 mL qid
Rondec DM Oral Drops	PE	CH	DM	0.75 to 1 mL qid
Rynatan	PE	CH	-	1-2 tabs q12h
Rynatan-P Pediatric	PE	CH	-	2.5-5 mL q12h*
Semprex-D	PS	AC	-	1cap q4-6h
Tanafed	PS	CH	-	10-20 mL q12h*
Tussionex ©III	-	CH	HY	5 mL q12h

AC=acrivastine	DL= desloratadine	FE=fexofenadine	PE=phenylephrine
BR=brompheniramine	DM=dextromethorphan	GU=guaifenesin	PR=promethazine
CH=chlorpheniramine	DBR=dexbrompheniramine	HY=hydrocodone	PS=pseudoephedrine
CO=codeine	DPH=diphenhydramine	LO=loratadine	TR=triprolidine

*5 mL/dose if 6-11 yo. 2.5 mL if 2-5 yo. †2.5 mL/dose if 6-11 yo. 1.25 mL if 2-5 yo. ‡Also contains acetaminophen.

Ear Preparations

AURALGAN (*benzocaine + antipyrine*) 2–4 drops in ear(s) tid-qid prn. [Generic/Trade: Otic soln 10 & 15 mL.] ▶Not absorbed ♀C ▶? $

CARBAMIDE PEROXIDE (*Debrox, Murine Ear*) 5–10 drops in ear(s) bid × 4 d. [OTC: Generic/Trade: Otic soln 6.5%, 15 & 30 mL.] ▶Not absorbed ♀? ▶? $

CIPRO HC OTIC (*ciprofloxacin + hydrocortisone*) ≥1 yo to adult: 3 drops in ear(s) bid × 7 d. [Trade only: Otic susp 10 mL.] ▶Not absorbed ♀C ▶- $$$$

CIPRODEX OTIC (*ciprofloxacin + dexamethasone*) ≥6 mo to adult: 4 drops in ear(s) bid × 7 d. [Trade only: Otic susp 5 & 7.5 mL.] ▶Not absorbed ♀C ▶- $$$$

CORTISPORIN OTIC (*hydrocortisone + polymyxin + neomycin, Pediotic*) 4 drops in ear(s) tid-qid up to 10 d of soln or susp. Peds: 3 drops in ear(s) tid-qid up to 10 d. Caveats with perforated TMs or tympanostomy tubes: (1) Risk of neomycin ototoxicity, especially if use prolonged or repeated; (2) Use susp rather than acidic soln. [Generic/Trade: Otic soln or susp 7.5 & 10 mL.] ▶Not absorbed ♀? ▶? $

CORTISPORIN TC OTIC (*hydrocortisone + neomycin + thonzonium + colistin*) 4–5 drops in ear(s) tid-qid up to 10 d. [Trade only: Otic susp, 10 mL.] ▶Not absorbed ♀? ▶? $$$

DOMEBORO OTIC (*acetic acid + aluminum acetate*) 4–6 drops in ear(s) q2–3h. Peds: 2–3 drops in ear(s) q3–4h. [Generic only: Otic soln 60 mL.] ▶Not absorbed ♀? ▶? $

FLUOCINOLONE—OTIC (*DermOtic*) 5 drops in affected ear(s) bid for 7–14 d. [Trade only: Otic oil 0.01% 20 mL.] ▶L ♀C ▶? $$

OFLOXACIN—OTIC (*Floxin Otic*) >12 yo: 10 drops in ear(s) bid. 1–12 yo: 5 drops in ear(s) bid. [Generic/Trade: Otic soln 0.3% 5, 10 mL. Trade only: "Singles": single-dispensing containers 0.25 mL (5 drops), 2 per foil pouch.] ▶Not absorbed ♀C ▶- $$$

SWIM-EAR (*isopropyl alcohol + anhydrous glycerins*) 4–5 drops in ears after swimming. [OTC: Trade only: Otic soln 30 mL.] ▶Not absorbed ♀? ▶? $

VOSOL HC (*acetic acid + propylene glycol + hydrocortisone*) 5 drops in ear(s) tid-qid. Peds >3 yo: 3–4 drops in ear(s) tid-qid. VoSoL HC adds hydrocortisone 1%. [Generic/Trade: Otic soln 2%-3%-1% 10 mL.] ▶Not absorbed ♀? ▶? $

Mouth & Lip Preparations

AMLEXANOX (*Aphthasol, OraDisc A*) Aphthous ulcers: Apply ¼ inch paste or mucoadhesive patch to affected area qid after oral hygiene for up to 10 d. Up to 3 patches may be applied at one time. [Trade only: Oral paste 5%, 5 g tube. Mucoadhesive patch 2 mg, #20.] ▶LK ♀B ▶? $

CEVIMELINE (*Evoxac*) Dry mouth due to Sjogren's syndrome: 30 mg PO tid. [Trade only: Caps 30 mg.] ▶L ♀C ▶- $$$$

CHLORHEXIDINE GLUCONATE (*Peridex, Periogard, ◆Denticare*) Rinse with 15 mL of undiluted soln for 30 sec bid. Do not swallow. Spit after rinsing. [Generic/Trade: Oral rinse 0.12% 473–480 mL bottles.] ▶Fecal excretion ♀B ▶? $

DEBACTEROL (*sulfuric acid + sulfonated phenolics*) Aphthous stomatitis, mucositis: Apply to dry ulcer. Rinse with water. [Trade only: 1 mL prefilled, single-use applicator.] ▶Not absorbed ♀C ▶+ $$

GELCLAIR (*maltodextrin + propylene glycol*) Aphthous ulcers, mucositis, stomatitis: Rinse mouth with 1 packet tid or prn. [Trade only: 21 packets/box.] ▶Not absorbed ♀+ ▶+ $$$

LIDOCAINE—VISCOUS (*Xylocaine*) Mouth or lip pain in adults only: 15–20 mL topically or swish & spit q3h. [Generic/Trade: soln 2%, 20 mL unit dose, 100 mL bottle.] ▶LK ♀B ▶+ $

MAGIC MOUTHWASH (*diphenhydramine + Mylanta + sucralfate*) 5 mL PO swish & spit or swish & swallow tid before meals and prn. [Compounded susp. A standard mixture is 30 mL diphenhydramine liquid (12.5 mg/5 mL)/60 mL Mylanta or Maalox/4 g Carafate.] ▶LK ♀B(- in 1st trimester) ▶- $$$

PILOCARPINE (*Salagen*) Dry mouth due to radiation of head & neck or Sjogren's syndrome: 5 mg PO tid-qid. [Generic/Trade: Tabs 5, 7.5 mg.] ▶L ♀C ▶- $$$$

Nasal Preparations—Corticosteroids

BECLOMETHASONE (*Vancenase, Vancenase AQ Double Strength, Beconase AQ*) Vancenase: 1 spray per nostril bid-qid. Beconase AQ: 1–2 spray(s) per nostril bid. Vancenase AQ Double Strength: 1–2 spray(s) per nostril daily. [Trade only: Vancenase 42 mcg/spray, 80 or 200 sprays/bottle. Beconase AQ 42 mcg/spray, 200 sprays/bottle. Vancenase AQ Double Strength 84 mcg/spray, 120 sprays/bottle.] ▶L ♀C ▶? $$$$

BUDESONIDE—NASAL (*Rhinocort Aqua*) 1–4 sprays per nostril daily. [Trade only: Nasal inhaler 120 sprays/bottle.] ▶L ♀B ▶? $$$

CICLESONIDE (*Omnaris*) 2 sprays per nostril daily. [Trade only: Nasal spray, 50 mcg/spray, 120 sprays/bottle.] ▶L ♀C ▶? $

FLUNISOLIDE (*Nasalide, Nasarel, ✚Rhinalar*) Start 2 sprays/nostril bid. Max 8 sprays/nostril/d. [Generic/Trade: Nasal soln 0.025%, 200 sprays/bottle. Nasalide with pump unit. Nasarel with meter pump & nasal adapter.] ▶L ♀C ▶? $$

FLUTICASONE—NASAL (*Flonase, Veramyst*) 2 sprays per nostril daily. [Generic/Trade: Nasal spray 0.05%, 120 sprays/bottle. Trade only: (Veramyst): Nasal spray susp: 27.5 mcg/spray, 120 sprays/bottle.] ▶L ♀C ▶? $$$

MOMETASONE—NASAL (*Nasonex*) Adult: 2 sprays/nostril daily. Peds 2–11 yo: 1 spray/nostril daily. [Trade only: Nasal spray, 120 sprays/bottle.] ▶L ♀C ▶? $$$

TRIAMCINOLONE—NASAL (*Nasacort AQ, Nasacort HFA, Tri-Nasal*) Nasacort HFA, Tri-Nasal: 2 sprays per nostril daily-bid. Max 4 sprays/nostril/d. Nasacort AQ: 2 sprays per nostril daily. [Trade only: Nasal inhaler 55 mcg/spray, 100 sprays/bottle (Nasacort HFA). Nasal spray, 55 mcg/spray, 120 sprays/bottle (Nasacort AQ). Nasal spray 50 mcg/spray, 120 sprays/bottle (Tri-Nasal).] ▶L ♀C ▶- $$$

Nasal Preparations—Other

AZELASTINE—NASAL (*Astelin*) Allergic/vasomotor rhinitis: 1–2 sprays/nostril bid. [Trade only: Nasal spray, 200 sprays/bottle.] ▶L ♀C ▶? $$$

CROMOLYN—NASAL (*NasalCrom*) 1 spray per nostril tid-qid. [OTC: Generic/Trade: Nasal inhaler 200 sprays/bottle 13 & 26 mL.] ▶LK ♀B ▶+ $

IPRATROPIUM—NASAL (*Atrovent Nasal Spray*) 2 sprays per nostril bid-qid. [Generic/Trade: Nasal spray 0.03%, 345 sprays/bottle & 0.06%, 165 sprays/bottle.] ▶L ♀B ▶? $$

LEVOCABASTINE—NASAL (*✦Livostin Nasal Spray*) Canada only. 2 sprays in each nostril bid, increase prn to tid-qid. [Trade only: nasal spray 0.5 mg/mL, plastic bottles of 15 mL. Each spray delivers 50 mcg.] ▶L (but minimal absorption) ♀C ▶- $$

OLOPATADINE—NASAL (*Patanase*) Allergic rhinitis: 2 sprays/nostril bid. [Trade only: Nasal spray, 240 sprays/bottle.] ▶L ♀C ▶? $$$

OXYMETAZOLINE (*Afrin, Dristan 12 Hr Nasal, Nostrilla, Vicks Sinex 12 Hr*) 2–3 drops/sprays per nostril bid prn rhinorrhea for ≤ 3 d. [OTC: Generic/Trade: Nasal spray 0.05% 15 & 30 mL, Nose drops 0.025% & 0.05% 20 mL with dropper.] ▶L ♀C ▶? $

PHENYLEPHRINE—NASAL (*Neo-Synephrine, Vicks Sinex*) 2–3 sprays/drops per nostril q4h prn × 3 d. [OTC: Generic/Trade: Nasal drops/spray 0.25, 0.5, 1% (15 mL).] ▶L ♀C ▶? $

SALINE NASAL SPRAY (*SeaMist, Entsol, Pretz, NaSal, Ocean, ✦HydraSense*) Nasal dryness: 1–3 sprays or drops per nostril prn. [Generic/Trade: Nasal spray 0.4, 0.5, 0.65, 0.75%, Nasal drops 0.4 & 0.65%. Trade only: Preservative Free-Nasal spray 3% (Entsol).] ▶Not metabolized ♀A ▶+ $

Other

CETACAINE (*benzocaine + tetracaine + butamben*) Topical anesthesia of mucous membranes: Spray: Apply for ≤1 sec. Liquid or gel: Apply with cotton applicator directly to site. [Trade only: (14%-2%-2%) Spray 56 mL. Topical liquid 56 mL. Topical gel 5 & 29 g.] ▶LK ♀C ▶? $$

GASTROENTEROLOGY

Antidiarrheals

BISMUTH SUBSALICYLATE (*Pepto-Bismol, Kaopectate*) 2 tabs or 30 mL (262 mg/15 mL) PO q 30 min–1 h up to 8 doses/ d. Peds: 10 mL (262 mg/15 mL) or 2/3 tab if 6–9 yo, 5 mL (262 mg/15 mL) or 1/3 tab if 3–6 yo. Risk of Reye's syndrome in children. [OTC Generic/Trade: chew tab 262 mg, susp 262, 525, 750 mg/15 mL. Generic only: susp 130 mg/15 mL. Trade only: caplets 262 mg (Pepto-Bismol), susp 87 mg/5 mL (Kaopectate Children's Liquid), caplets 750 mg (Kaopectate).] ▶K ♀D ▶? $

IMODIUM ADVANCED (*loperamide + simethicone*) 2 caplets PO initially, then 1 caplet PO after each unformed stool to a max of 4 caplets/24 h. Peds: 1 caplet PO initially, then ½ caplet PO after each unformed stool to a max of 2 caplets/d (if 6–8 yo or 48–59 lbs) or 3 caplets/d (if 9–11 yo or 60–95 lbs). [OTC Generic/trade: caplet & chew tab 2 mg loperamide/125 mg simethicone.] ▶L ♀B ▶+ $

LOMOTIL (*diphenoxylate + atropine*) 2 tabs or 10 mL PO qid. [Generic/Trade: soln 2.5/0.025 mg diphenoxylate/atropine per 5 mL, tab 2.5/0.025 mg.] ▶L ♀C ▶– ©V $

LOPERAMIDE (*Imodium, Imodium AD, ✦Loperacap, Diarr-eze*) 4 mg PO initially, then 2 mg PO after each unformed stool to a max of 16 mg/d. Peds: 2 mg PO tid if >30 kg, 2 mg bid if 20–30 kg, 1 mg tid if 13–20 kg. [Rx Generic/Trade: cap 2 mg, tab 2 mg. OTC Generic/Trade: tab 2 mg, liquid 1 mg/5 mL.] ▶L ♀B ▶+ $

MOTOFEN (*difenoxin + atropine*) 2 tabs PO initially, then 1 after each loose stool q3–4 h prn. Max of 8 tabs/24 h. [Trade only: tab difenoxin 1 mg + atropine 0.025 mg.] ▶L ♀C ▶– ©IV $

OPIUM (*opium tincture, paregoric*) 5–10 mL paregoric PO daily-qid or 0.3–0.6 mL PO opium tincture qid. [Trade only: opium tincture 10% (deodorized opium tincture, 10 mg morphine equivalent per mL). Generic only: paregoric (camphorated opium tincture, 2 mg morphine equivalent/5 mL).] ▶L ♀B (D with long-term use) ▶? ©II (opium tincture), III (paregoric) $$

Antiemetics—5-HT3 Receptor Antagonists

DOLASETRON (*Anzemet*) Nausea with chemo: 1.8 mg/kg up to 100 mg IV/PO single dose. Post-op nausea: 12.5 mg IV in adults and 0.35 mg/kg IV in children as single dose. Alternative for prevention 100 mg (adults) or 1.2 mg/kg (children) PO 2 h before surgery. [Trade only: Tab 50,100 mg.] ▶LK ♀B ▶? $$$

GRANISETRON (*Kytril*) Nausea with chemo: 10 mcg/kg IV over 5 min, 30 min prior to chemo. Oral: 1 mg PO bid × 1 d only. Radiation-induced N/V: 2 mg PO 1 h before first irradiation fraction of each d. [Generic/Trade: Tab 1 mg. Oral soln 2 mg/10 mL (30 mL).] ▶L ♀B ▶? $$$

ONDANSETRON (*Zofran*) Nausea with chemo (≥6 mo old): 32 mg IV over 15 min, or 0.15 mg/kg doses 30 min prior to chemo and repeated at 4 & 8 h after first dose. Oral dose if ≥12 yo: 8 mg PO and repeated 8 h later. If 4–11 yo: 4 mg PO 30 min prior to chemo and repeated at 4 & 8 h. Prevention of post-op nausea: 4 mg IV over 2–5 min or 4 mg IM or 16 mg PO 1 h before anesthesia. If 1 mo–12 yo: 0.1 mg/kg IV over 2–5 min × 1 if ≤40 kg; 4 mg IV over 2–5 min × 1 if >40 kg. Prevention of N/V associated with radiotherapy: 8 mg PO tid. [Generic/Trade: Tab 4, 8, 24 mg, orally disintegrating tab 4, 8 mg, solution 4 mg/5 mL. Generic only: Tab 16 mg, orally disintegrating tab 16, 24 mg.] ▶L ♀B ▶? $$$$$

PALONOSETRON (*Aloxi*) Nausea with chemo: 0.25 mg IV over 30 sec, 30 min prior to chemo. Prevention of postoperative N/V: 0.075 mg IV over 10 sec just prior to anesthesia. ▶L ♀B ▶? $$$$$

Antiemetics—Other

APREPITANT (*Emend, fosaprepitant*) Prevention of nausea with moderately to highly emetogenic chemo, in combination with dexamethasone and ondansetron: 125 mg PO on d 1 (1 h prior to chemo), then 80 mg PO qam on d 2 & 3. Alternative for first dose only is 115 mg IV (fosaprepitant form) over 15 min given 30 min prior to chemo. Prevention of postoperative N/V: 40 mg PO

(cont.)

within 3 h prior to anesthesia. [Trade only (aprepitant): cap 40, 80, 125 mg. IV prodrug form is fosaprepitant.] ▶L ♀B ▶? $$$$$

DICLECTIN (**doxylamine + pyridoxine**) Canada only. 2 tabs PO qhs. May add 1 tab in am and 1 tab in afternoon, if needed. [Trade only: delayed-release tab doxylamine 10 mg + pyridoxine 10 mg.] ▶LK ♀A ▶? $

DIMENHYDRINATE (**Dramamine, ♣Gravol**) 50–100 mg PO/IM/IV q4–6h prn. [OTC: Generic/Trade: Tab 50 mg. Trade only: chew tab 50 mg. Generic only: solution 12.5 mg/5 mL.] ▶LK ♀B ▶- $

DOMPERIDONE (**♣Motilium**) Canada only. Postprandial dyspepsia: 10–20 mg PO tid-qid, 30 min before a meal. [Canada only. Trade/generic: tabs 10, 20 mg.] ▶L ♀? ▶?

DOXYLAMINE (**Unisom Nighttime Sleep Aid, others**) 12.5 mg PO bid; often used in combination with pyridoxine. [OTC Generic/Trade: tab 25 mg.] ▶L ♀A ▶? $

DRONABINOL (**Marinol**) Nausea with chemo: 5 mg/m2 PO 1–3 h before chemo then 5 mg/m2/dose q2–4h after chemo for 4–6 doses/d. Anorexia associated with AIDS: Initially 2.5 mg PO bid before lunch and dinner. [Trade only: cap 2.5, 5, 10 mg.] ▶L ♀C ▶- ©III $$$$$

DROPERIDOL (**Inapsine**) 0.625–2.5 mg IV or 2.5 mg IM. May cause fatal QT prolongation, even in patients with no risk factors. Monitor ECG before, ▶L ♀C ▶? $

METOCLOPRAMIDE (**Reglan, ♣Maxeran**) 10 mg IV/IM q2–3h prn. 10–15 mg PO qid, 30 min before meals and qhs. [Generic/Trade: tabs 5,10 mg, Generic only: soln 5 mg/5 mL.] ▶K ♀B ▶? $

NABILONE (**Cesamet**) 1 to 2 mg PO bid, 1 to 3 h before chemotherapy. [Trade only: cap 1 mg].] ▶L ♀C ▶- ©II $$$$

PHOSPHORATED CARBOHYDRATES (**Emetrol**) 15–30 mL PO q15 min prn, max 5 doses. Peds: 5–10 mL. [OTC Generic/Trade: Solution containing dextrose, fructose, and phosphoric acid.] ▶L ♀A ▶+ $

PROCHLORPERAZINE (**Compazine, ♣Stemetil**) 5–10 mg IV over at least 2 min. 5–10 mg PO/IM tid-qid. 25 mg PR q12h. Sustained release: 15 mg PO qam or 10 mg PO q12h. Peds: 0.1 mg/kg/dose PO/PR tid-qid or 0.1–0.15 mg/kg/dose IM tid-qid. [Generic/Trade: tabs 5, 10, 25 mg, supp 25 mg. Trade only: extended-release caps (Compazine Spansules) 10, 15, 30 mg, supp 2.5, 5 mg, liquid 5 mg/5 mL.] ▶LK ♀C ▶? $

PROMETHAZINE (**Phenergan**) Adults: 12.5–25 mg PO/IM/PR q4–6h. Peds: 0.25–1 mg/kg PO/IM/PR q4–6h. Contraindicated if <2 yo; caution in older children. IV use common but not approved. [Generic/Trade: tab/supp 12.5, 25, 50 mg. Generic only: syrup 6.25 mg/5 mL.] ▶LK ♀C ▶- $

SCOPOLAMINE (**Transderm-Scop, Scopace, ♣Transderm-V**) Motion sickness: Apply 1 disc (1.5 mg) behind ear 4h prior to event; replace q3d. Tab: 0.4 to 0.8 mg PO 1 h before travel and q8h prn. [Trade only: topical disc 1.5 mg/72h, box of 4. Oral tab 0.4 mg.] ▶L ♀C ▶+ $$

THIETHYLPERAZINE (**Torecan**) 10 mg PO/IM 1–3 times/d. [Trade only: tab 10 mg.] ▶L ♀? ▶? $

TRIMETHOBENZAMIDE (**Tigan**) 250 mg PO q6–8h, 200 mg IM/PR q6–8h. Peds: 100–200 mg/dose PO/PR q6–8h if 13.6–40.9 kg; 100 mg PR q6–8h if <13.6 kg (not newborns). [Generic/Trade: Caps 300 mg. Generic only: Caps 250 mg.] ▶LK ♀C but + ▶? $

Antiulcer—Antacids

ALKA-SELTZER (*aspirin + citrate + bicarbonate*)   2 regular strength tabs in 4 oz water q4h PO prn, max 8 tab (<60 yo) or 4 tabs (>60 yo) in 24h or 2 extra-strength tabs in 4 oz water q6h PO prn, max 7 tabs (<60 yo) or 4 tabs (>60 yo) in 24h. [OTC Trade only: regular strength, original: ASA 325 mg + citric acid 1000 mg + sodium bicarbonate 1916 mg. Regular strength lemon lime and cherry: 325 mg + 1000 mg + 1700 mg. Extra-strength: 500 mg + 1000 mg + 1985 mg. Not all forms of Alka Seltzer contain aspirin (eg, Alka Seltzer Heartburn Relief).] ▶LK ♀? (- 3rd trimester) ▶? $

ALUMINUM HYDROXIDE (*Alternagel, Amphojel, Alu-Tab, Alu-Cap, ✦Basalgel, Mucaine*)   5–10 mL or 1–2 tabs PO up to 6 times daily. Constipating. [OTC Generic/Trade: cap 475 mg, susp 320 & 600 mg/5 mL. Trade only: cap 400 mg (Alu-Cap)] ▶K ♀+ (? 1st trimester) ▶? $

CITROCARBONATE (*bicarbonate + citrate*)   1–2 teaspoonfuls in cold water PO 15 min to 2 h after meals prn. [OTC Trade only: sodium bicarbonate 0.78 g + sodium citrate anhydrous 1.82 g in each 1 teaspoonful dissolved in water, 150, 300 g.] ▶K ♀? ▶? $

GAVISCON (*aluminum hydroxide + magnesium carbonate*)   2–4 tabs or 15–30 mL (regular strength) or 10 mL (extra strength) PO qid prn. [OTC Trade only: Tab: regular strength (Al hydroxide 80 mg + Mg trisilicate 20 mg), extra strength (Al hydroxide 160 mg + Mg carbonate 105 mg). Liquid: regular strength (Al hydroxide 95 mg + Mg carbonate 358 mg per 15 mL), extra strength (Al hydroxide 508 mg + Mg carbonate 475 mg per 30 mL) ▶K ♀? ▶? $

MAALOX (*aluminum hydroxide + magnesium hydroxide*)   10–20 mL or 1–4 tab PO prn. [OTC Generic/Trade: regular strength chew tab (Al hydroxide + Mg hydroxide 200/200 mg), susp (225/200 mg per 5 mL).] ▶K ♀+ (? 1st trimester) ▶? $

MAGALDRATE (*Riopan*)   5–10 mL PO prn. [OTC Trade only: susp 540 mg/5 mL. Riopan Plus (with simethicone) available as susp 540/20 mg/5 mL, chew tab 540/20 mg.] ▶K ♀+ (? 1st trimester) ▶? $

MYLANTA (*aluminum hydroxide + magnesium hydroxide + simethicone*)   2–4 tab or 10–45 mL PO prn. [OTC Generic/Trade: Liquid, double strength liquid, tab, double strength tab. Trade only: tab sodium + sugar + dye free.] ▶K ♀+ (? 1st trimester) ▶? $

ROLAIDS (*calcium carbonate + magnesium hydroxide*)   2–4 tabs PO q1h prn, max 12 tabs/d (regular strength) or 10 tabs/d (extra-strength). [OTC Trade only: Tab: regular strength (Ca carbonate 550 mg, Mg hydroxide 110 mg), extra-strength (Ca carbonate 675 mg, Mg hydroxide 135 mg).] ▶K ♀? ▶? $

Antiulcer—H2 Antagonists

CIMETIDINE (*Tagamet, Tagamet HB*)   300 mg IV/IM/PO q6–8h, 400 mg PO bid, or 400–800 mg PO qhs. Erosive esophagitis: 800 mg PO bid or 400 mg PO qid. Continuous IV infusion 37.5–50 mg/h (900–1200 mg/d). [Rx Generic/Trade: tab 200, 300, 400, 800 mg. Rx Generic liquid 300 mg/5 mL. OTC Generic/Trade: tab 200 mg.] ▶LK ♀B ▶+ $$$

FAMOTIDINE (*Pepcid, Pepcid AC, Max Strength Pepcid AC*) 20 mg IV q12h. 20–40 mg PO qhs, or 20 mg PO bid. [Generic/Trade: tab 10 mg (OTC, Pepcid AC Acid Controller), 20 (Rx and OTC, Max Strength Pepcid AC), 30, 40 mg. Rx Trade only: susp.40 mg/5 mL.] ▶LK ♀B ▶? $$

NIZATIDINE (*Axid, Axid AR*) 150–300 mg PO qhs, or 150 mg PO bid. [OTC Trade only (Axid AR): tabs 75 mg Rx Trade only: oral solution 15 mg/mL (120, 480 mL). Rx Generic/Trade: cap 150, 300 mg.] ▶K ♀B ▶? $$$$

PEPCID COMPLETE (*famotidine + calcium carbonate + magnesium hydroxide*) Treatment of heartburn: 1 tab PO prn. Max 2 tabs/d. [OTC: Trade only: chew tab famotidine 10 mg with calcium carbonate 800 mg & magnesium hydroxide 165 mg.] ▶LK ♀B ▶? $

RANITIDINE (*Zantac, Zantac 25, Zantac 75, Zantac 150, Peptic Relief*) 150 mg PO bid or 300 mg PO qhs. 50 mg IV/IM q8h, or continuous infusion 6.25 mg/h (150 mg/d). [Generic/Trade: tabs 75 mg (OTC, Zantac 75, Zantac 150), 150,300 mg, syrup 75 mg/5 mL. Rx Trade only: effervescent tab 25,150 mg. Rx Generic only: caps 150,300 mg.] ▶K ♀B ▶? $$$

Antiulcer—Helicobacter pylori Treatment

HELIDAC (*bismuth subsalicylate + metronidazole + tetracycline*) 1 dose PO qid for 2 wk. To be given with an H2 antagonist. [Trade only: Each dose: bismuth subsalicylate 524 (2 × 262 mg) chewable tab + metronidazole 250 mg tab + tetracycline 500 mg cap.] ▶LK ♀D ▶- $$$$

PREVPAC (*lansoprazole + amoxicillin + clarithromycin, ✦HP-Pac*) 1 dose PO bid × 10–14 d. [Trade only: lansoprazole 30 mg × 2 + amoxicillin 1 g (2 × 500 mg) × 2, clarithromycin 500 mg × 2.] ▶LK ♀C ▶? $$$$$

PYLERA (*biskalcitrate + metronidazole + tetracycline*) 3 caps PO qid (after meals and at bedtime) × 10 d. To be given with omeprazole 20 mg PO bid. [Trade only: Each cap: biskalcitrate 140 mg + metronidazole 125 mg + tetracycline 125 mg.] ▶LK ♀D ▶- $$$$$

Antiulcer—Proton Pump Inhibitors

ESOMEPRAZOLE (*Nexium*) Erosive esophagitis: 20–40 mg PO daily × 4–8 wk. Maintenance of erosive esophagitis: 20 mg PO daily. Zollinger-Ellison: 40 mg PO bid × 4–8 wk, may repeat for additional 4–8 wk. GERD: 20 mg PO daily × 4 wk. GERD with esophagitis: 20–40 mg IV daily × 10 d until taking PO. Prevention of NSAID-associated gastric ulcer: 20–40 mg PO daily × up to 6 mo. H pylori eradication: 40 mg PO daily with amoxicillin 1000 mg PO bid & clarithromycin 500 mg PO bid × 10 d. [Trade only: Delayed release cap 20, 40 mg. Delayed release granules for oral susp 10, 20, 40 mg per packet.] ▶L ♀B ▶? $$$$

LANSOPRAZOLE (*Prevacid, Prevacid NapraPac*) Duodenal ulcer or maintenance therapy after healing of duodenal ulcer, erosive esophagitis, NSAID-induced gastric ulcer: 30 mg PO daily × 8 wk (treatment), 15 mg PO daily for up to 12 wk (prevention). GERD: 15 mg PO daily. Gastric ulcer: 30 mg PO daily. Erosive esophagitis: 30 mg PO daily or 30 mg IV daily × 7 d or until taking PO. [Trade only: Cap 15, 30 mg. Susp 15, 30 mg packets. Orally

HELICOBACTER PYLORI THERAPY

Triple therapy PO × 7-14 d: clarithromycin 500 mg bid + amoxicillin 1 g bid (or metronidazole 500 mg bid) + a proton pump inhibitor

Quadruple therapy PO × 14 d: bismuth subsalicylate 525 mg (or 30 mL) tid-qid + metronidazole 500 mg tid-qid + tetracycline 500 mg tid-qid + a proton pump inhibitor or a H2 blocker

PPI's: esomeprazole 40 mg qd, lansoprazole 30 mg bid, omeprazole 20 mg bid, pantoprazole 40 mg bid, rabeprazole 20 mg bid.

H2 blockers: cimetidine 400 mg bid, famotidine 20 mg bid, nizatidine 150 mg bid, ranitidine 150 mg bid.

Adapted from *The Medical Letter Treatment Guidelines* 2004:10.

disintegrating tab 15, 30 mg. Prevacid NapraPac: 7 lansoprazole 15 mg caps packaged with 14 naproxen tabs 375 mg or 500 mg.] ▶L ♀B ▶? $$$$
OMEPRAZOLE (*Prilosec, ✦Losec*) GERD, duodenal ulcer, erosive esophagitis: 20 mg PO daily. Heartburn (OTC): 20 mg PO daily × 14 d. Gastric ulcer: 40 mg PO daily. Hypersecretory conditions: 60 mg PO daily. [Rx Generic/Trade: Cap 10, 20 mg. Trade only: Cap 40 mg, granules for susp 2.5 mg, 10 mg. OTC: Cap 20 mg.] ▶L ♀C ▶? OTC $, Rx $$$$
PANTOPRAZOLE (*Protonix, ✦Pantoloc*) GERD: 40 mg PO daily. Zollinger-Ellison syndrome: 80 mg IV q8–12h × 6 d until taking PO. GERD associated with a history of erosive esophagitis: 40 mg IV daily × 7–10 d until taking PO. [Generic/Trade: Tabs 20, 40 mg. Trade only: Granules for susp 40 mg/packet.] ▶L ♀B ▶? $$$$
RABEPRAZOLE (*AcipHex, ✦Pariet*) 20 mg PO daily. [Generic/Trade: Tab 20 mg.] ▶L ♀B ▶? $$$$
ZEGERID (*omeprazole + bicarbonate*) Duodenal ulcer, GERD, erosive esophagitis: 20 mg PO daily × 4–8 wk. Gastric ulcer: 40 mg PO once daily × 4–8 wk. Reduction of risk of upper GI bleed in critically ill (susp only): 40 mg PO, then 40 mg 6–8 h later, then 40 mg once daily thereafter × 14 d. [Trade only: Caps 20/1,100 & 40/1,100 mg omeprazole/sodium bicarbonate, powder packets for susp 20/1,680 & 40/1,680 mg.] ▶L ♀C ▶? $$$$

Antiulcer—Other

DICYCLOMINE (*Bentyl, Bentylol, Antispas, ✦Formulex, Protylol, Lomine*) 10–20 mg PO/IM up to 40 mg PO qid. [Generic/Trade: Tab 20 mg, cap 10 mg, syrup 10 mg/5 mL. Generic only: Cap 20 mg.] ▶LK ♀B ▶- $
DONNATAL (*phenobarbital + atropine + hyoscyamine + scopolamine*) 1–2 tabs/caps or 5–10 mL PO tid-qid. 1 extended release tab PO q8–12h. [Generic/Trade: Phenobarbital 16.2 mg + hyoscyamine 0.1 mg + atropine 0.02 mg + scopolamine 6.5 mcg in each tab, cap or 5 mL. Extended-release tab 48.6 + 0.3111 + 0.0582 + 0.0195 mg.] ▶LK ♀C ▶- $
GI COCKTAIL (*Green Goddess*) Acute GI upset: mixture of Maalox/Mylanta 30 mL + viscous lidocaine (2%) 10 mL + Donnatal 10 mL administered PO in a single dose. ▶LK ♀See individual ▶See individual $

HYOSCINE (*✦Buscopan*) Canada: GI or bladder spasm: 10–20 mg PO/IV up to 60 mg daily (PO) or 100 mg daily (IV). [Canada: Trade: Tab 10 mg.] ▶LK ♀C ▶? ?

HYOSCYAMINE (*Anaspaz, A-spaz, Cystospaz, ED Spaz, Hyosol, Hyospaz, Levbid, Levsin, Levsinex, Medispaz, NuLev, Spacol, Spasdel, Symax*) Bladder spasm, control gastric secretion, GI hypermotility, irritable bowel syndrome: 0.125–0.25 mg PO/SL q4h or prn. Extended release: 0.375–0.75 mg PO q12h. Max 1.5 mg/d. [Generic/Trade: Tab 0.125. Sublingual Tab 0.125 mg. Extended release Tab 0.375 mg. Extended release Cap 0.375 mg. Elixir 0.125 mg/ 5 mL. Drops 0.125 mg/1 mL. Trade: Tab 0.15 mg (Hyospaz, Cystospaz). Tab, orally disintegrating 0.125 (NuLev).] ▶LK ♀C ▶- $

MEPENZOLATE (*Cantil*) 25–50 mg PO tid-qid, with meals and qhs. [Trade only: Tab 25 mg]. ▶LK ♀B ▶? $$$$$

MISOPROSTOL (*PGE1, Cytotec*) Prevention of NSAID-induced gastric ulcers: Start 100 mcg PO bid, then titrate as tolerated up to 200 mcg PO qid. Cervical ripening: 25 mcg intravaginally q3–6h (or 50 mcg q6h). First-trimester pregnancy failure: 800 mcg intravaginally, repeat on q 3 if expulsion incomplete. [Generic/Trade: Oral tabs 100 & 200 mcg.] ▶LK ♀X ▶- $

PROPANTHELINE (*Pro-Banthine, ✦Propanthel*) 7.5–15 mg PO 30 min ac & qhs. [Generic/Trade: Tab 15 mg. Trade only: Tab 7.5 mg.] ▶LK ♀C ▶- $$$

SIMETHICONE (*Mylicon, Gas-X, Phazyme, ✦Ovol*) 40–160 mg PO qid prn. Infants: 20 mg PO qid prn [OTC: Generic/Trade: Tab 60,95 mg, chew tab 40,80,125 mg, cap 125 mg, drops 40 mg/0.6 mL.] ▶Not absorbed ♀C but + ▶? $

SUCRALFATE (*Carafate, ✦Sulcrate*) 1 g PO 1 h before meals (2 h before other medications) and qhs. [Generic/Trade: Tab 1 g, susp 1 g/10 mL.] ▶Not absorbed ♀B ▶? $$$

Laxatives—Bulk-Forming

METHYLCELLULOSE (*Citrucel*) 1 heaping tablespoon in 8 oz. water PO daily-tid. [OTC Trade only: regular & sugar-free packets and multiple use canisters, clear-mix solution, caplets 500 mg.] ▶Not absorbed ♀ + ▶? $

POLYCARBOPHIL (*FiberCon, Fiberall, Konsyl Fiber, Equalactin*) Laxative: 1 g PO qid prn. Diarrhea: 1 g PO q30 min. Max daily dose 6 g. [OTC Generic/Trade: Tab 500,625 mg, chew tab 500,1000 mg.] ▶Not absorbed ♀ + ▶? $

PSYLLIUM (*Metamucil, Fiberall, Konsyl, Hydrocil, ✦Prodium Plain*) 1 tsp in liquid, 1 packet in liquid or 1–2 wafers with liquid PO daily-tid. [OTC: Generic/Trade: regular and sugar-free powder, granules, caps, wafers, including various flavors and various amounts of psyllium.] ▶Not absorbed ♀ + ▶? $

Laxatives—Osmotic

GLYCERIN (*Fleet*) One adult or infant supp PR prn. [OTC Generic/Trade: supp infant & adult, solution (Fleet Babylax) 4 mL/applicator.] ▶Not absorbed ♀C ▶? $

LACTULOSE (*Chronulac, Cephulac, Kristalose*) Constipation: 15–30 mL (syrup) or 10–20 g (powder for oral solution) PO daily. Hepatic encephalopathy: 30–45 mL (syrup) PO tid-qid, or 300 mL retention enema. [Generic/Trade: syrup 10 g/15 mL. Trade only (Kristalose): 10, 20 g packets for oral solution.] ▶Not absorbed ♀B ▶? $$

MAGNESIUM CITRATE (*◆Citro-Mag*) 150-300 mL PO divided daily-bid. Children <6 yo: 2–4 mL/kg/24 h. [OTC Generic only: solution 300 mL/bottle. Low sodium & sugar-free available.] ▶K ♀+ ▶? $

MAGNESIUM HYDROXIDE (*Milk of Magnesia*) Laxative: 30–60 mL regular strength liquid PO. Antacid: 5–15 mL regular strength liquid or 622–1244 mg PO qid prn. [OTC Generic/Trade: susp 400 mg/5 mL. Trade only: chew tab 311 mg. Generic only: susp (concentrated) 1200 mg/5 mL, sugar-free 400 mg/5 mL.] ▶K ♀+ ▶? $

POLYETHYLENE GLYCOL (*MiraLax, GlycoLax*) 17 g (1 heaping tablespoon) in 4–8 oz water, juice, soda, coffee, or tea PO daily. [OTC Generic/Trade: powder for oral solution 17 g/scoop. Rx Trade only: 17 g packets for oral solution.] ▶Not absorbed ♀C ▶? $

POLYETHYLENE GLYCOL WITH ELECTROLYTES (*GoLytely, Colyte, TriLyte, NuLytely, Moviprep, HalfLytely and Bisacodyl Tab Kit, ◆Klean-Prep, Electropeg, Peg-Lyte*) Bowel prep: 240 mL q10 min PO or 20–30 mL/min per NG until 4 L is consumed. Moviprep: Follow specific instructions. [Generic/Trade: powder for oral solution in disposable jug 4 L or 2 L (Moviprep). Also, as a kit of 2 L bottle of polyethylene glycol with electrolytes and 2 or 4 bisacodyl tabs 5 mg (HalfLytely and Bisacodyl Tab Kit). Trade only (GoLytely): packet for oral solution to make 3.785 L.] ▶Not absorbed ♀C ▶? $

SODIUM PHOSPHATE (*Fleet enema, Fleet Phospho-Soda, Accu-Prep, Visicol, ◆Enemol, Phoslax*) 1 adult or pediatric enema PR or 20–30 mL of oral soln PO prn (max 45 mL/24 h). Visicol: Evening before colonoscopy: 3 tabs with 8 oz clear liquid q15 min until 20 tabs are consumed. Day of colonoscopy: starting 3–5 h before procedure, 3 tabs with 8 oz clear liquid q15 min until 20 tabs are consumed. [OTC Trade only: pediatric & adult enema, oral solution. Rx Trade only: Visicol tab (trade $$$): 1.5 g.] ▶Not absorbed ♀C ▶? $

SORBITOL 30–150 ML (*of 70% solution*) PO or 120 mL (of 25–30% solution) PR as a single dose. Cathartic: 1–2 mL/kg PO. [Generic only: solution 70%.] ▶Not absorbed ♀+ ▶? $

Laxatives—Stimulant

BISACODYL (*Correctol, Dulcolax, Feen-a-Mint*) 10–15 mg PO prn, 10 mg PR prn, 5–10 mg PR prn if 2–11 yo. [OTC Generic/Trade: tab 5 mg, supp 10 mg.] ▶L ♀+ ▶? $

CASCARA 325 mg PO qhs prn or 5 mL of aromatic fluid extract PO qhs prn. [OTC Generic only: tab 325 mg, liquid aromatic fluid extract.] ▶L ♀C ▶+ $

CASTOR OIL (*Purge, Fleet Flavored Castor Oil*) 15–60 mL of castor oil or 30–60 mL emulsified castor oil PO qhs, 5–15 mL/dose of castor oil PO or 7.5–30 mL emulsified castor oil PO for child. [OTC Generic/Trade: liquid 30,60,120,480 mL, emulsified susp 45,60,90,120 mL.] ▶Not absorbed ♀– ▶? $

SENNA (*Senokot, SenokotXTRA, Ex-Lax, Fletcher's Castoria, ✦Glysennid*) 2 tabs or 1 tsp granules or 10–15 mL syrup PO. Max 8 tabs, 4 tsp granules, 30 mL syrup per d. Take granules with full glass of water. [OTC Generic/Trade (All dosing is based on sennosides content; 1 mg sennosides = 21.7 mg standardized senna concentrate): granules 15 mg/tsp, syrup 8.8 mg/5 mL, liquid 3 mg/mL (Fletcher's Castoria), tab 8.6, 15, 17, 25 mg , chewable tab 15 mg.] ▶L ♀C ▶+ $

Laxatives—Stool Softener

DOCUSATE (*Colace, Surfak, Kaopectate Stool Softener*) Docusate calcium: 240 mg PO daily. Docusate sodium: 50–500 mg/d PO divided in 1–4 doses. Peds: 10–40 mg/d if <3 yo, 20–60 mg/d if 3–6 yo, 40–150 mg/d if 6–12 yo. Cerumen impaction: Instill 1 mL in affected ear. [Docusate calcium OTC Generic/Trade: cap 240 mg. Docusate sodium OTC Generic/Trade: cap 50,100, 250 mg, tab 50,100 mg, liquid 10 & 50 mg/5 mL, syrup 16.75 & 20 mg/5 mL.] ▶L ♀+ ▶? $

Laxatives—Other or Combinations

LUBIPROSTONE (*Amitiza*) Chronic idiopathic constipation: 24 mcg PO bid with meals. Irritable bowel syndrome with constipation in women >18 yo: 8 mcg PO bid. [Trade only: 8, 24 mcg caps.] ▶Gut ♀C ▶? $$$$$
MINERAL OIL (*Kondremul, Fleet Mineral Oil Enema, ✦Lansoyl*) 15–45 mL PO. Peds: 5–15 mL/dose PO. Mineral oil enema: 60–150 mL PR. Peds 30–60 mL PR. [OTC Generic/Trade: plain mineral oil, mineral oil emulsion (Kondremul).] ▶Not absorbed ♀C ▶? $
PERI-COLACE (*docusate + sennosides*) 2–4 tabs PO once daily or in divided doses prn. [OTC Generic/Trade: tab 50 mg docusate + 8.6 mg sennosides.] ▶L ♀C ▶? $
SENOKOT-S (*senna + docusate*) 2 tabs PO daily. [OTC Generic/Trade: tab 8.6 mg senna concentrate/50 mg docusate.] ▶L ♀C ▶+ $

Ulcerative Colitis

BALSALAZIDE (*Colazal*) 2.25 g PO tid × 8–12 wk. [Generic/Trade: cap 750 mg.] ▶Minimal absorption ♀B ▶? $$$$$
MESALAMINE (*5-aminosalicylic acid, 5-ASA, Asacol, Lialda, Pentasa, Canasa, Rowasa, ✦Mesasal, Salofalk*) Asacol: 800–1600 mg PO tid. Pentasa: 1000 mg PO qid. Lialda: 2.4–4.8 g PO daily with a meal. Canasa: 500 mg PR bid-tid or 1000 mg PR qhs. [Trade only: delayed-release tab 400 mg (Asacol), controlled-release cap 250 & 500 mg (Pentasa), delayed-release tab 1200 mg (Lialda), rectal supp 1000 mg (Canasa). Generic/Trade: rectal susp 4 g/60 mL (Rowasa).] ▶Gut ♀B ▶? $$$$$
OLSALAZINE (*Dipentum*) Ulcerative colitis: 500 mg PO bid. [Trade only: cap 250 mg.] ▶L ♀C ▶- $$$$

SULFASALAZINE (*Azulfidine, Azulfidine EN-tabs, ◆Salazopyrin En-tabs, S.A.S.*) Colitis: 500–1000 mg PO qid. Peds: 30–60 mg/kg/d divided q4-6h. RA: 500 mg PO daily-bid after meals up to 1 g PO bid. May turn body fluids, contact lenses or skin orange-yellow. [Generic/Trade: Tabs 500 mg, scored. Enteric coated, Delayed-release (EN-Tabs) 500 mg.] ▶L ♀B ▶- $$

Other GI Agents

ALOSETRON (*Lotronex*) Diarrhea-predominant IBS in women who have failed conventional therapy: 0.5 mg PO twice daily for 4 wk; in patients who become constipated, decrease to 0.5 mg PO once daily. If well tolerated after 4 wk, may increase to 1 mg PO bid. Discontinue if symptoms not controlled in 4 wk on 1 mg PO bid. [Trade only: tab 0.5, 1 mg.] ▶L ♀B ▶? $$$$$

ALPHA-GALACTOSIDASE (*Beano*) 5 drops per ½ cup gassy food, 3 tabs PO (chew, swallow, crumble) or 15 drops per typical meal. [OTC Trade only: drops 150 GalU/5 drops, tab 150 GalU.] ▶Minimal absorption ♀? ▶? $

ALVIMOPAN (*Entereg*) Short-term (up to 15 doses) in hospitalized patients undergoing partial large or small bowel resection surgery with primary anastomosis: 12 mg PO 30 min to 0.5 h prior to surgery, then 12 mg bid for up to 7 d [Trade only: Cap: 12 mg.] ▶Intestinal flora ♀B ▶? ?

BUDESONIDE (*Entocort EC*) 9 mg PO daily × 8 wk (remission induction) or 6 mg PO daily × 3 mo (maintenance). [Trade only: cap 3 mg.] ▶L ♀C ▶? $$$$$

CERTOLIZUMAB (*Cimzia*) Crohn's: 400 mg SQ at 0, 2, and 4 wk. If response occurs, then 400 mg SQ every 4 wk. [Trade: 400 mg kit.] ▶Plasma, K ♀B ▶? $$$$$

CHLORDIAZEPOXIDE-CLIDINIUM 1 cap PO tid-qid. [Generic only: cap clidinium 2.5 mg + chlordiazepoxide 5 mg.] ▶K ♀D ▶- $

GLYCOPYRROLATE (*Robinul, Robinul Forte*) 0.1 mg/kg PO bid-tid, max 8 mg/d. [Generic/Trade: Tab 1, 2 mg.] ▶K ♀B ▶? $$$$

LACTASE (*Lactaid*) Swallow or chew 3 caplets (Original strength), 2 caplets (Extra strength), 1 caplet (Ultra) with first bite of dairy foods. Adjust dose based on response. [OTC Generic/Trade: caplets, chew tab.] ▶Not absorbed ♀+ ▶+ $

LIBRAX (*chlordiazepoxide + methscopolamine*) 1 cap PO tid-qid. [Trade only: cap methscopolamine 2.5 mg + chlordiazepoxide 5 mg.] ▶K ♀D ▶- $$$$$

METHYLNALTREXONE (*Relistor*) 38 to <62 kg: 8 mg SC qod, 62 to 114 kg: 12 mg SC qod. All others: 0.15 mg/kg SC qod. [Injectable solution 12 mg/0.6 mL.] ▶unchanged ♀B ▶? ?

NEOMYCIN—ORAL (*Mycifradin, Neo-Fradin*) Hepatic encephalopathy: 4–12 g/d PO divided q6–8h. Peds: 50–100 mg/kg/d PO divided q6–8h. [Generic only: tab 350, 500 mg. Trade only (Neo-Fradin): solution 125 mg/5 mL.] ▶Minimally absorbed ♀D ▶? $$$

OCTREOTIDE (*Sandostatin, Sandostatin LAR*) Variceal bleeding: Bolus 50–100 mcg IV followed by infusion 25–50 mcg/h. AIDS diarrhea: 100–500 mcg SC tid. [Generic/Trade: injection vials 0.05, 0.1, 0.2, 0.5, 1 mg. Trade only: long-acting injectable susp (Sandostatin LAR) 10,20,30 mg.] ▶LK ♀B ▶? $$$$$

ORLISTAT (*Alli, Xenical*) Weight loss: 120 mg PO tid with meals. [Trade only: Caps 60 (OTC), 120 (Rx) mg.] ▶Gut ♀B ▶? $$$$$

PANCREATIN (*Creon, Donnazyme, Ku-Zyme, ✦Entozyme*) 8,000–24,000 units lipase (1–2 tab/cap) PO with meals and snacks. [Tab, cap with varying amounts of pancreatin, lipase, amylase and protease.] ▶Gut ♀C ▶? $$$

PANCRELIPASE (*Viokase, Pancrease, Pancrecarb, Cotazym, Ku-Zyme HP*) 4,000–33,000 units lipase (1–3 tab/cap) PO with meals and snacks. [Tab, cap, powder with varying amounts of lipase, amylase and protease.] ▶Gut ♀C ▶? $$$

PINAVERIUM (*✦Dicetel*) Canada only. 50–100 mg PO tid. [Trade only: tabs 50, 100 mg.] ▶? ♀C ▶- $$$

SECRETIN (*SecreMax*) Test dose 0.2 mcg IV. If tolerated, 0.2–0.4 mcg/kg IV over 1 min. ▶Serum ♀C ▶? $$$$$

URSODIOL (*Actigall, Ursofalk, URSO, URSO Forte*) Gallstone dissolution (Actigall); 8–10 mg/kg/d PO divided bid-tid. Prevention of gallstones associated with rapid weight loss (Actigall): 300 mg PO bid. Primary biliary cirrhosis (URSO): 13–15 mg/kg/d PO divided in 2–4 doses. [Generic/Trade: cap 300 mg. Trade only: tab 250 mg (URSO), 500 mg scored (URSO Forte).] ▶Bile ♀B ▶? $$$$

HEMATOLOGY

Anticoagulants—Heparin, LMW Heparins, & Fondaparinux

NOTE *See cardiovascular section for antiplatelet drugs & thrombolytics.*

DALTEPARIN (*Fragmin*) DVT prophylaxis, acute medical illness with restricted mobility: 5,000 units SC daily. DVT prophylaxis, abdominal surgery: 2,500 units SC 1–2 h preop & daily postop. DVT prophylaxis, abdominal surgery in patients with malignancy: 5,000 units SC evening before surgery and daily postop, or 2,500 units 1–2 h preop and 12 h later, then 5,000 units daily. DVT prophylaxis, hip replacement: Pre-op start: 2,500 units SC given 2 h preop, 4–8 h postop, then 5,000 units daily starting ≥6 h after second dose, or 5,000 units 10–14 h preop, 4–8 h postop, then daily (approximately 24 h between doses). Postop start: 2,500 units 4–8 h postop, then 5,000 units daily starting ≥6 h after first dose. Treatment of DVT/PE in cancer: 200 units/kg SC daily × 1 mo, then 150 units/kg SC daily × 5 mo; max 18,000 units/d. Unstable angina or non-Q-wave MI: 120 units/kg up to 10,000 units SC q12h with aspirin (75–165 mg/d PO) until clinically stable. [Trade only: Single-dose syringes 2,500 & 5,000 anti-Xa units/0.2 mL, 7500 anti-Xa/0.3 mL, 10,000 anti-Xa units/1 mL, 12,500 anti-Xa units/0.5 mL, 15,000 anti-Xa units/0.6 mL, 18,000 anti-Xa units/0.72 mL; multi-dose vial 10,000 units/mL, 9.5 mL and 25,000 units/mL, 3.8 mL.] ▶KL ♀B ▶+ $$$$$

ENOXAPARIN (*Lovenox*) DVT prophylaxis, acute medical illness with restricted mobility: 40 mg SC daily (CrCl <30 mL/min): 30 mg SC daily). Hip/knee replacement: 30 mg SC q12h starting 12–24 h postop (CrCl <30 mL/min: 30 mg SC daily). Alternative for hip replacement: 40 mg SC daily starting 12 h preop. Abdominal surgery: 40 mg SC daily starting 2 h preop (CrCl <30

(cont.)

mL/min: 30 mg SC daily). Outpatient treatment of DVT without pulmonary embolus: 1 mg/kg SC q12h. Continue for ≥5 d and until therapeutic oral anticoagulation established. Inpatient treatment of DVT with/without pulmonary embolus: 1 mg/kg SC q12h or 1.5 mg/kg SC q24h (CrCl <30 mL/min: 1 mg/kg SC daily). Continue for ≥5 d and until therapeutic oral anticoagulation established. Unstable angina or non-Q-wave MI: 1 mg/kg SC q12h with aspirin (100–325 mg PO daily) for ≥2 d and until clinically stable (CrCl <30 mL/min: 1 mg/kg SC daily). Acute ST-elevation MI: if ≤75 yo: 30 mg IV bolus followed 15 min later by 1 mg/kg SC dose then 1 mg/kg SC q12 h (max 100 mg/dose for the first two doses) SC q12 h (CrCl <30 mL/min: 30 mg IV bolus followed 15 min later by 1 mg/kg SC dose then 1 mg/kg SC daily); if >75 yo: 0.75 mg/kg (max 75 mg/dose for the first two doses, no bolus) SC q12 h (CrCl <30 mL/min: 1 mg/kg SC daily, no bolus). [Trade only: Multi-dose vial 300 mg; Syringes 30,40 mg; graduated syringes 60,80,100,120,150 mg. Concentration is 100 mg/mL except for 120,150 mg which are 150 mg/mL.] ▶KL ♀B ▶+ $$$$$

FONDAPARINUX (Arixtra) DVT prophylaxis, hip/knee replacement or hip fracture surgery, abdominal surgery: 2.5 mg SC daily starting 6–8 h postop. DVT / PE treatment based on weight: 5 mg (if <50 kg), 7.5 mg (if 50–100 kg), 10 mg (if >100 kg) SC daily for ≥5 d & therapeutic oral anticoagulation. [Trade only: Pre-filled syringes 2.5 mg/0.5 mL, 5 mg/0.4 mL, 7.5 mg/0.6 mL, 10 mg/0.8 mL.] ▶K ♀B ▶? $$$$$

HEPARIN (*Hepalean*) Venous thrombosis/pulmonary embolus treatment: Load 80 units/kg IV, then initiate infusion at 18 units/kg/h. Adjust based on coagulation testing (PTT). DVT prophylaxis: 5,000 units SC q8–12h. Peds: Load 50 units/kg IV, then infuse 25 units/kg/h. [Generic only: 1000, 2500, 5000, 7500, 10,000, 20,000 units/mL in various vial and syringe sizes.] ▶Reticuloendothelial system ♀C but + ▶+ $

TINZAPARIN (Innohep) DVT with/without pulmonary embolus: 175 units/kg SC daily for ≥6 d and until adequate anticoagulation with warfarin. [Trade only: 20,000 anti-Xa units/mL, 2 mL multi-dose vial.] ▶K ♀B ▶+ $$$$$

WEIGHT-BASED HEPARIN DOSING FOR DVT/PE*

Initial dose: 80 units/kg IV bolus, then 18 units/kg/h. Check PTT in 6 h.
PTT <35 sec (<1.2 × control): 80 units/kg IV bolus, then ↑ infusion rate by 4 units/kg/h.
PTT 35–45 sec (1.2–1.5 × control): 40 units/kg IV bolus, then ↑ infusion rate by 2 units/kg/h.
PTT 46–70 sec (1.5–2.3 × control): No change.
PTT 71–90 sec (2.3–3 × control): ↑ infusion rate by 2 units/kg/h.
PTT >90 sec (>3 × control): Hold infusion for 1 h, then ↑ infusion rate by 3 units/kg/h.

*PTT = Activated partial thromboplastin time. Reagent-specific target PTT may differ; use institutional nomogram when available. Consider establishing a max bolus dose/max initial infusion rate or use an adjusted body weight in obesity. Monitor PTT 6 h after heparin initiation and 6 h after each dosage adjustment. When PTT is stable within therapeutic range, monitor every morning. Therapeutic PTT range corresponds to anti-factor Xa activity of 0.3-0.7 units/mL. Check platelets between d 3 and 5. Can begin warfarin on 1st d of heparin; continue heparin for ≥4 to 5 d of combined therapy. Adapted from Ann Intern Med 1993;119:874; Chest 2008:133:463S-464S, Circulation 2001; 103:2994.

Anticoagulants—Other

ARGATROBAN Heparin-induced thrombocytopenia: Start 2 mcg/kg/min IV infusion. Get PTT at baseline and 2 h after starting infusion. Adjust dose (not >10 mcg/kg/min) until PTT is 1.5–3 times baseline (not >100 sec). ▶L ♀B▶- $$$$$

BIVALIRUDIN (*Angiomax*) Anticoagulation during PCI (including patients with or at risk of heparin-induced thrombocytopenia or heparin-induced thrombocytopenia and thrombosis syndrome: 0.75 mg/kg IV bolus prior to intervention, then 1.75 mg/kg/h for duration of procedure (with provisional Gp IIb/IIIa inhibition). For CrCl <30 mL/min, reduce infusion dose to 1 mg/kg/h after bolus. Use with aspirin 300–325 mg PO daily. Additional bolus of 0.3 mg/kg if activated clotting time <225 sec. ▶proteolysis/K ♀B ▶? $$$$$

LEPIRUDIN (*Refludan*) Anticoagulation in heparin-induced thrombocytopenia and associated thromboembolic disease: Bolus 0.4 mg/kg up to 44 mg IV over 15–20 sec, then infuse 0.15 mg/kg/h up to 16.5 mg/h. Adjust dose to maintain APTT ratio of 1.5–2.5. ▶K ♀B ▶? $$$$$

WARFARIN (*Coumadin, Jantoven*) Start 2–5 mg PO daily × 1–2 d, then adjust dose to maintain therapeutic PT/INR. [Generic/Trade: Tabs 1, 2, 2.5, 3, 4, 5, 6, 6.5, 7.5, 10 mg]. ▶L ♀X ▶+ $

Colony Stimulating Factors

DARBEPOETIN (*Aranesp, NESP*) Anemia of chronic renal failure: 0.45 mcg/kg IV/SC once weekly, or q2 wk in some patients. Cancer chemo anemia: 2.25 mcg/kg SC q wk, or 500 mcg SC every 3 wk. Adjust dose based on Hb. [Trade only: All forms are available with or without albumin. Single-dose vials 25, 40, 60, 100, 200, 300, 500 mcg/1 mL. Single-dose 150 mcg/0.75 mL. Single-dose prefilled syringes or autoinjectors - 25 mcg/0.42 mL, 40 mcg/0.4 mL, 60 mcg/0.3 mL, 100 mcg/0.5 mL, 150 mcg/0.3 mL, 200 mcg/0.4 mL, 300 mcg/0.6 mL, 500 mcg/1 mL.] ▶cellular sialidases, L ♀C ▶? $$$$$

EPOETIN ALFA (*Epogen, Procrit, erythropoietin alpha, ✚Eprex*) Anemia: 1 dose IV/SC 3 times/wk. Initial dose if renal failure = 50–100 units/kg, Zidovudine-induced anemia = 100 units/kg, or chemo-associated anemia = 150 units/kg. Alternate for chemo-associated anemia: 40,000 units SC once/wk. Adjust dose based on Hb. [Trade only: Single-dose 1 mL vials 2,000, 3,000, 4,000, 10,000, 40,000 units/mL. Multi-dose vials 10,000 units/mL 2 mL & 20,000 units/mL 1 mL.] ▶L ♀C ▶? $$$$$

THERAPEUTIC GOALS FOR ANTICOAGULATION

INR Range*	Indication
2.0–3.0	Atrial fibrillation, deep venous thrombosis†, pulmonary embolism†, bio-prosthetic heart valve, mechanical prosthetic heart valve (aortic position, bileaflet or tilting disk with normal sinus rhythm and normal left atrium)
2.5–3.5	Mechanical prosthetic heart valve: (1) mitral position, (2) aortic position with atrial fibrillation, (3) caged ball or caged disk

*Aim for an INR in the middle of the INR range (eg, 2.5 for range of 2–3 and 3.0 for range of 2.5–3.5).
Adapted from: *Chest* 2008; 133: 456-7S, 459S, 547S, 594-5S; see this manuscript for additional information and other indications. †For first-event unprovoked DVT/PE, after 3 mo of therapy at goal INR 2-3, may consider low-intensity therapy (INR range 1.5-2.0) in patients with strong preference for less frequent INR testing.

FILGRASTIM (*G-CSF, Neupogen*) Neutropenia: 5 mcg/kg SC/IV daily. [Trade only: Single-dose vials 300 mcg/1 mL, 480 mcg/1.6 mL. Single-dose syringes 300 mcg/0.5 mL, 480 mcg/0.8 mL.] ▶L ♀C ▶? $$$$$

OPRELVEKIN (*Neumega*) Chemotherapy-induced thrombocytopenia in adults: 50 mcg/kg SC daily. [Trade only: 5 mg single-dose vials with diluent.] ▶K ♀C ▶? $$$$$

PEGFILGRASTIM (*Neulasta*) 6 mg SC once each chemo cycle. [Trade only: Single-dose syringes 6 mg/0.6 mL.] ▶Plasma ♀C ▶? $$$$$

SARGRAMOSTIM (*GM-CSF, Leukine*) Specialized dosing for marrow transplant. ▶L ♀C ▶? $$$$$

Other Hematological Agents

NOTE *See endocrine section for vitamins and minerals.*

AMINOCAPROIC ACID (*Amicar*) Hemostasis: 4–5 g PO/IV over 1 h, then 1 g/h prn. [Generic/Trade: Syrup or oral soln 250 mg/mL, tabs 500 mg.] ▶K ♀D ▶? $$

ANAGRELIDE (*Agrylin*) Thrombocythemia due to myeloproliferative disorders: Start 0.5 mg PO qid or 1 mg PO bid, then after 1 wk adjust to lowest effective dose. Max 10 mg/d. [Generic/Trade: Caps, 0.5, 1 mg.] ▶LK ♀C ▶? $$$$$

HYDROXYUREA (*Hydrea, Droxia*) Sickle cell anemia (Droxia): Start 15 mg/ kg PO daily while monitoring CBC q 2 wk. If no marrow depression, then increase dose q 12 wk by 5 mg/kg/d (max 35 mg/kg/d). Give concomitant folic acid 1 mg/d. Chemotherapy: doses vary by indication. [Generic/Trade: Cap 500 mg. Trade only: (Droxia) Caps 200, 300, 400 mg.] ▶LK ♀D ▶- $ varies by therapy

PROTAMINE Reversal of heparin: 1 mg antagonizes ~100 units heparin. Reversal of low molecular weight heparin: 1 mg protamine per 100 anti-Xa units of dalteparin or tinzaparin. 1 mg protamine per 1 mg enoxaparin. Give IV (max 50 mg) over 10 min. May cause allergy/anaphylaxis. ▶Plasma ♀C ▶? $

HERBAL & ALTERNATIVE THERAPIES

NOTE *In the US, herbal and alternative therapy products are regulated as dietary supplements, not drugs. Premarketing evaluation and FDA approval are not required unless specific therapeutic claims are made. Since these products are not required to demonstrate efficacy, it is unclear whether many of them have health benefits. In addition, there may be considerable variability in content from lot to lot or between products. See www.tarascon.com/herbals for the evidence-based efficacy ratings used by Tarascon editorial staff.*

ALOE VERA (*acemannan, burn plant*) Topical: Efficacy unclear for seborrheic dermatitis, psoriasis, genital herpes, skin burns. Gel possibly effective for oral lichen planus. Do not apply to surgical incisions; impaired healing reported. Oral: Mild to moderate active ulcerative colitis (possibly effective): 100 mL PO bid. Efficacy unclear for type 2 diabetes. OTC laxatives containing aloe were removed from US market due to possible increased risk of colon cancer. [Not

(cont.)

by prescription.] ▶L, peripheral conversion to estrogens & androgens ♀- ▶- $ ▶LK ♀oral- topical +? ▶oral- topical +? $

ANDROSTENEDIONE (*andro*) Marketed as anabolic steroid to enhance athletic performance. May cause androgenic (primarily in women) and estrogenic (primarily in men) side effects. FDA warned manufacturers to stop marketing as dietary supplement in 2004. [Not by prescription.]

ARISTOLOCHIC ACID (*Aristolochia, Asarum, Bragantia*) Nephrotoxic & carcinogenic; do not use. Was promoted for weight loss. [Not by prescription.] ▶? ♀- ▶- $

ARNICA (*Arnica montana, leopard's bane, wolf's bane*) Do not take by mouth. Topical promoted for treatment of skin wounds, bruises, aches, and sprains; but insufficient data to assess efficacy. Do not use on open wounds. [Not by prescription.] ▶? ♀- ▶- $

ARTICHOKE LEAF EXTRACT (*Cynara-SL, Cynara scolymus*) May reduce total cholesterol, but clinical significance is unclear. Cynara-SL is promoted as digestive aid (possibly effective for dyspepsia) at a dose of 1–2 caps PO daily (320 mg dried artichoke leaf extract/cap). [Not by prescription.] ▶? ♀? ▶? $

ASTRAGALUS (*Astragalus membranaceus, huang qi, vetch*) Used in combination with other herbs in traditional Chinese medicine, but efficacy unclear for CHD, CHF, chronic kidney disease, viral infections, and URIs. Possibly effective for improving survival and performance status with platinum-based chemotherapy for non-small cell lung cancer. [Not by prescription.] ▶? ♀? ▶? $

BILBERRY (*Vaccinium myrtillus, huckleberry, Tegens, VMA extract*) Cataracts (efficacy unclear): 160 mg PO bid of 25% anthocyanosides extract. Insufficient data to evaluate efficacy for macular degeneration. Does not appear effective for improving night vision. [Not by prescription.] ▶Bile, K ♀- ▶- $

BITTER MELON (*Momordica charantia, ampalaya, karela*) Efficacy unclear for type 2 diabetes. Dose unclear; juice may be more potent than dried fruit powder. Hypoglycemic coma reported in 2 children ingesting tea. Seeds can cause hemolytic anemia in G6PD deficiency. [Not by prescription.] ▶? ♀- ▶- $$

BITTER ORANGE (*Citrus aurantium, Seville orange, Acutrim Natural AM, Dexatrim Natural Ephedrine Free*) Sympathomimetic similar to ephedra; safety and efficacy not established. Case reports of stroke and MI in patients taking bitter orange with caffeine. Do not use with MAOIs. [Not by prescription.] ▶K ♀- ▶- $

BLACK COHOSH (*Cimicifuga racemosa, Remifemin, Menofem*) Ineffective for relief of menopausal symptoms. [Not by prescription.] ▶? ♀- ▶- $

BUTTERBUR (*Petesites hybridus, Petadolex, Petaforce, Tesalin, ZE 339*) Migraine prophylaxis (possibly effective): Petadolex 50–75 mg PO bid. Allergic rhinitis prophylaxis (possibly effective): Petadolex 50 mg PO bid or Tesalin 1 tab PO qid or 2 tabs tid. Efficacy unclear for asthma or allergic skin disease. [Not by prescription. Standardized pyrrolizidine-free extracts: Petadolex (7.5 mg of petasin & isopetasin/50 mg tab). Tesalin (ZE 339; 8 mg petasin/tab).] ▶? ♀- ▶- $

CHAMOMILE (*Matricaria recutita—German chamomile, Anthemis nobilis—Roman chamomile*) Promoted as a sedative or anxiolytic, to relieve GI distress, for skin infections or inflammation, many other indications. Efficacy unclear for any indication. [Not by prescription.] ▶? ♀-▶? $

CHAPARRAL (*Larrea divaricata, creosote bush*) Hepatotoxic; do not use. Promoted as cancer cure. [Not by prescription.] ▶? ♀-▶ $

CHASTEBERRY (*Vitex agnus castus fruit extract, Femaprin*) Premenstrual syndrome (possibly effective): 20 mg PO daily of extract ZE 440. [Not by prescription.] ▶? ♀-▶ $

CHONDROITIN Does not appear effective for relief of knee osteoarthritis pain, but possibly reduces joint space narrowing. Glucosamine/Chondroitin Arthritis Intervention Trial (GAIT) did not find overall improvement in pain of knee OA with chondroitin 400 mg PO tid +/- glucosamine. Chondroitin + glucosamine improved pain in subgroup of patients with moderate to severe knee OA. [Not by prescription.] ▶K ♀? ▶? $

COENZYME Q10 (*CoQ-10, ubiquinone*) Heart failure: 100 mg/d PO divided bid-tid (conflicting clinical trials; Am Heart Assoc does not recommend). Statin-induced muscle pain: 100–200 mg PO daily (conflicting clinical trials). Parkinson's disease: 1200 mg/d PO divided qid ($$$$; efficacy unclear; might slow progression slightly, but Am Acad Neurol does not recommend). Efficacy unclear for improving athletic performance. Appears ineffective for diabetes. [Not by prescription.] ▶Bile ♀-▶- $

COMFREY (*Symphytum officinale*) May cause hepatic cancer; do not use, even topically. [Not by prescription.] ▶? ♀-▶ $

CRANBERRY (*Cranactin, Vaccinium macrocarpon*) Prevention of UTI (possibly effective): 300 mL/d PO cranberry juice cocktail. Usual dose of cranberry juice extract caps/tabs is 300–400 mg PO bid. Insufficient data to assess efficacy for treatment of UTI. [Not by prescription.] ▶? ♀? ▶? $

CREATINE Promoted to enhance athletic performance. No benefit for endurance exercise; modest benefit for intense anaerobic tasks lasting <30 sec. Usual loading dose of 20 g/d PO × 5 d, then 2–5 g/d divided bid. [Not by prescription.] ▶LK ♀-▶- $

DEHYDROEPIANDROSTERONE (*DHEA, Aslera, Fidelin, Prasterone*) Does not improve cognition, quality of life, or sexual function in elderly. To improve well-being in women with adrenal insufficiency: 50 mg PO daily (possibly effective; conflicting clinical trials). [Not by prescription.] ▶Peripheral conversion to estrogens and androgens ♀-▶- $

DEVIL'S CLAW (*Harpagophytum procumbens, Phyto Joint, Doloteffin, Harpadol*) Osteoarthritis, acute exacerbation of chronic low back pain (possibly effective): 2400 mg extract/d (50—100 mg harpagoside/d) PO divided bid-tid. [Not by prescription. Extracts standardized to harpagoside (iridoid glycoside) content.] ▶? ♀-▶- $

DONG QUAI (*Angelica sinensis*) Appears ineffective for postmenopausal symptoms; North American Menopause Society recommends against use. May increase bleeding risk with warfarin; avoid concurrent use. [Not by prescription.] ▶? ♀-▶- $

ECHINACEA (*E. purpurea, E. angustifolia, E. pallida, cone flower, EchinaGuard, Echinacin Madaus*)   Conflicting clinical trials for prevention or treatment of upper respiratory infections. [Not by prescription.] ▶? ♀- ▶- $

ELDERBERRY (*Sambucus nigra, Rubini, Sambucol, Sinupret*)   Efficacy unclear for influenza, sinusitis, and bronchitis. [Not by prescription.] ▶? ♀- ▶- $

EPHEDRA (*Ephedra sinica, ma huang, Metabolife 356, Biolean, Ripped Fuel, Xenadrine*)   Little evidence of efficacy for obesity, other than modest short-term weight loss. Traditional use as bronchodilator. [Not by prescription.] ▶K ♀- ▶- $

EVENING PRIMROSE OIL (*Oenothera biennis*)   Appears ineffective for pre-menstrual syndrome, postmenopausal symptoms, atopic dermatitis. [Not by prescription.] ▶? ♀? ▶? $

FENUGREEK (*Trigonelle foenum-graecum*)   Efficacy unclear for diabetes or hyperlipidemia. [Not by prescription.] ▶? ♀- ▶? $$

FEVERFEW (*Chrysanthemum parthenium, MIG-99, Migra-Lief, MigraSpray, Tanacetum parthenium L.*)   Prevention of migraine (possibly effective): 50–100 mg extract PO daily; 2–3 fresh leaves PO with or after meals daily; 50–125 mg freeze-dried leaf PO daily. May take 1–2 mo to be effective. Inadequate data to evaluate efficacy for acute migraine. [Not by prescription.] ▶? ♀- ▶- $

FLAVOCOXID (*Limbrel, UP446*)   Osteoarthritis (efficacy unclear): 250–500 mg PO bid. [Caps 250,500 mg. Marketed as medical food by prescription only (not all medical foods require a prescription). Medical foods are intended to be given under physician supervision to meet distinctive nutritional needs of a disease, but they do not undergo an approval process to establish safety and efficacy.] ▶? ♀- ▶- $$$

GARCINIA (*Garcinia cambogia, Citri Lean*)   Appears ineffective for weight loss. [Not by prescription.] ▶? ♀- ▶- $

GARLIC SUPPLEMENTS (*Allium sativum, Kwai, Kyolic*)   Ineffective for hyperlipidemia. Small reductions in BP, but efficacy in HTN unclear. Does not appear effective for diabetes. Cytochrome P450 3A4 inducer. Significantly decreases saquinavir levels. May increase bleeding risk with warfarin with/without increase in INR. [Not by prescription.] ▶LK ♀- ▶- $

GINGER (*Zingiber officinale*)   Prevention of motion sickness (efficacy unclear): 500–1000 mg powdered rhizome PO single dose 1 h before exposure. American College of Obstetrics and Gynecology considers ginger 250 mg PO qid a nonpharmacologic option for N/V of pregnancy. Does not appear effective for postop N/V. [Not by prescription.] ▶? ♀? ▶? $

GINKGO BILOBA (*EGb 761, Ginkgold, Ginkoba, Quanterra Mental Sharpness*)   Dementia (efficacy unclear): 40 mg PO tid of standardized extract containing 24% ginkgo flavone glycosides and 6% terpene lactones. Am Psychiatric Assn and others find evidence too weak to support use for Alzheimers or other dementias. Does not appear to improve memory in people with normal cognitive function. Does not appear effective for prevention of acute altitude sickness. Limited benefit in intermittent claudication. [Not by prescription.] ▶K ♀- ▶- $

GINSENG—AMERICAN (*Panax quinquefolius L.*) Reduction of postprandial glucose in type 2 diabetes (possibly effective): 3 g PO taken with or up to 2 h before meal . [Not by prescription.] ▶K ♀ - ▶ - $

GINSENG—ASIAN (*Panax ginseng, Ginsana, Ginsai, G115, Korean red ginseng*) Promoted to improve vitality and well-being: 200 mg PO daily. Ginsana: 2 caps PO daily or 1 cap PO bid. Ginseng Sport: 1 cap PO daily. Preliminary evidence of efficacy for erectile dysfunction. Efficacy unclear for improving physical or psychomotor performance, diabetes, herpes simplex infections, cognitive or immune function. American College of Obstetrics and Gynecologists and North American Menopause Society recommend against use for postmenopausal hot flashes . [Not by prescription.] ▶? ♀ - ▶ - $

GINSENG—SIBERIAN (*Eleutherococcus senticosus, Ci-wu-jia*) Does not appear effective for improving athletic endurance, or chronic fatigue syndrome. May interfere with FPIA and MEIA digoxin assays. [Not by prescription.] ▶? ♀ - ▶ - $

GLUCOSAMINE (*Aflexa, Cosamin DS, Dona, Flextend, Promotion*) Efficacy for osteoarthritis is unclear (conflicting data). Glucosamine/Chondroitin Arthritis Intervention Trial (GAIT) did not find overall improvement in pain of knee OA with glucosamine HCl 500 mg +/- chondroitin 400 mg both PO tid. Glucosamine + chondroitin did improve pain in subgroup of patients with moderate to severe OA. Some earlier studies reported improved pain with glucosamine sulfate (Dona 1500 mg PO once daily). Glucosamine sulfate was ineffective for hip OA in GOAL study. [Not by prescription.] ▶L ♀ - ▶ - $

GOLDENSEAL (*Hydrastis canadensis*) Often used in attempts to achieve false-negative urine test for illicit drug use (efficacy unclear). Often combined with echinacea in cold remedies; but insufficient data to assess efficacy for common cold or URIs. [Not by prescription.] ▶? ♀ - ▶ - $

GRAPE SEED EXTRACT (*Vitis vinifera L., procyanidolic oligomers, PCO*) Small clinical trials suggest benefit in chronic venous insufficiency. No benefit in single study of seasonal allergic rhinitis. [Not by prescription.] ▶? ♀? ▶? $

GREEN TEA (*Camellia sinensis*) Efficacy unclear for cancer prevention, weight loss, hypercholesterolemia. Large doses might decrease INR with warfarin due to vitamin K content. Contains caffeine. [Not by prescription. Green tea extract available in caps standardized to polyphenol content.] ▶? ♀ + in moderate amount in food, - in supplements ▶ + in moderate amount in food, - in supplements $

GUARANA (*Paullinia cupana*) Marketed as an ingredient in weight-loss dietary supplements. Seeds contain caffeine. Guarana in weight loss dietary supplements may provide high doses of caffeine. [Not by prescription.] ▶? ♀ + in food, - in supplements ▶ + in food, - in supplements $

GUGGULIPID (*Commiphora mukul extract, guggul*) Does not appear effective for hyperlipidemia. [Not by prescription.] ▶? ♀ - ▶ - $$

HAWTHORN (*Crataegus laevigata, monogyna, oxyacantha, standardized extract WS 1442—Crataegutt novo, HeartCare*) Mild heart failure (possibly effective): 80 mg PO bid to 160 mg PO tid of standardized extract (19% oligomeric procyanidins; WS 1442; HeartCare 80 mg tabs). [Not by prescription.] ▶? ♀ - ▶ - $

HONEY (*Medihoney*) Topical for burn/wound (including diabetic foot, statis leg ulcers, pressure ulcers, 1st and 2nd degree partial thickness burns): Apply Medihoney for 12–24 h/d. Oral for nocturnal cough due to upper respiratory tract infection (efficacy unclear): Give PO within 30 min before sleep. Dose is ½ tsp for 2–5 yo, 1 tsp for 6–11 yo, 2 tsp for 12–18 yo. Do not feed honey to children <1 yo due to risk of infant botulism. [Mostly not by prescription. Medihoney is FDA approved product.] ▶? ♀+ ▶+ $ for PO $$$ for Medihoney

HORSE CHESTNUT SEED EXTRACT (*Aesculus hippocastanum, HCE50, Venastat*) Chronic venous insufficiency (effective): 1 cap Venastat (16% aescin standardized extract) PO bid with water before meals. [Not by prescription.] ▶? ♀- ▶- $

KAVA (*Piper methysticum, One-a-d Bedtime & Rest, Sleep-Tite*) Promoted as anxiolytic (possibly effective) or sedative. Do not use due to hepatotoxicity. [Not by prescription.] ▶K ♀- ▶- $

KOMBUCHA TEA (*Manchurian or Kargasok tea*) Do not use. No proven benefit for any indication; may cause severe acidosis. [Not by prescription.] ▶? ♀- ▶- $

LICORICE (*Cankermelt, Glycyrrhiza glabra, Glycyrrhiza uralensis*) Insufficient data to assess efficacy for postmenopausal vasomotor symptoms. Chronic high doses can cause pseudo-primary aldosteronism (with HTN, edema, hypokalemia). Cankermelt (dissolving oral patch); efficacy unclear for aphthous ulcers): Apply patch to ulcer for 16 h/d until healed. [Not by prescription.] ▶Bile ♀- ▶- $

MELATONIN (*N-acetyl-5-methoxytryptamine*) To reduce jet lag after flights over >5 time zones (possibly effective): 0.5–5 mg PO qhs × 3–6 nights starting on d of arrival. [Not by prescription.] ▶L ♀- ▶- $

METHYLSULFONYLMETHANE (*MSM, dimethyl sulfone, crystalline DMSO2*) Insufficient data to assess efficacy of oral and topical MSM for arthritis pain. [Not by prescription.] ▶? ♀- ▶- $

MILK THISTLE (*Silybum marianum, Legalon, silymarin, Thisylin*) Hepatic cirrhosis (possibly effective): 100–200 mg PO tid of standardized extract with 70–80% silymarin. [Not by prescription.] ▶LK ♀- ▶- $

NETTLE ROOT (*stinging nettle, Urtica dioica radix*) Efficacy unclear for treatment of BPH. [Not by prescription.] ▶? ♀- ▶- $

NONI (*Morinda citrifolia*) Promoted for many medical disorders; but insufficient data to assess efficacy. Potassium content comparable to orange juice; hyperkalemia reported in chronic renal failure. Case reports of hepatotoxicity. [Not by prescription.] ▶? ♀- ▶- $$$

POLICOSANOL (*One-a-Day Cholesterol Plus, CholeRx, Cholest Response, Cholesstor, Cholestin*) Ineffective for hyperlipidemia. A Cuban formulation (unavailable in US) reduced LDL cholesterol in studies by a single group of researchers, but studies by other groups found no benefit. Clinical study of a US formulation (Cholesstor) also found no benefit. [Not by prescription.] ▶? ♀- ▶- $

PROBIOTICS (*Acidophilus, Align, Bifantis, Bifidobacteria, Lactobacillus, Bacid, Culturelle, Florastor, IntestiFlora, Lactinex, LiveBac, Power-Dophilus, Primadophilus, Probiotica, Saccharomyces boulardii, VSL#3*) Prevention of antibiotic-associated diarrhea (effective): Forastor (Saccharomyces boulardii) 2

(cont.)

caps PO bid for adults; 1 cap PO bid for peds. Culturelle (Lactobacillus GG) 1 cap PO once daily or bid for peds. Give 2 h before/after antibiotic. Peds rotavirus gastroenteritis (effective): Lactobacillus GG ≥10 billion cells/d PO started early in illness. VSL#3 (approved as medical food) for ulcerative colitis or pouchitis: 1–8 packets/d or 4–32 caps/d for adults; peds dose based on weight and number of bowel movements. Irritable bowel syndrome: VSL#3 either ½ - 1 packet PO daily or 2–4 caps PO daily to relieve gas/bloating. Align 1 cap PO once daily to relieve abdominal pain/bloating. Safety and efficacy of probiotics unclear for prevention of recurrant C difficile diarrhea. [Not by prescription. Culturelle contains Lactobacillus GG 10 billion cells/cap. Florastor contains Saccharomyces boulardii 5 billion cells/250 mg cap. Probiotica contains Lactobacillus reuteri 100 million cells/chew tab. VSL#3 contains 450 billion cells/packet, 225 billion cells/2 caps (Bifidobacterium breve, longum, infantis; Lactobacillus acidophilus, plantarum, casei, bulgaricus; Streptococcus thermophilus). Align contains Bifidobacterium infantis 35624, 1 billion cells/cap. VSL#3 is marketed as non-prescription medical food. Medical foods are to be given under physician —supervision to meet distinctive nutritional needs of a disease, but they do not undergo an approval process to establish safety and efficacy.] ▶? ♀+ ▶+ $

PYCNOGENOL (French maritime pine tree bark)   Promoted for many medical disorders; but efficacy unclear for chronic venous insufficiency, hypertension, sperm dysfunction, melasma, osteoarthritis, diabetes, and ADHD. [Not by prescription.] ▶L ♀? ▶? $

PYGEUMAFRICANUM (African plum tree, Prostata, Prostatonin, Provol)   BPH (may have modest efficacy): 50–100 mg PO bid or 100 mg PO daily of standardized extract containing 14% triterpenes. Prostatonin (also contains Urtica dioica): 1 cap PO bid with meals up to 6 wk for full response. [Not by prescription.] ▶? ♀- ▶- $

RED CLOVER ISOFLAVONE EXTRACT (Trifolium pratense, trefoil, Promensil, Rimostil, Supplifem, Trinovin)   Postmenopausal vasomotor symptoms (conflicting evidence exists; does not appear to be effective overall, but may have modest benefit for severe symptoms): Promensil 1 tab PO daily-bid with meals. [Not by prescription. Isoflavone content (genistein, daidzein, biochanin, formononetin) is 40 mg/tab in Promensil and Trinovin, 57 mg/tab in Rimostil.] ▶Gut, L, K ♀- ▶- $$

RED YEAST RICE (Monascus purpureus, Xuezhikang, Zhibituo, Hypocol, Lipolysar)   Efficacy of currently available US products for hyperlipidemia is unclear. Some products were removed from the market because they contained up to 10 mg/d of lovastatin. Others, such as Cholestin, were reformulated with policosanol (ineffective for hyperlipidemia). Cases of myopathy have been reported with red yeast rice supplements. [Not by prescription. Xuezhikang marketed in Asia, Norway (HypoCol), Italy (Lipolysar).] ▶L ♀- ▶- $$

S-ADENOSYLMETHIONINE (SAM-e, sammy)   Depression (possibly effective): 400–1600 mg/d PO. Osteoarthritis (possibly effective): 400–1200 mg/d PO. Onset of response in OA in 2–4 wk. [Not by prescription.] ▶L ♀? ▶? $$$

SAINT JOHN'S WORT (Alterra, Hypericum perforatum, Kira, Movana, One-a-d Tension & Mood, LI-160, St John's wort)   Mild depression (effective): 300 mg PO tid of standardized extract (0.3% hypericin). Conflicting clinical

(cont.)

trials for moderate major depression. Does not appear effective for attention-deficit/hyperactivity disorder. May decrease efficacy of many drugs (eg, oral contraceptives) by inducing liver metabolism. May cause serotonin syndrome with SSRIs, MAOIs. [Not by prescription.] ▶L ♀- ▶- $

SAW PALMETTO (*Serenoa repens, One-a-d Prostate Health, Quanterra*) BPH (possibly effective for mild to moderate; appears ineffective for moderate to severe): 160 mg PO bid or 320 mg PO daily of standardized liposterolic extract. Take with food. Brewed teas may not be effective. [Not by prescription.] ▶?
♀- ▶- $

SHARK CARTILAGE (*BeneFin, Cancenex, Cartilade*) Appears ineffective for palliative care of advanced cancer. [Not by prescription.] ▶? ♀- ▶- $$$$$

SILVER—COLLOIDAL (*mild & strong silver protein, silver ion*) Promoted as anti-microbial; unsafe and ineffective for any use. Silver accumulates in skin (leads to grey tint), conjunctiva, and internal organs with chronic use. [Not by prescription. May come as silver chloride, cyanide, iodide, oxide, or phosphate.] ▶? ♀- ▶- $

SOY (*Genisoy, Healthy Woman, Novasoy, Phytosoya, Supro*) Cardiovascular risk reduction: ≥25 g/d soy protein (50 mg/d isoflavones) PO. Hypercholesterolemia: ~50 g/d soy protein PO reduces LDL cholesterol by ~3%; no apparent benefit for isoflavone supplements. Postmenopausal vasomotor symptoms (modest benefit if any): 20–60 g/d soy protein PO (40–80 mg/d isoflavones). Conflicting clinical trials for postmenopausal bone loss. [Not by prescription.] ▶Gut, L, K ♀+ for food, ? for supplements ▶+ for food, ? for supplements $

STEVIA (*Stevia rebaudiana*) Leaves traditionally used as sweetener. Efficacy unclear for treatment of type 2 diabetes or hypertension. [Not by prescription.] ▶L ♀- ▶- $

TEA TREE OIL (*melaleuca oil, Melaleuca alternifolia*) Not for oral use; CNS toxicity reported. Efficacy unclear for onychomycosis, tinea pedis, acne vulgaris, dandruff, pediculosis. [Not by prescription.] ▶? ♀- ▶- $

VALERIAN (*Valeriana officinalis, Alluna, One-a-d Bedtime & Rest, Sleep-Tite*) Insomnia (possibly effective; conflicting clinical trials): 400–900 mg of standardized extract PO 30 min before bedtime. Alluna: 2 tabs PO 1 h before bedtime. [Not by prescription.] ▶? ♀- ▶- $

WILD YAM (*Dioscorea villosa*) Ineffective as topical "natural progestin." Was used historically to synthesize progestins, cortisone, and androgens; it is not converted to them or DHEA in the body. [Not by prescription.] ▶L ♀? ▶? $

WILLOW BARK EXTRACT (*Salix alba, Salicis cortex, Assalix, salicin*) Osteoarthritis, low back pain (possibly effective): 60 to 240 mg/d salicin PO divided bid-tid. [Not by prescription. Some products standardized to 15% salicin content.] ▶K ♀- ▶- $

YOHIMBE (*Corynanthe yohimbe, Pausinystalia yohimbe, Potent V*) Nonprescription yohimbe promoted for impotence and as aphrodisiac, but these products rarely contain much yohimbine. FDA considers yohimbe bark in herbal remedies an unsafe herb. [Yohimbine is the primary alkaloid in the bark of the yohimbe tree. Yohimbine HCl is a prescription drug in the US; yohimbe bark is available without prescription. Yohimbe bark (not by prescription) and prescription yohimbine HCl are not interchangeable.] ▶L ♀- ▶- $

IMMUNOLOGY

Immunizations

NOTE *For vaccine info see CDC website (www.cdc.gov).*

AVIAN INFLUENZA VACCINE H5N1—Inactivated injection 1 mL IM × 2 doses, separated by 21–35 d. ▶Immune system ♀C ▶??

BCG VACCINE (*Tice BCG, ✦Oncotice, Immucyst*) 0.2–0.3 mL percutaneously. ▶Immune system ♀C ▶? $$$$

COMVAX (*Haemophilus B vaccine + hepatitis B vaccine*) Infants born of HBsAg (−) mothers: 0.5 mL IM × 3 doses at 2, 4, and 12–15 mo of age. ▶Immune system ♀C ▶? $$$

DIPHTHERIA TETANUS AND ACELLULAR PERTUSSIS VACCINE (*DTaP, Tdap, Tripedia, Infanrix, Daptacel, Boostrix, Adacel, ✦Tripacel*) 0.5 mL IM. Do not use Boostrix or Adacel for primary childhood vaccination series. ▶Immune system ♀C ▶- $$

DIPHTHERIA-TETANUS TOXOID (*Td, DT, ✦D2T5*) 0.5 mL IM. [Injection DT (pediatric: 6 wk–6 yo). Td (adult and children: ≥7 yr).] ▶Immune system ♀C ▶? $

HAEMOPHILUS B VACCINE (*ActHIB, HibTITER, PedvaxHIB*) 0.5 mL IM. Dosing schedule varies depending on formulation used and age of child at first dose. ▶Immune system ♀C ▶? $$

HEPATITIS A VACCINE (*Havrix, Vaqta, ✦Avaxim, Epaxal*) Adult formulation 1 mL IM, repeat in 6–12 mo. Peds ≥1 yo: 0.5 mL IM, repeat 6–18 mo later. [Single dose vial (specify pediatric or adult).] ▶Immune system ♀C ▶+ $$$

HEPATITIS B VACCINE (*Engerix-B, Recombivax HB*) Adults: 1 mL IM, repeat in 1 and 6 mo. Separate pediatric formulations and dosing. ▶Immune system ♀C ▶+ $$$

HUMAN PAPILLOMAVIRUS RECOMBINANT VACCINE (*Gardasil*) 0.5 mL IM at 0, 2 and 6 mo. ▶Immune system ♀B ▶? $$$$$

INFLUENZA VACCINE—INACTIVATED INJECTION (*Afluria, Fluarix, FluLaval, Fluzone, Fluvirin, ✦Fluviral, Vaxigrip*) 0.5 mL IM. Fluarix and FluLaval not indicated if <18 yo, Fluvirin not indicated if <4 yo. ▶Immune system ♀C ▶+ $$

INFLUENZA VACCINE—LIVE INTRANASAL (*FluMist*) 1 dose (0.2 mL) intranasally. ▶Immune system ♀C ▶+ $

JAPANESE ENCEPHALITIS VACCINE (*JE-Vax*) 1.0 mL SC × 3 doses on d 0, 7, and 30. ▶Immune system ♀C ▶? $$$$

MEASLES MUMPS & RUBELLA VACCINE (*M-M-R II, ✦Priorix*) 0.5 mL (1 vial) SC. ▶Immune system ♀C ▶+ $$$

MENINGOCOCCAL VACCINE (*Menomune-A/C/Y/W-135, Menactra, ✦Menjugate*) 0.5 mL SC (Menomune) or IM (Menactra). ▶Immune system ♀C ▶? $$$$

PEDIARIX (*diphtheria tetanus and acellular pertussis vaccine + hepatitis B vaccine + polio vaccine*) 0.5 mL at 2, 4, 6 mo IM. ▶Immune system ♀C ▶? $$$

PLAGUE VACCINE Age 18–61 yo: 1 mL IM × 1 dose, then 0.2 mL IM 1–3 mo after the 1st injection, then 0.2 mL IM 5–6 mo later. ▶Immune system ♀C ▶+ $

PNEUMOCOCCAL 23-VALENT VACCINE (*Pneumovax*, ✦*Pneumo 23*) 0.5 mL IM/SC. ▶Immune system ♀C ▶+ $$

PNEUMOCOCCAL 7-VALENT CONJUGATE VACCINE (*Prevnar*) 0.5 mL IM × 3 doses 6–8 wk apart starting at 2–6 mo of age, followed by a fourth dose at 12–15 mo. ▶Immune system ♀C ▶? $$$

POLIO VACCINE (*IPOL*) 0.5 mL IM or SC. ▶Immune system ♀C ▶? $$

PROQUAD (*measles mumps & rubella vaccine + varicella vaccine, MMRV*) 12 mo–12 yr: 0.5 mL (1 vial) SC. ▶Immune system ♀C ▶? $$$$

RABIES VACCINE (*RabAvert, Imovax Rabies, BioRab, Rabies Vaccine Adsorbed*) 1 mL IM in deltoid region on d 0, 3, 7, 14, 28. ▶Immune system ♀C ▶? $$$$$

ROTAVIRUS VACCINE (*RotaTeq, Rotarix*) RotaTeq: Give the first dose (2 mL PO) between 6–12 wk of age, and then the 2nd & 3rd doses at 4–10 wk intervals thereafter (last dose no later than 32 wk). Rotarix: Give first dose (1 mL) at 6 wk of age, and second dose (1 mL) at least 4 wk later, and prior to 24 wk of age. [Trade only: Oral susp 2 mL (RotaTeq), 1 mL (Rotarix).] ▶Immune system ♀ ▶? $$$$$

TETANUS TOXOID 0.5 ML IM/SC. ▶Immune system ♀C ▶+ $

TRIHIBIT (*Haemophilus B vaccine + diphtheria tetanus and acellular pertussis vaccine*) 4th dose only, 15–18 mo: 0.5 mL IM. ▶Immune system ♀C ▶- $$$

TWINRIX (*hepatitis A vaccine + hepatitis B vaccine*) Adults: 1 mL IM in deltoid, repeat in 1 & 6 mo. Accelerated dosing schedule: 0, 7, 21–30 d and booster dose at 12 mo. ▶Immune system ♀C ▶? $$$

TYPHOID VACCINE—INACTIVATED INJECTION (*Typhim Vi*, ✦*Typherix*) 0.5 mL IM × 1 dose. May revaccinate q2–5 yr if high risk. ▶Immune system ♀C ▶? $$

TYPHOID VACCINE—LIVE ORAL (*Vivotif Berna*) 1 cap qod × 4 doses. May revaccinate q2–5 yr if high risk. [Trade only: Caps ▶Immune system ♀C ▶? $$

VARICELLA VACCINE (*Varivax*, ✦*Varilrix*) Children 1 to 12 yo: 0.5 mL SC × 1 dose. Age ≥13: 0.5 mL SC, repeat 4–8 wk later.] ▶Immune system ♀C ▶+ $$$

YELLOW FEVER VACCINE (*YF-Vax*) 0.5 mL SC. ▶Immune system ♀C ▶+ $$$

ZOSTER VACCINE—LIVE (*Zostavax*) Adults ≥60 yo: 0.65 mL SC × 1. ▶Immune system ♀C ▶? $$$$

Immunoglobulins

ANTIVENIN—CROTALIDAE IMMUNE FAB OVINE POLYVALENT (*CroFab*) Rattlesnake envenomation: Give 4–6 vials IV infusion over 60 min, within 6 h of bite if possible. Administer 4–6 additional vials if no initial control of envenomation syndrome, then 2 vials q6h for up to 18 h (3 doses) after initial control has been established. ▶? ♀C ▶? $$$$$

BOTULISM IMMUNE GLOBULIN (*BabyBIG*) Infant botulism <1 yo: 1 mL (50 mg)/kg IV. ▶L ♀? ▶? $$$$$

CHILDHOOD IMMUNIZATION SCHEDULE*

Age	Birth	1	2	4	6	12	15	18	2	4-6	11-12
						Months				**Years**	
Hepatitis B	HB	HB				HB					
Rotavirus			Rota	Rota	Rota						
DTP			DTaP	DTaP	DTaP		DTaP			DTaP	DTaP
H influenza b			Hib	Hib	Hib	Hib					
Pneumococci			PCV	PCV	PCV	PCV					
Polio			IPV	IPV		IPV				IPV	
Influenza†						Influenza (yearly)†					
MMR						MMR				MMR	
Varicella						Varicella				Vari	
Hepatitis A¶						Hep A × 2¶					
Papillomavirus§											HPV × 3§
Meningococcal											MCV

*2007 schedule from the CDC, ACIP, AAP, & AAFP, see CDC website (www.cdc.gov).
†If ≥5 yo and healthy can use intranasal form. If <9 yo receiving for first time, should get 2 doses ≥4 weeks apart for injected form and ≥6 weeks apart for intranasal.
¶Two doses at least 6 months apart.
§Second and third doses 2 and 6 months after first dose.

HEPATITIS B IMMUNE GLOBULIN (*H-BIG, HyperHep B, HepaGam B, NABI-HB*) 0.06 mL/kg IM within 24 h of needlestick, ocular, or mucosal exposure, repeat in 1 mo. ▶L ♀C ▶? $$$

IMMUNE GLOBULIN—INTRAMUSCULAR (*Baygam, ✦Gamastan*) Hepatitis A prophylaxis: 0.02–0.06 mL/kg IM depending on length of stay. Measles (within 6 d post-exposure): 0.2–0.25 mL/kg IM. ▶L ♀C ▶? $$$$

IMMUNE GLOBULIN—INTRAVENOUS (*Carimune, Polygam, Panglobulin, Octagam, Flebogamma, Gammagard, Gamunex, Iveegam, Privigen, Venoglobulin*) IV dosage varies by indication and product. ▶L ♀C ▶? $$$$$

IMMUNE GLOBULIN—SUBCUTANEOUS (*Vivaglobulin*) 100–200 mg/kg SC weekly. ▶L ♀C ▶? $$$$$

LYMPHOCYTE IMMUNE GLOBULIN (*Atgam*) Specialized dosing. ▶L ♀C ▶? $$$$$

RABIES IMMUNE GLOBULIN HUMAN (*Imogam Rabies-HT, HyperRAB S/D*) 20 units/kg, as much as possible infiltrated around bite, the rest IM. ▶L ♀C ▶? $$$$$

RSV IMMUNE GLOBULIN (*RespiGam*) IV infusion for RSV. ▶Plasma ♀C ▶? $$$$$

TETANUS IMMUNE GLOBULIN (*BayTet, ✦Hypertet*) Prophylaxis: 250 units IM. ▶L ♀C ▶? $$$$

VARICELLA-ZOSTER IMMUNE GLOBULIN (*VariZIG, VZIG*) Specialized dosing. ▶L ♀C ▶? $$$$$

TETANUS WOUND CARE (www.cdc.gov)		
	Uncertain or<3 prior tetanus immunizations	≥3 prior tetanus immunizations
Non tetanus-prone wound (e.g., clean and minor)	Td (DT if <7 yo)	Td if >10 yr since last dose
Tetanus-prone wound (e.g., dirt, contamination, punctures, crush components)	Td (DT if <7 yo) and tetanus immune globulin 250 units IM at site other than dT	Td if >5 yr since last dose

Immunosuppression (Specialized dosing for organ transplantation.)

BASILIXIMAB (*Simulect*) Specialized dosing for organ transplantation. ▶Plasma ♀B ▶? $$$$$

CYCLOSPORINE (*Sandimmune, Neoral, Gengraf*) Specialized dosing for organ transplantation, RA, and psoriasis. [Generic/Trade: microemulsion Caps 25, 100 mg. Generic/Trade: Caps (Sandimmune) 25, 100 mg, solution (Sandimmune) 100 mg/mL, microemulsion solution (Neoral, Gengraf) 100 mg/mL.] ▶L ♀C ▶- $$$$$

DACLIZUMAB (*Zenapax*) Specialized dosing for organ transplantation. ▶L ♀C ▶? $$$$$

MYCOPHENOLATE MOFETIL (*Cellcept, Myfortic*) Specialized dosing for organ transplantation. [Trade only (CellCept): caps 250 mg, tabs 500 mg, oral susp 200 mg/mL. Trade (Myfortic): tab, extended-release: 180, 360 mg.] ▶? ♀D ▶? $$$$$

SIROLIMUS (*Rapamune*) Specialized dosing for organ transplantation. [Trade only: oral solution 1 mg/mL (60 mL). Tab 1, 2 mg.] ▶L ♀C ▶- $$$$$

TACROLIMUS (*Prograf, FK 506*) Specialized dosing for organ transplantation. [Trade only: Caps 0.5, 1, 5 mg.] ▶L ♀C ▶- $$$$$

Other

HYMENOPTERA VENOM Specialized desensitization dosing protocol. ▶Serum ♀C ▶? $$$$

TUBERCULIN PPD (*Aplisol, Tubersol, Mantoux, PPD*) 5 TU (0.1 mL) intradermally, read 48–72 h later. ▶L ♀C ▶+ $

NEUROLOGY

Alzheimer's Disease—Cholinesterase Inhibitors

DONEPEZIL (*Aricept*) Start 5 mg PO qhs. May increase to 10 mg PO qhs in 4–6 wk. For severe disease (MMSE ≤10), the recommended dose is 10 mg/d. [Generic/Trade: Tabs 5,10 mg. Trade only: Orally disintegrating tabs 5,10 mg.] ▶LK ♀C ▶? $$$$

GALANTAMINE (*Razadyne, Razadyne ER, ✦Reminyl*) Extended release: Start 8 mg PO q am with food; increase to 16 mg q am after 4 wk. May increase
(cont.)

to 24 mg q am after another 4 wk. Immediate release: Start 4 mg PO bid with food; increase to 8 mg bid after 4 wk. May increase to 12 mg bid after another 4 wk. [Trade only: Tabs (Razadyne) 4, 8, 12 mg; oral solution 4 mg/mL. Extended release caps (Razadyne ER) 8, 16, 24 mg. Prior to April 2005 was called Reminyl.] ▶LK ♀B ▶? $$$$

RIVASTIGMINE (*Exelon, Exelon Patch*) Alzheimer's disease: Start 1.5 mg PO bid with food. Increase to 3 mg bid after 2 wk. Max 12 mg/d. Patch: Start 4.6 mg/24 h once daily; may increase after ≥1 mo to max 9.5 mg/24 h. Dementia associated with Parkinson's disease: Start 1.5 mg PO bid with food. Increase by 3 mg/d at intervals >4 wk to max 12 mg/d. Patch: Start 4.6 mg/24 h once daily; may increase after ≥1 mo to max 9.5 mg/24 h. Trade only: Caps 1.5, 3, 4.5, 6 mg. Trade only: Oral solution 2 mg/mL (120 mL). Transdermal patch: 4.6 mg/24 h (9 mg/patch), 9.5 mg/24 h (18 mg/patch). ▶K ♀B ▶? $$$$$

Alzheimer's Disease—NMDA Receptor Antagonists

MEMANTINE (*Namenda, ✦Ebixa*) Start 5 mg PO daily. Increase by 5 mg/d at weekly intervals to max 20 mg/d. Doses >5 mg/d should be divided bid. [Trade only: Tabs 5, 10 mg. Oral soln 2 mg/mL.] ▶KL ♀B ▶? $$$$

Anticonvulsants

CARBAMAZEPINE (*Tegretol, Tegretol XR, Carbatrol, Epitol, Equetro*) Epilepsy: 200–400 mg PO bid-qid. Extended-release: 200 mg PO bid. Age 6–12 yo: 100 mg PO bid or 50 mg PO qid; increase by 100 mg/d at weekly intervals divided tid-qid (regular release), bid (extended-release), or qid (susp). Age <6 yo: 10–20 mg/kg/d PO divided bid-qid. Bipolar disorder, acute manic/mixed episodes (Equetro): Start 200 mg PO bid; increase by 200 mg/d to max 1,600 mg/d. Aplastic anemia, agranulocytosis, many drug interactions. [Generic/Trade: Tabs 200 mg, chew tabs 100 mg, susp 100 mg/5 mL. Generic Only: Tabs 100,300,400 mg, chew tabs 200 mg. Trade only: Extended-release tabs (Tegretol XR): 100, 200, 400 mg. Extended-release caps (Carbatrol & Equetro): 100, 200, 300 mg.] ▶LK ♀D ▶+ $$

CLOBAZAM (*✦Frisium*) Canada only. Adults: Start 5–15 mg PO daily. Increase prn to max 80 mg/d. Children <2 yo: 0.5–1 mg/kg PO daily. Children 2–16 yo: Start 5 mg PO daily. May increase prn to max 40 mg/d. [Generic/Trade: Tabs 10 mg.] ▶L ♀X (*first trimester*) D (2nd/3rd trimesters) ▶- $

ETHOSUXIMIDE (*Zarontin*) Absence seizures, age 3–6 yo: Start 250 mg PO daily (or divided bid). Age >6 yo: Start 500 mg PO daily (or divided bid). Max 1.5 g/d. [Generic/Trade: Caps 250 mg. Syrup 250 mg/5 mL.] ▶LK ♀C ▶+ $$$$

FELBAMATE (*Felbatol*) Start 400 mg PO tid. Max 3,600 mg/d. Peds: Start 15 mg/kg/d PO divided tid-qid. Max 45 mg/kg/d. Aplastic anemia, hepatotoxicity. Not first line. Requires written informed consent. [Trade only: Tabs 400, 600 mg. Susp 600 mg/5 mL.] ▶KL ♀C ▶- $$$$$

FOSPHENYTOIN (*Cerebyx*) Load: 15–20 mg "phenytoin equivalents" (PE) per kg IM/IV no faster than 150 PE mg/min. Maintenance: 4–6 PE/kg/d. ▶L ♀D ▶+ $$$$$

GABAPENTIN (*Neurontin*) Partial seizures, adjunctive therapy: Start 300 mg PO qhs. Increase gradually to 300–600 mg PO tid. Max 3,600 mg/d. Postherpetic neuralgia: Start 300 mg PO on d 1; increase to 300 mg bid on d 2, and to 300 mg tid on d 3. Max 1,800 mg/d. Partial seizures, initial monotherapy: Titrate as above. Usual effective dose is 900–1,800 mg/d. [Generic only: Tabs 100, 300, 400 mg. Generic/Trade: Caps 100, 300, 400 mg. Tabs (scored) 600, 800 mg. Soln 50 mg/mL.] ▶K ♀C ▶? $$$$

LAMOTRIGINE (*Lamictal, Lamictal CD*) Partial seizures, Lennox-Gastaut syndrome, or generalized tonic-clonic seizures, adjunctive therapy with a single enzyme-inducing anticonvulsant. Age >12 yo: 50 mg PO daily × 2 wk, then 50 mg bid × 2 wk, then gradually increase to 150–250 mg PO bid. Age 2–12 yo: dosing based on weight and concomitant meds (see package insert). Also approved for conversion to monotherapy (age ≥16 yo): see package insert. Drug interaction with valproate (see package insert for adjusted dosing guidelines). Potentially life-threatening rashes reported in 0.3% of adults 0.8% of children; discontinue at first sign of rash. [Generic/Trade: Chewable dispersible tabs 5, 25 mg. Trade only: Tabs 25, 100, 150, 200 mg. Chewable dispersible tabs (Lamictal CD) 2 mg not available in pharmacies; obtain through manufacturer representative or call 1–888-825–5249.] ▶LK ♀C ▶- $$$$

LEVETIRACETAM (*Keppra*) Partial seizures, juvenile myoclonic epilepsy (JME), or primary generalized tonic-clonic seizures (GTC), adjunctive: Start 500 mg PO/IV bid; increase by 1,000 mg/d q2 wk prn to max 3,000 mg/d (partial seizures) or to target dose of 3,000 mg/d (JME or GTC). IV route not approved if <16 yo. [Trade only: Tabs 250, 500, 750, 1,000 mg. Oral solution 100 mg/mL.] ▶K ♀C ▶? $$$$$

OXCARBAZEPINE (*Trileptal*) Start 300 mg PO bid. Titrate to 1,200 mg/d (adjunctive) or 1,200–2,400 mg/d (monotherapy). Peds 2–16 yo: Start 8–10 mg/kg/d divided bid. Life-threatening rashes & hypersensitivity reported. [Generic/Trade: Tabs (scored) 150, 300, 600 mg. Trade only: Oral susp 300 mg/5 mL.] ▶LK ♀C ▶- $$$$$

PHENOBARBITAL (*Luminal*) Load: 20 mg/kg IV at rate ≤60 mg/min. Maintenance: 100–300 mg/d PO given once daily or divided bid; peds 3–5 mg/kg/d PO divided bid-tid. Many drug interactions. [Generic only: Tabs 15, 16.2, 30, 32.4, 60, 100 mg. Elixir 20 mg/5 mL.] ▶L ♀D ▶- ©IV $

PHENYTOIN (*Dilantin, Phenytek*) Status epilepticus: Load 10–15 mg/kg IV no faster than 50 mg/min, then 100 mg IV/PO q6–8h. Epilepsy: Oral load: 400 mg PO initially, then 300 mg in 2 h and 4 h. Maintenance: 5 mg/kg (or 300 mg PO) given once daily (extended-release) or divided tid (standard release) and titrated to a therapeutic level. [Generic/Trade: Extended-release caps 30, 100 mg (Dilantin). Susp 125 mg/5 mL. Chew tabs 50 mg. Trade only: Extended-release caps 200, 300 mg (Phenytek). Chew tabs 50 mg (Dilantin Infatabs).] ▶L ♀D ▶+ $$

PREGABALIN (*Lyrica*) Painful diabetic peripheral neuropathy: Start 50 mg PO tid; may increase within 1 wk to max 100 mg PO tid. Postherpetic neuralgia: Start 150 mg/d PO divided bid-tid. May increase within 1 wk to 300 mg/d PO divided bid-tid; max 600 mg/d. Partial seizures (adjunctive): Start

(cont.)

150 mg/d PO divided bid-tid; increase prn to max 600 mg/d divided bid-tid. Fibromyalgia: Start 75 mg PO bid; may increase to 150 mg bid within 1 wk; max 225 mg bid. [Trade only: Caps 25, 50, 75, 100, 150, 200, 225, 300 mg.] ▶K ♀C ▶? ©V $$$$$

PRIMIDONE (Mysoline) Start 100–125 mg PO qhs. Increase over 10 d to 250 mg tid-qid. Max 2 g/d. Metabolized to phenobarbital. [Generic/Trade: Tabs 50, 250 mg.] ▶LK ♀D ▶- $$$$

TIAGABINE (Gabitril) Start 4 mg PO daily. Increase by 4–8 mg/d at weekly intervals prn to max 32 mg (children ≥12 yo) or 56 mg/d (adults) divided bid-qid. Avoid off-label use. [Trade only: Tabs 2, 4, 12, 16 mg.] ▶L ♀C ▶? $$$$$

TOPIRAMATE (Topamax) Partial seizures or primary generalized tonic-clonic seizures, monotherapy (age >10 yo): Start 25 mg PO bid (wk 1), 50 mg bid (wk 2), 75 mg bid (wk 3), 100 mg bid (wk 4), 150 mg bid (wk 5), then 200 mg bid as tolerated. Partial seizures, primary generalized tonic-clonic seizures, or Lennox Gastaut Syndrome, adjunctive therapy: Start 25–50 mg PO qhs. Increase weekly by 25–50 mg/d to usual effective dose of 200 mg PO bid. Doses >400 mg/d not shown to be more effective. Migraine prophylaxis: 50 mg PO bid. [Trade only: Tabs 25, 50, 100, 200 mg. Sprinkle Caps 15, 25 mg.] ▶K ♀C ▶? $$$$$

VALPROIC ACID (Depakene, Depakote, Depakote ER, Depacon, Stavzor, divalproex, sodium valproate, ✛Epival, Deproic) Epilepsy: 10–15 mg/kg/d PO/IV divided bid-qid (standard release, delayed release, or IV) or given once daily (Depakote ER). Titrate to max 60 mg/kg/d. Use rate ≤20 mg/min when given IV. Migraine prophylaxis: Start 250 mg PO bid (Depakote or Stavzor) or 500 mg PO daily (Depakote ER) × 1 wk, then increase to max 1,000 mg/d PO divided bid (Depakote or Stavzor) or given once daily (Depakote ER). [Generic/Trade: Immediate release caps 250 mg (Depakene), syrup (Depakene, valproic acid) 250 mg/5 mL. Trade only (Depakote): Delayed release sprinkle caps 125 mg, delayed release tabs 125, 250, 500 mg; extended release tabs (Depakote ER) 250, 500 mg. Trade only (Stavzor): Delayed release caps 125, 250, 500 mg.] ▶L ♀D ▶+ $$$$

ZONISAMIDE (Zonegran) Start 100 mg PO daily. Titrate q2 wk to 200–400 mg/d given once daily or divided bid. Max 600 mg/d. Drug interactions. Contraindicated in sulfa allergy. [Generic/Trade: Caps 25, 50, 100 mg.] ▶LK ♀C ▶? $$$$

Migraine Therapy—Triptans (5-HT1 Receptor Agonists)

NOTE May cause vasospasm. Avoid in ischemic or vasospastic heart disease, cerebrovascular syndromes, peripheral arterial disease, uncontrolled HTN, and hemiplegic or basilar migraine. Do not use within 24 h of ergots or other triptans. Risk of serotonin syndrome if used with SSRIs or MAOIs.

ALMOTRIPTAN (Axert) 6.25–12.5 mg PO. May repeat in 2 h prn. Max 25 mg/d. Avoid MAOIs. [Trade only: Tabs 6.25, 12.5 mg.] ▶LK ♀C ▶? $$

ELETRIPTAN (Relpax) 20–40 mg PO. May repeat in >2 h prn. Max 40 mg/ dose or 80 mg/d. Drug interactions. Avoid MAOIs. [Trade only: Tabs 20, 40 mg.] ▶LK ♀C ▶? $$

FROVATRIPTAN (*Frova*)   2.5 mg PO. May repeat in 2 h prn. Max 7.5 mg/24 h. [Trade only: Tabs 2.5 mg.] ▶LK ♀C ▶? $

NARATRIPTAN (*Amerge*)   1–2.5 mg PO. May repeat in 4 h prn. Max 5 mg/24 h. [Trade only: Tabs 1, 2.5 mg.] ▶KL ♀C ▶? $$$

RIZATRIPTAN (*Maxalt, Maxalt MLT*)   5–10 mg PO. May repeat in 2 h prn. Max 30 mg/24 h. MLT form dissolves on tongue without liquids. Avoid MAOIs. [Trade only: Tabs 5, 10 mg. Orally disintegrating tabs (MLT) 5, 10 mg.] ▶LK ♀C ▶? $$

SUMATRIPTAN (*Imitrex*)   4–6 mg SC. May repeat in 1 h prn. Max 12 mg/24 h. Tabs: 25–100 mg PO (50 mg most common). May repeat q2 h prn with 25–100 mg doses. Max 200 mg/24 h. Intranasal spray: 5–20 mg q2 h. Max 40 mg/24 h. Avoid MAOIs. [Trade only: Tabs 25, 50, 100 mg. Nasal spray 5, 20 mg/spray. Injection (single-dose vial) 6 mg/0.5 mL. Injection (STATdose System) 4, 6 mg prefilled cartridges.] ▶LK ♀C ▶+ $$

TREXIMET (*sumatriptan + naproxen*)   1 tab PO at onset; may repeat in ≥2 h. Max 2 tabs/24 h. [Trade only: Tabs 85 mg sumatriptan + 500 mg naproxen sodium.] ▶LK ♀C ▶- $$$$

ZOLMITRIPTAN (*Zomig, Zomig ZMT*)   1.25–2.5 mg PO q2h. Max 10 mg/24 h. Orally disintegrating tabs (ZMT) 2.5 mg PO. May repeat in 2 h prn. Max 10 mg/24 h. Nasal spray: 5 mg (1 spray) in one nostril. May repeat in 2 h. Max 10 mg/24 h. [Trade only: Tabs 2.5, 5 mg. Orally disintegrating tabs (ZMT) 2.5, 5 mg. Nasal spray 5 mg/spray.] ▶L ♀C ▶? $$

Migraine Therapy—Other

CAFERGOT (*ergotamine + caffeine*)   2 tabs (1/100 mg each) PO at onset, then 1 tab q30 min prn. Max 6 tabs/attack or 10/wk. Drug interactions. Fibrotic complications. [Trade only: Tabs 1/100 mg ergotamine/caffeine.] ▶L ♀X ▶- $

DIHYDROERGOTAMINE (*D.H.E. 45, Migranal*)   Solution (DHE 45) 1 mg IV/IM/SC. May repeat in 1 h prn. Max 2 mg (IV) or 3 mg (IM/SC) per d. Nasal spray (Migranal): 1 spray in each nostril. May repeat in 15 min prn. Max 6 sprays/24 h or 8 sprays/wk. Drug interactions. Fibrotic complications. [Trade only: Nasal spray 0.5 mg/spray (Migranal). Self-injecting solution (D.H.E 45): 1 mg/mL.] ▶L ♀X ▶- $$

FLUNARIZINE (*♣Sibelium*)   Canada only. 10 mg PO qhs. [Generic/Trade: Caps 5 mg.] ▶L ♀C ▶- $$

MIDRIN (*isometheptene + dichloralphenazone + acetaminophen*)(*Amidrine, Durdrin, Migquin, Migratine, Migrazone, Va-Zone*)   Tension and vascular headache treatment: 1–2 caps PO q4h. Max 8 caps/d. Migraine treatment: 2 caps PO × 1, then 1 cap q1h prn to max 5 caps/12 h. [Generic only: Caps (isometheptene / dichloralphenazone / acetaminophen) 65/100/325 mg.] ▶L ♀? ▶? ©IV $

Multiple sclerosis

GLATIRAMER (*Copaxone*)   Multiple sclerosis: 20 mg SC daily. [Trade only: Injection 20 mg single dose vial.] ▶Serum ♀B ▶? $$$$$

Dermatomes

MOTOR FUNCTION BY NERVE ROOTS

Level	Motor Function
C3/C4/C5	Diaphragm
C5/C6	Deltoid/biceps
C7/C8	Triceps
C8/T1	Finger flexion/intrinsics
T1–T12	Intercostal/abd muscles
L2/L3	Hip flexion
L2/L3/L4	Hip adduction/quads
L4/L5	Ankle dorsiflexion
S1/S2	Ankle plantarflexion
S2/S3/S4	Rectal tone

LUMBOSACRAL NERVE ROOT COMPRESSION	Root	Motor	Sensory	Reflex
	L4	quadriceps	medial foot	knee-jerk
	L5	dorsiflexors	dorsum of foot	medial hamstring
	S1	plantarflexors	lateral foot	ankle-jerk

GLASGOW COMA SCALE

Eye Opening	Verbal Activity	Motor Activity
4. Spontaneous	5. Oriented	6. Obeys commands
3. To command	4. Confused	5. Localizes pain
2. To pain	3. Inappropriate	4. Withdraws to pain
1. None	2. Incomprehensible	3. Flexion to pain
	1. None	2. Extension to pain
		1. None

INTERFERON BETA-1A (*Avonex, Rebif*) Multiple sclerosis: Avonex-30 mcg (6 million units) IM q wk. Rebif- start 8.8 mcg SC three times weekly; titrate over 4 wk to maintenance dose of 44 mcg three times weekly. Suicidality, hepatotoxicity, blood dyscrasias. Follow LFTs and CBC. [Trade only: Avonex: Injection 30 mcg single dose vial with & without albumin. Pre-filled syringe 30 mcg. Rebif: Starter kit 20 mcg pre-filled syringe. Pre-filled syringe 22, 44 mcg.] ▶L ♀C ▶? $$$$$

INTERFERON BETA-1B (*Betaseron*) Multiple sclerosis: Start 0.0625 mg SC qod; titrate over six wk to 0.25 mg (8 million units) SC qod. Suicidality, hepatotoxicity. Follow LFTs. [Trade only: Injection 0.3 mg (9.6 million units) single dose vial.] ▶L ♀C ▶? $$$$$

Myasthenia Gravis

EDROPHONIUM (*Tensilon*) Evaluation for myasthenia gravis: 2 mg IV over 15–30 sec (test dose) while on cardiac monitor, then 8 mg IV after 45 sec. Atropine should be readily available in case of cholinergic reaction. Duration of effect is 5–10 min.] ▶Plasma ♀C ▶? $

NEOSTIGMINE (*Prostigmin*) 15–375 mg/d PO in divided doses, or 0.5 mg IM/SC. [Trade only: Tabs 15 mg.] ▶L ♀C ▶? $$$

PYRIDOSTIGMINE (*Mestinon, Mestinon Timespan, Regonal*) Myasthenia gravis: 60–200 mg PO tid (standard release) or 180 mg PO daily or divided bid (extended release). [Generic/Trade: Tabs 60 mg. Trade only: Extended release tabs 180 mg. Syrup 60 mg/5 mL.] ▶Plasma, K ♀C ▶+ $$

Parkinsonian Agents—Anticholinergics

BENZTROPINE MESYLATE (*Cogentin*) Parkinsonism: 0.5–2 mg IM/PO/IV given once daily or divided bid. Drug-induced extrapyramidal disorders: 1–4 mg PO/IM/IV given once daily or divided bid. [Generic only: Tabs 0.5, 1, 2 mg.] ▶LK ♀C ▶? $

BIPERIDEN (*Akineton*) 2 mg PO tid-qid, max 16 mg/d. [Trade only: Tabs 2 mg.] ▶LK ♀C ▶? $$$

TRIHEXYPHENIDYL (*Artane*) Start 1 mg PO daily. Gradually increase to 6–10 mg/d divided tid. Max 15 mg/d. [Generic only: Tabs 2, 5 mg. Elixir 2 mg/5 mL.] ▶LK ♀C ▶? $

Parkinsonian Agents—COMT Inhibitors

ENTACAPONE (*Comtan*) Start 200 mg PO with each dose of carbidopa/levodopa. Max 8 tabs (1,600 mg)/d. [Trade only: Tabs 200 mg.] ▶L ♀C ▶? $$$$$

Parkinsonian Agents—Dopaminergic Agents & Combinations

APOMORPHINE (*Apokyn*) Start 0.2 mL SC prn. May increase in 0.1 mL increments every few d. Monitor for orthostatic hypotension after initial dose and with dose escalation. Max 0.6 mL/dose or 2 mL/d. Potent emetic - pretreat with trimethobenzamide 300 mg PO tid starting 3d prior to use, and continue for ≧2 mo. Contains sulfites. [Trade only: Cartridges (for injector pen, 10 mg/mL) 3 mL. Ampules (10 mg/mL) 2 mL.] ▶L ♀C ▶? $$$$$

CARBIDOPA-LEVODOPA (*Sinemet, Sinemet CR, Parcopa*) Start 1 tab (25/100 mg) PO tid. Increase q1–4 d as needed. Sustained release: Start 1 tab (50/200 mg) PO bid; increase q 3d as needed. [Generic/Trade: Tabs (carbidopa/levodopa) 10/100, 25/100, 25/250 mg. Tabs, sustained release (Sinemet CR, carbidopa-levodopa ER) 25/100, 50/200 mg. Trade only: orally disintegrating tab (Parcopa) 10/100, 25/100, 25/250.] ▶L ♀C ▶? $$$$$

PRAMIPEXOLE (*Mirapex*) Parkinson's disease: Start 0.125 mg PO tid. Gradually increase to 0.5–1.5 mg PO tid. Restless legs syndrome: Start 0.125 mg PO 2–3 h prior to bedtime. May increase q4–7 d to max 0.5 mg/dose. [Generic/Trade: Tabs 0.125, 0.25, 0.5, 1, 1.5 mg. Trade only: Tabs 0.75 mg.] ▶K ♀C ▶? $$$$$

ROPINIROLE (*Requip, Requip XL*) Parkinson's disease: Start 0.25 mg PO tid, then gradually increase to 1 mg PO tid. Extended-release: Start 2 mg PO daily, then gradually titrate dose at ≧ weekly intervals. Max 24 mg/d. Restless legs syndrome: Start 0.25 mg PO 1–3 h before sleep for 2 d, then increase to 0.5 mg/d on d 3–7. Increase by 0.5 mg/d at weekly intervals prn to max 4 mg/d given 1–3 h before sleep. [Generic/Trade: Tabs 0.25, 0.5, 1, 2, 3, 4 mg. Trade only: Tabs 5 mg, Extended-release caps 2, 3, 4, 8 mg.] ▶L ♀C ▶? $$$$$

STALEVO (*carbidopa + levodopa + entacapone*) Parkinson's disease (conversion from carbidopa-levodopa +/- entacapone): Start Stalevo tab that contains the same amount of carbidopa-levodopa as the patient was previously taking, and titrate to desired response. May need to reduce levodopa dose if not already taking entacapone. [Trade only: Tabs (carbidopa/levodopa/entacapone): Stalevo 50 (12.5/50/200 mg), Stalevo 100 (25/100/200 mg), Stalevo 150 (37.5/150/200 mg), Stalevo 200 (50/200/200 mg).] ▶L ♀C ▶ - $$$$$

Parkinsonian Agents—Monoamine Oxidase Inhibitors (MAOIs)

RASAGILINE (*Azilect*) Parkinson's disease, monotherapy: 1 mg PO qam. Parkinson's disease, adjunctive: 0.5 mg PO qam. Max 1 mg/d. MAOI diet. [Trade only: Tabs 0.5, 1 mg.] ▶L ♀C ▶? $$$$$

SELEGILINE (*Eldepryl, Zelapar*) 5 mg PO q am at noon, max 10 mg/d. Zelapar ODT: 1.25–2.5 mg q am, max 2.5 mg/d. [Generic/Trade: Caps 5 mg. Tabs 5 mg. Trade only: Oral disintegrating tabs (Zelapar ODT) 1.25 mg.] ▶LK ♀C ▶? $$$$

Other Agents

BOTULINUM TOXIN TYPE A (*Botox, Botox Cosmetic*) Dose varies based on indication. [Trade only: 100 unit single-use vials.] ▶Not absorbed ♀C ▶? $$$$$

MANNITOL (*Osmitrol, Resectisol*) Intracranial HTN: 0.25–2 g/kg IV over 30–60 min. ▶K ♀C ▶? $$

NIMODIPINE (*Nimotop*) Subarachnoid hemorrhage: 60 mg PO q4h × 21 d. [Generic/Trade: Caps 30 mg.] ▶L ♀C ▶ - $$$$$

OXYBATE (*Xyrem, GHB, gamma hydroxybutyrate*) Narcolepsy-associated cataplexy or excessive daytime sleepiness: 2.25 g PO qhs. Repeat in 2.5–4h. May increase by 1.5 g/d at > 2 wk intervals to max 9 g/d. From a centralized pharmacy. [Trade only: Solution 180 mL (500 mg/mL) supplied with measuring device and child-proof dosing cups.] ▶L ♀B ▶? ©III $$$$$

RILUZOLE (*Rilutek*) ALS: 50 mg PO q12h. Monitor LFTs. [Trade only: Tabs 50 mg.] ▶LK ♀C ▶ - $$$$$

TETRABENAZINE (*Xenazine, +Nitoman*) Start 12.5 mg PO qam. Increase after 1 wk to 12.5 mg PO bid. May increase by 12.5 mg/d ≥ weekly. For doses > 37.5-50 mg/d divide doses tid. For doses > 50 mg/d genotype for CYP2D6 and titrate by 12.5 mg/d weekly and divide tid to max 100 mg/d and 37.5 mg/ dose (extensive/intermediate metabolizers) or 50 mg/d and 25 mg/dose (poor metabolizers). ▶L ♀? ▶ - $$$$

OB/GYN

Contraceptives (Oral contraceptives table on page 119.)

ETONOGESTREL (*Implanon*) Contraception: 1 subdermal implant every three yr. [Trade only: Single rod implant, 68 mg etonogestrel.] ▶L ♀X ▶+ $$$$$

LEVONORGESTREL (*Plan B*) Emergency contraception: 1 tab PO ASAP but within 72 h of intercourse. 2nd tab 12 h later. [OTC: Trade only: Kit contains 2 tabs 0.75 mg.] ▶L ♀X ▶ - $$

NUVARING (*ethinyl estradiol vaginal ring + etonogestrel*) Contraception: 1 ring intravaginally × 3 wk each mo. [Trade only: Flexible intravaginal ring, 15 mcg ethinyl estradiol/0.120 mcg etonogestrel/d. 1 and 3 rings/box.] ▶L ♀X ▶- $$$

ORTHO EVRA (*norelgestromin + ethinyl estradiol transdermal, ✦Evra*) Contraception: 1 patch q wk × 3 wk, then 1 wk patch-free. [Trade only: Transdermal patch: 150 mcg norelgestromin + 20 mcg ethinyl estradiol/d. 1 and 3 patches/box.] ▶L ♀X ▶- $$$

Estrogens

NOTE *See also Hormone Combinations.*

ESTERIFIED ESTROGENS (*Menest*) 0.3 to 1.25 mg PO daily. [Trade only: Tabs 0.3, 0.625, 1.25, 2.5 mg.] ▶L ♀X ▶- $$

ESTRADIOL (*Estrace, Gynodiol*) 1–2 mg PO daily. [Generic/Trade: Tabs, micronized 0.5, 1, 2 mg, scored. Trade only: 1.5 mg (Gynodiol).] ▶L ♀X ▶- $

ESTRADIOL ACETATE (*Femtrace*) 0.45–1.8 mg PO daily. [Trade only: Tabs, 0.45, 0.9, 1.8 mg.] ▶L ♀X ▶- $$

ESTRADIOL ACETATE VAGINAL RING (*Femring*) Menopausal atrophic vaginitis & vasomotor symptoms: Insert & replace after 90 d. [Trade only: 0.05 mg/d and 0.1 mg/d.] ▶L ♀X ▶- $$

ESTRADIOL CYPIONATE (*Depo-Estradiol*) 1–5 mg IM q 3–4 wk. ▶L ♀X ▶- $

ESTRADIOL GEL (*Divigel, Estrogel, Elestrin*) Thinly apply contents of one complete pump depression to one entire arm (Estrogel) or upper arm (Elestrin) or contents of one foil packet (Divigel) to one upper thigh. [Trade only: Gel 0.06% in non-aerosol, metered-dose pump with #64 or #32 - 1.25 g doses (Estrogel) & #100 - 0.87 g doses (Elestrin). Gel 0.1% in single dose foil packets of 0.25, 0.5 & 1.0 g, carton of 30.] ▶L ♀X ▶- $$$

ESTRADIOL TOPICAL EMULSION (*Estrasorb*) Rub contents of 1 pouch each to left or right legs (spread & thighs & calves) qam. Daily dose: two 1.74 g pouches. [Trade only: Topical emulsion, 56 pouches/carton.] ▶L ♀X ▶- $$

ESTRADIOL TRANSDERMAL PATCH (*Alora, Climara, Esclim, Estraderm, FemPatch, Menostar, Vivelle, Vivelle Dot, ✦Estradot, Oesclim*) Apply one patch/wk (Climara, FemPatch, Estradiol, Menostar) or 2/wk (Esclim, Estraderm, Vivelle, Vivelle Dot, Alora). [Generic/Trade: Transdermal patches doses in mg/d: Climara (q wk) 0.025, 0.0375, 0.05, 0.06, 0.075, 0.1. Trade only: FemPatch (q wk) 0.025. Esclim (twice/wk) 0.025, 0.0375, 0.05, 0.075, 0.1. Vivelle, Vivelle Dot (twice/wk) 0.025, 0.0375, 0.05, 0.075, 0.1. Estraderm (twice/wk) 0.05, & 0.1. Alora (twice/wk) 0.025, 0.05, 0.075, 0.1.] ▶L ♀X ▶- $$

ESTRADIOL TRANSDERMAL SPRAY (*Evamist*) 1–3 sprays daily to forearm. [Trade only: Spray: 1.53 mg estradiol per 90 mcL spray, 56 sprays per metered-dose pump.] ▶L ♀X ▶- $$$

ESTRADIOL VAGINAL RING (*Estring*) Menopausal atrophic vaginitis: Insert & replace after 90 d. [Trade only: 2 mg ring single pack.] ▶L ♀X ▶- $$$

ESTRADIOL VAGINAL TAB (*Vagifem*) Menopausal atrophic vaginitis: 1 tab vaginally daily × 2 wk, then 1 tab vaginally 2×/wk. [Trade only: Vaginal tab: 25 mcg in disposable single-use applicators, 8 & 18/pack.] ▶L ♀X ▶- $-$$

ESTRADIOL VALERATE (*Delestrogen*) 10–20 mg IM q4 wk. ▶L ♀X ▶- $

ESTROGEN VAGINAL CREAM (*Premarin, Estrace*) Menopausal atrophic vaginitis: Premarin: 0.5–2 g daily. Estrace: 2–4 g daily × 2 wk, then reduce. [Trade only: Vaginal cream. Premarin: 0.625 mg conjugated estrogens/g in 42.5 g with or w/o calibrated applicator. Estrace: 0.1 mg estradiol/g in 42.5 g w/ calibrated applicator.] ▶L ♀X ▶? $$$$

ESTROGENS CONJUGATED (*Premarin, C.E.S., Congest*) 0.3 to 1.25 mg PO daily. Abnormal uterine bleeding: 25 mg IV/IM. Repeat in 6–12 h if needed. [Trade only: Tabs 0.3, 0.45, 0.625, 0.9, 1.25 mg.] ▶L ♀X ▶- $$

ESTROGENS SYNTHETIC CONJUGATED A (*Cenestin*) 0.3 to 1.25 mg PO daily. [Trade only: Tabs 0.3, 0.45, 0.625, 0.9, 1.25 mg.] ▶L ♀X ▶- $$$

ESTROGENS SYNTHETIC CONJUGATED B (*Enjuvia*) 0.3 to 1.25 mg PO daily. [Trade only: Tabs 0.3, 0.45, 0.625, 0.9, 1.25 mg.] ▶L ♀X ▶- $$

ESTROPIPATE (*Ogen, Ortho-Est*) 0.75 to 6 mg PO daily. [Generic/Trade: Tabs 0.75, 1.5, 3, 6 mg of estropipate.] ▶L ♀X ▶- $

Hormone Combinations

NOTE *See also estrogens.*

ACTIVELLA (*estradiol + norethindrone*) 1 tab PO daily. [Trade only: Tab 1/0.5 mg and 0.5/0.1 mg estradiol/norethindrone acetate in calendar dial pack dispenser.] ▶L ♀X ▶- $$

ANGELIQ (*estradiol + drospirenone*) 1 tab PO daily. [Trade only: Tabs 1 mg estradiol/0.5 mg drospirenone.] ▶L ♀X ▶- $$

CLIMARA PRO (*estradiol + levonorgestrel*) 1 patch weekly. [Trade only: Transdermal 0.045/0.015 estradiol/levonorgestrel in mg/d, 4 patches/box.] ▶L ♀X ▶- $$

COMBIPATCH (*estradiol + norethindrone*) (✦*Estalis*) 1 patch twice weekly. [Trade only: Transdermal patch 0.05 estradiol/ 0.14 norethindrone & 0.05 estradiol/0.25 norethindrone in mg/d, 8 patches/box.] ▶L ♀X ▶- $$$

ESTRATEST (*esterified estrogens + methyltestosterone*) 1 tab PO daily. [Trade only: Tabs 1.25 mg esterified estrogens/2.5 mg methyltestosterone.] ▶L ♀X ▶- $$$$

ESTRATEST H.S. (*esterified estrogens + methyltestosterone*) 1 tab PO daily. [Trade only: Tabs 0.625 mg esterified estrogens/1.25 mg methyltestosterone.] ▶L ♀X ▶- $$$

FEMHRT (*ethinyl estradiol + norethindrone*) 1 tab PO daily. [Trade only: Tabs 5/1 and 2.5/0.5 mcg ethinyl estradiol/mg norethindrone, 28/blister card.] ▶L ♀X ▶- $$

EMERGENCY CONTRACEPTION within 72 h of unprotected sex: Take 1st dose ASAP, then identical dose 12 h later. *Plan B* kit contains 2 levonorgestrel 0.75 mg tabs. Each dose is 1 pill. Progestin-only method causes less nausea & may be more effective. Alternate regimens: Each dose is either 2 pills of *Ovral* or *Ogestrel*, 4 pills of *Cryselle, Levlen, Levora, Lo/Ovral, Nordette, Tri-Levlen*, Triphasil*, Trivora*,* or *Low Ogestrel*, or 5 pills of *Alesse, Aviane, Lessina,* or *Levlite*. If vomiting occurs within 1 h of taking either dose, consider whether to repeat dose with antiemetic 1h prior. More info at: www.not-2-late.com.

---

*Use 0.125 mg levonorgestrel/30 mcg ethinyl estradiol tabs.

ORAL CONTRACEPTIVES* ▶L ♀X *Monophasic*	Estrogen (mcg)	Progestin (mg)
Norinyl 1+50, Ortho-Novum 1/50, Necon 1/50	50 mestranol	1 norethindrone
Ovcon-50		
Demulen 1/50, Zovia 1/50E	50 eth estradiol	1 ethynodiol
Ovral, Ogestrel		0.5 norgestrel
Norinyl 1+35, Ortho-Novum 1/35, Necon 1/35, Nortrel 1/35		1 norethindrone
Brevicon, Modicon, Necon 0.5/35, Nortrel 0.5/35		0.5 norethindrone
Ovcon-35, Femcon Fe, Balziva	35 eth estradiol	0.4 norethindrone
Previfem		0.18 norgestimate
Ortho-Cyclen, MonoNessa, Sprintec-28		0.25 norgestimate
Demulen 1/35, Zovia 1/35E, Kelnor 1/35		1 ethynodiol
Loestrin 21 1.5/30, Loestrin Fe 1.5/30, Junel 1.5/30, Junel Fe 1.5/30, Microgestin Fe 1.5/30		1.5 norethindrone
Cryselle, Lo/Ovral, Low-Ogestrel		0.3 norgestrel
Apri, Desogen, Ortho-Cept, Reclipsen	30 eth estradiol	0.15 desogestrel
Levlen, Levora, Nordette, Portia, Seasonale, Seasonique†, Quasense		0.15 levonorgestrel
Yasmin		3 drospirenone
Loestrin 21 1/20, Loestrin Fe 1/20, Loestin 24 Fe, Junel 1/20, Junel Fe 1/20, Microgestin Fe 1/20		1 norethindrone
Alesse, Aviane, Lessina, Levlite, Lutera, Lo Seasonique††	20 eth estradiol	0.1 levonorgestrel
Lybrel		0.09 levonorgestrel
Yaz		3 drospirenone
Kariva, Mircette	20/10 eth estrad	0.15 desogestrel
Progestin-only		
Micronor, Nor-Q.D., Camila, Errin, Jolivette, Nora-BE	none	0.35 norethindrone
Biphasic (estrogen & progestin contents vary)		
Ortho Novum 10/11, Necon 10/11	35 eth estradiol	0.5/1 norethindrone
Triphasic (estrogen & progestin contents vary)		
Cyclessa, Velivet	25 eth estradiol	0.100/0.125/0.150 desogestrel
Ortho-Novum 7/7/7, Necon 7/7/7, Nortrel 7/7/7	35 eth estradiol	0.5/0.75/1 norethindr
Tri-Norinyl, Leena, Aranelle		0.5/1/0.5 norethindr
Enpresse, Tri-Levlen, Triphasil, Trivora-28	30/40/30 eth estradiol	0.5/0.75/0.125 levonorgestrel
Ortho Tri-Cyclen, Trinessa, Tri-Sprintec, Tri-Previfem	35 eth estradiol	0.18/0.215/0.25 norgestimate
Ortho Tri-Cyclen Lo	25 eth estradiol	
Estrostep Fe, Tri-Legest, Tri-Legest Fe	20/30/35 eth estr	1 norethindrone

*All: Not recommended in smokers. Increase risk of thromboembolism, stroke, MI, hepatic neoplasia & GB disease. Nausea, breast tenderness, & breakthrough bleeding are common transient side effects. Effectiveness reduced by hepatic enzyme-inducing drugs such as certain anticonvulsants & barbiturates, rifampin, rifabutin, griseofulvin, & protease inhibitors. Coadmin with St. John's wort may decrease efficacy. Vomiting or diarrhea may also increase risk of contraceptive failure. Consider additional form of birth control in above circumstances. See product insert for instructions on missing doses. Most available in 21 and 28 day packs. **Progestin only:** Must be taken same time every d. Because most literature on OC adverse effects pertains to estrogen/progestin combinations, extent to which progestin-only contraceptives cause these effects unclear. No significant interaction found with broad-spectrum antibiotics. Effect of St. John's wort unclear. No placebo days, start new pack immediately after finishing current one. Available in 28 d packs. Useful website: www.managingcontraception.com. †84 light blue-green active pills followed by 7 yellow pills w/ 10 mcg ethinyl estradiol. ††84 orange active pills followed by 7 yellow pills w/ 10mcg ethinyl estradiol

PREFEST (*estradiol + norgestimate*) 1 pink tab PO daily × 3 d followed by 1 white tab PO daily × 3 d, sequentially throughout the mo. [Trade only: Tabs in 30-d blister packs 1 mg estradiol (15 pink) & 1 mg estadiol/0.09 mg norgestimate (15 white).] ▶L ♀X ▶- $$$

PREMPHASE (*estrogens conjugated + medroxyprogesterone*) 1 tab PO daily. [Trade only: Tabs in 28-d EZ-Dial dispensers: 0.625 mg conjugated estrogens (14) & 0.625 mg/5 mg conjugated estrogens/medroxyprogesterone (14).] ▶L ♀X ▶- $$$

PREMPRO (*estrogens conjugated + medroxyprogesterone, ✦Premplus*) 1 tab PO daily. [Trade only: Tabs in 28-d EZ-Dial dispensers: 0.625 mg/5 mg, 0.625 mg/2.5 mg, 0.45 mg/1.5 mg (Prempro low dose), or 0.3 mg/1.5 mg conjugated estrogens/medroxyprogesterone.] ▶L ♀X ▶- $$$

SYNTEST D.S. (*esterified estrogens + methyltestosterone*) 1 tab PO daily. [Trade only: Tabs 1.25 mg esterified estrogens/2.5 mg methyltestosterone.] ▶L ♀X ▶- $$

SYNTEST H.S. (*esterified estrogens + methyltestosterone*) 1 tab PO daily. [Trade only: Tabs 0.625 mg esterified estrogens/1.25 mg methyltestosterone.] ▶L ♀X ▶- $$

Labor Induction/Cervical Ripening

DINOPROSTONE (*PGE2, Prepidil, Cervidil, Prostin E2*) Cervical ripening: One syringe of gel placed directly into the cervical os for cervical ripening or one insert in the posterior fornix of the vagina. [Trade only: Gel (Prepidil) 0.5 mg/3 g syringe. Vaginal insert (Cervidil) 10 mg. Vaginal supp (Prostin E2) 20 mg.] ▶Lung ♀C ▶? $$$$$

OXYTOCIN (*Pitocin*) Labor induction: 10 units in 1000 mL NS (10 milliunits/mL), start at 6–12 mL/h (1–2 milliunits/min). Postpartum bleeding: 10 units IM or 10–40 units in 1000 mL NS IV, infuse 20–40 milliunits/min. ▶LK ♀? ▶- $

Ovulation Stimulants

CLOMIPHENE (*Clomid, Serophene*) Specialized dosing for ovulation induction. [Generic/Trade: Tabs 50 mg, scored.] ▶L ♀D ▶? $$

Progestins

HYDROXYPROGESTERONE CAPROATE Amenorrhea, dysfunctional uterine bleeding, metrorrhagia: 375 mg IM. Production of secretory endometrium & desquamation: 125–250 mg IM on 10th d of the cycle, repeat q7d until suppression no longer desired. ▶L ♀X ▶? $

MEDROXYPROGESTERONE (*Provera, Amen*) 10 mg PO daily for last 10–12 d of mo, or 2.5–5 mg PO daily. Secondary amenorrhea, abnormal uterine bleeding: 5–10 mg PO daily × 5–10 d. Endometrial hyperplasia: 10–30 mg PO daily. [Generic/Trade: Tabs 2.5, 5, & 10 mg, scored.] ▶L ♀X ▶-

MEDROXYPROGESTERONE—INJECTABLE (*Depo-Provera, depo-subQ provera 104*) Contraception/Endometriosis: 150 mg IM in deltoid or gluteus maximus or 104 mg SC in anterior thigh or abdomen q13 wk. ▶L ♀X ▶+ $

MEGESTROL (*Megace, Megace ES*) Endometrial hyperplasia: 40–160 mg PO daily × 3–4 mo. AIDS anorexia: 800 mg (20 mL) susp PO daily or 625 mg (5 mL) ES daily. [Generic/Trade: Tabs 20 & 40 mg. Susp 40 mg/mL in 240 mL. Trade only: Megace ES susp 125 mg/mL (150 mL).] ▶L ♀D ▶? $$$$$

NORETHINDRONE (*Aygestin, Micronor, Nor-Q.D., Camila, Errin, Jolivette, Nora-BE*) Amenorrhea, abnormal uterine bleeding: 2.5–10 mg PO daily × 5–10 d during the second half of the menstrual cycle. Endometriosis: 5 mg PO daily × 2 wk. Increase by 2.5 mg q 2 wk to 15 mg. [Generic/Trade: Tabs 5 mg, scored. Trade only: 0.35 mg tabs.] ▶L ♀D/X ▶

PROGESTERONE GEL (*Crinone, Prochieve*) Secondary amenorrhea: 45 mg (4%) intravaginally qod up to 6 doses. If no response, use 90 mg (8%) qod up to 6 doses. Infertility: special dosing. [Trade only: 4%, 8% single-use, prefilled applicators.] ▶Plasma ♀- ▶? $$$

PROGESTERONE MICRONIZED (*Prometrium*) 200 mg PO qhs 10–12 d/ mo or 100 mg qhs daily. Secondary amenorrhea: 400 mg PO qhs × 10 d. Contraindicated in peanut allergy. [Trade only: Caps 100 & 200 mg.] ▶L ♀B ▶+ $$

PROGESTERONE VAGINAL INSERT (*Endometrin*) Infertility: special dosing. [Trade only: 100 mg vaginal insert.] ▶Plasma ♀- ▶? $$$$

Selective Estrogen Receptor Modulators

RALOXIFENE (*Evista*) Osteoporosis prevention/treatment, breast cancer prevention: 60 mg PO daily. [Trade only: Tabs 60 mg.] ▶L ♀X ▶- $$$$

TAMOXIFEN (*Nolvadex, Soltamox, Tamone, ✦Tamofen*) Breast cancer prevention: 20 mg PO daily × 5 yr. Breast cancer: 10–20 mg PO bid. [Generic/Trade: Tabs 10 & 20 mg, Trade only (Soltamox): sugar-free soln 10 mg/5 mL (150 mL).] ▶L ♀D ▶- $$$$

Uterotonics

CARBOPROST (*Hemabate, 15-methyl-prostaglandin F2 alpha*) Refractory postpartum uterine bleeding: 250 mcg deep IM. ▶LK ♀C ▶? $$$

METHYLERGONOVINE (*Methergine*) Refractory postpartum uterine bleeding: 0.2 mg IM/PO tid-qid prn. [Trade only: Tabs 0.2 mg.] ▶LK ♀C ▶? $

Vaginitis Preparations

NOTE *See also STD/vaginitis table in antimicrobial section.*

BORIC ACID Resistant vulvovaginal candidiasis: 1 vag supp qhs × wk. [No commercial preparation; must be compounded by pharmacist. Vaginal suppositories 600 mg in gelatin caps.] ▶Not absorbed ♀? ▶- $

BUTOCONAZOLE (*Gynazole, Mycelex-3*) Vulvovaginal candidiasis: Mycelex 3: 1 applicatorful qhs × 3–6 d. Gynazole-1: 1 applicatorful intravaginally qhs × 1. [OTC: Trade only (Mycelex 3): 2% vaginal cream in 5 g pre-filled applicators (3s) & 20 g tube with applicators. Rx: Trade only (Gynazole-1): 2% vaginal cream in 5 g pre-filled applicator.] ▶LK ♀C ▶? $(OTC), $$$(Rx)

DRUGS GENERALLY ACCEPTED AS SAFE IN PREGNANCY (selected)

Analgesics: acetaminophen, codeine*, meperidine*, methadone*. **Antimicrobials:** penicillins, cephalosporins, erythromycin (not estolate), azithromycin, nystatin, clotrimazole, metronidazole, nitrofurantoin***, Nix. **Antivirals:** acyclovir, valacyclovir, famciclovir. **CV:** labetalol, methyldopa, hydralazine, nifedipine. **Derm:** erythromycin, clindamycin, benzoyl peroxide. **Endo:** insulin, liothyronine, levothyroxine. **ENT:** chlorpheniramine, diphenhydramine, dimenhydrinate, dextromethorphan, guaifenesin, nasal steroids, nasal cromolyn. **GI:** trimethobenzamide, antacids*, simethicone, cimetidine, famotidine, ranitidine, nizatidine, psyllium, metoclopramide, bisacodyl, docusate, doxylamine, meclizine. **Heme:** Heparin, low molecular weight heparins. **Psych:** desipramine, doxepin. **Pulmonary:** short-acting inhaled beta-2 agonists, cromolyn, nedocromil, beclomethasone, budesonide, theophylline, prednisone**. *Except if used long-term or in high dose at term. **Except 1st trimester. ***Contraindicated at term & during labor & delivery.

APGAR SCORE		0. Absent	1. <100	2. >100
	Heart rate	0. Absent	1. <100	2. >100
	Respirations	0. Absent	1. Slow/irreg	2. Good/crying
	Muscle tone	0. Limp	1. Some flexion	2. Active motion
	Reflex irritability	0. No response	1. Grimace	2. Cough/sneeze
	Color	0. Blue	1. Blue extremities	2. Pink

CLINDAMYCIN—VAGINAL (Cleocin, Clindesse, ✚Dalacin) Bacterial vaginosis: Cleocin: 1 applicatorful cream qhs × 7d or one vaginal supp qhs × 3d. Clindesse: 1 applicatorful cream × 1. [Generic/Trade: 2% vaginal cream in 40 g tube with 7 disposable applicators (Cleocin). Vag supp (Cleocin Ovules) 100 mg (3) w/applicator. 2% vaginal cream in a single-dose prefilled applicator (Clindesse).] ▶L ♀− ▶+ $$

CLOTRIMAZOLE—VAGINAL (Mycelex 7, Gyne-Lotrimin, ✚Canesten, Clotrimaderm) Vulvovaginal candidiasis: 1 applicatorful 1% cream qhs × 7 d. 1 applicatorful 2% cream qhs × 3 d. 1 vag supp 100 mg qhs × 7 d. 200 mg supp qhs × 3 d [OTC Generic/Trade: 1% vaginal cream with applicator (some pre-filled). 2% vaginal cream with applicator and 1% topical cream in some combination packs. OTC Trade only (Gyne-Lotrimin): Vaginal suppositories 100 mg (7) & 200 mg (3) with applicators.] ▶LK ♀B ▶? $

METRONIDAZOLE—VAGINAL (MetroGel-Vaginal, Vandazole) Bacterial vaginosis: 1 applicatorful qhs or bid × 5 d. [Generic/Trade: 0.75% gel in 70 g tube with applicator.] ▶LK ♀B ▶? $$

MICONAZOLE (Monistat, Femizol-M, M-Zole, Micozole, Monazole) Vulvovaginal candidiasis: 1 applicatorful qhs × 3 (4%) or 7 (2%) d. 100 mg vag supp qhs × 7 d. 400 mg vag supp qhs × 3 d. 1200 mg vag supp × 1. [OTC: Generic/Trade: 2% vaginal cream in 45 g with 1 applicator or 7 disposable applicators. Vaginal suppositories 100 mg (7) OTC: Trade only: 400 mg (3) & 1200 mg (1) with applicator. Generic/Trade: 4% vaginal cream in 25 g tubes or 3 prefilled applicators. Some in combination packs with 2% miconazole cream for external use.] ▶LK ♀+ ▶? $

NYSTATIN—VAGINAL (Mycostatin, ✚Nilstat, Nyaderm) Vulvovaginal candidiasis: 1 vag tab qhs × 14 d. [Generic/Trade: Vaginal Tabs 100,000 units in 15s & 30s with or without applicator(s).] ▶Not metabolized ♀A ▶? $$

TERCONAZOLE (*Terazol*) Vulvovaginal candidiasis: 1 applicatorful of 0.4% cream qhs × 7 d, or 1 applicatorful of 0.8% cream qhs × 3 d, or 80 mg vag supp qhs × 3 d. [All forms supplied with applicators: Generic/Trade: Vag cream 0.4% (Terazol 7) in 45 g tube, 0.8% (Terazol 3) in 20 g tube. Vag supp (Terazol 3) 80 mg (#3).] ▶LK ♀C ▶- $$

TIOCONAZOLE (*Monistat 1-Day, Vagistat-1*) Vulvovaginal candidiasis: 1 applicatorful of 6.5% ointment intravaginally qhs single-dose. [OTC: Trade only: Vaginal ointment: 6.5% (300 mg) in 4.6 g prefilled single-dose applicator.] ▶Not absorbed ♀C ▶- $

Other OB/GYN Agents

DANAZOL (*Danocrine, ✦Cyclomen*) Endometriosis: Start 400 mg PO bid, then titrate downward to maintain amenorrhea × 3–6 mo. Fibrocystic breast disease: 100–200 mg PO bid × 4–6 mo. [Generic only: Caps 50, 100, 200 mg.] ▶L ♀X ▶- $$$$$

MIFEPRISTONE (*Mifeprex, RU-486*) 600 mg PO × 1 followed by 400 mcg misoprostol on d 3, if abortion not confirmed. [Trade only: Tabs 200 mg.] ▶L ♀X ▶? $$$$$

PREMESIS-RX (*pyridoxine + folic acid + cyanocobalamin + calcium carbonate*) Pregnancy-induced nausea: 1 tab PO daily. [Trade only: Tabs 75 mg vitamin B6 (pyridoxine), sustained-release, 12 mcg vitamin B12 (cyanocobalamin), 1 mg folic acid, and 200 mg calcium carbonate.] ▶L ♀A ▶+ $

RHO IMMUNE GLOBULIN (*HyperRHO S/D, MICRhoGAM, RhoGAM, Rhophylac, WinRho SDF*) 300 mcg vial IM to mother at 28 wk gestation followed by a 2nd dose ≤72 h of delivery (if mother Rh- and baby is or might be Rh+). Microdose (50 mcg, MICRhoGAM) OK if spontaneous abortion <12 wk gestation. ▶L ♀C ▶? $$$$$

ONCOLOGY

ALKYLATING AGENTS altretamine (*Hexalen*), bendamustine (*Treanda*), busulfan (*Mylean, Busulfex*), carmustine (*BCNU, BiCNU, Gliadel*), chlorambucil (*Leukeran*), cyclophosphamide (*Cytoxan, Neosar*), dacarbazine (*DTIC-Dome*), ifosfamide (*Ifex*), lomustine (*CeeNu, CCNU*), mechlorethamine (*Mustargen*), melphalan (*Alkeran*), procarbazine (*Matulane*), streptozocin (*Zanosar*), temozolomide (*Temodar, ✦Temodal*), thiotepa (*Thioplex*). Antibiotics: bleomycin (*Blenoxane*), dactinomycin (*Cosmegen*), daunorubicin (*DaunoXome, Cerubidine*), doxorubicin liposomal (*Doxil, ✦Caelyx, Myocet*), doxorubicin non-liposomal (*Adriamycin, Rubex*), epirubicin (*Ellence, ✦Pharmorubicin*), idarubicin (*Idamycin*), mitomycin (*Mutamycin, Mitomycin-C*), mitoxantrone (*Novantrone*), valrubicin (*Valstar, ✦Valtaxin*). Antimetabolites: azacitidine (*Vidaza*), capecitabine (*Xeloda*), cladribine (*Leustatin, chlorodeoxyadenosine*), clofarabine (*Clolar*), cytarabine (*Cytosar-U, Tarabine, Depo-Cyt, AraC*), decitabine (*Dacogen*), floxuridine (*FUDR*), fludarabine (*Fludara*), fluorouracil (*Adrucil, 5-FU*), gemcitabine (*Gemzar*), hydroxyurea (*Hydrea, Droxia*), mercaptopurine (*6-MP, Purinethol*), nelarabine (*Arranon*), pemetrexed (*Alimta*), pentostatin (*Nipent*), thioguanine (*Tabloid*, ✦*Lanvis*). Cytoprotective Agents: amifostine (*Ethyol*), dexrazoxane (*Zinecard*), mesna (*Mesnex*, ✦*Uromitexan*), palifermin (*Kepivance*). Hormones: abarelix (*Plenaxis*), anastrozole (*Arimidex*), bicalutamide (*Casodex*), cyproterone (*Androcur, Androcur Depot*), estramustine (*Emcyt*), exemestane (*Aromasin*), flutamide (*Eulexin*, ✦*Euflex*), fulvestrant (*Faslodex*), goserelin (*Zoladex*), histrelin (*Vantas, Supprelin LA*), letrozole (*Femara*), leuprolide (*Eligard, Lupron, Lupron Depot, Oaklide, Viadur*), nilutamide (*Nilandron*), toremifene (*Fareston*), triptorelin (*Trelstar Depot*). Immunomodulators: aldesleukin (*Proleukin, interleukin-2*), alemtuzumab (*Campath*, ✦*MabCampath*), BCG (*Bacillus of Calmette & Guerin, Pacis, TheraCys, Tice BCG*, ✦*Oncotice, Immucyst*), bevacizumab (*Avastin*), cetuximab (*Erbitux*), dasatinib (*Sprycel*), denileukin (*Ontak*), erlotinib (*Tarceva*), gemtuzumab (*Mylotarg*), ibritumomab (*Zevalin*), imatinib (*Gleevec*), interferon alfa-2a (*Roferon-A*), lapatinib (*Tykerb*), nilotinib (*Tasigna*), panitumumab (*Vectibix*), rituximab (*Rituxan*), sunitinib (*Sutent*), temsirolimus (*Torisel*), tositumomab (*Bexxar*), trastuzumab (*Herceptin*). Mitotic Inhibitors: docetaxel (*Taxotere*), etoposide (*VP-16, Etopophos, Toposar, VePesid*), ixabepilone (*Ixempra*), paclitaxel (*Taxol, Abraxane, Onxol*), teniposide (*Vumon, VM-26*), vinblastine (*Velban, VLB*), vincristine (*Oncovin, Vincasar, VCR*), vinorelbine (*Navelbine*). Platinum-Containing Agents: carboplatin (*Paraplatin*), cisplatin (*Platinol-AQ*), oxaliplatin (*Eloxatin*). Radiopharmaceuticals: samarium 153 (*Quadramet*), strontium-89 (*Metastron*). Miscellaneous: arsenic trioxide (*Trisenox*), asparaginase (*Elspar*, ✦*Kidrolase*), bexarotene (*Targretin*), bortezomib (*Velcade*), dexrazoxane (*Totect*), gefitinib (*Iressa*), irinotecan (*Camptosar*), lenalidomide (*Revlimid*), leucovorin (*Wellcovorin, folinic acid*), levoleucovorin (*Fusilev*), mitotane (*Lysodren*), pegaspargase (*Oncaspar*), porfimer (*Photofrin*), sorafenib (*Nexavar*), thalidomide (*Thalomid*), topotecan (*Hycamtin*), tretinoin (*Vesanoid*), vorinostat (*Zolinza*).

OPHTHALMOLOGY

NOTE: *Most eye medications can be administered 1 drop at a time despite common manufacturer recommendations of 1-2 drops concurrently. Even a single drop is typically more than the eye can hold and thus a second drop is both wasteful and increases the possibility of systemic toxicity. If twice the medication is desired separate single drops by at least 5 minutes.*

Antiallergy—Decongestants & Combinations

NAPHAZOLINE (*Albalon, All Clear, AK-Con, Naphcon, Clear Eyes*) 1 gtt qid prn for up to 4 d. [OTC Generic/Trade: solution 0.012, 0.03% (15, 30 mL). Rx Generic/Trade: 0.1% (15 mL).] ▶? ♀C ▶? $

NAPHCON-A (*naphazoline + pheniramine, Visine-A*) 1 gtt qid prn for up to 4 d. [OTC Trade only: solution 0.025% + 0.3% (15 mL).] ▶L ♀C ▶? $

VASOCON-A (*naphazoline + antazoline*) 1 gtt qid prn for up to 4 d. [OTC Trade only: solution 0.05% + 0.5% (15 mL).] ▶L ♀C ▶? $

Antiallergy—Dual Antihistamine & Mast Cell Stabilizer

AZELASTINE—OPHTHALMIC (*Optivar*) 1 gtt bid. [Trade only: solution 0.05% (6 mL).] ▶L ♀C ▶? $$$
EPINASTINE (*Elestat*) 1 gtt bid. [Trade only: solution 0.05% (5 mL).] ▶K ♀C ▶? $$$
KETOTIFEN—OPHTHALMIC (*Alaway, Zaditor*) 1 gtt in each eye q8–12h. [OTC-Generic/Trade: solution 0.025% (5 mL).] ▶Minimal absorption ♀C ▶? $
OLOPATADINE (*Pataday, Patanol*) 1 gtt of 0.1% solution in each eye bid (Patanol) or 1 gtt of 0.2% solution in each eye daily (Pataday). [Trade only: solution 0.1% (5 mL, Patanol), 0.2% (2.5 mL, Pataday).] ▶K ♀C ▶? $$$

Antiallergy—Pure Antihistamines

EMEDASTINE (*Emadine*) 1 gtt up to qid. [Trade only: solution 0.05% (5 mL).] ▶L ♀B ▶? $$$
LEVOCABASTINE—OPHTHALMIC (*Livostin*) 1 gtt up to qid for 2 wk. [Trade only: susp 0.05% (5,10 mL).] ▶Minimal absorption ♀C ▶? $$$

Antiallergy—Pure Mast Cell Stabilizers

CROMOLYN—OPHTHALMIC (*Crolom, Opticrom*) 1–2 gtts in each eye 4–6 times per d. [Generic/Trade: solution 4% (10 mL).] ▶LK ♀B ▶? $$
LODOXAMIDE (*Alomide*) 1–2 gtts in each eye qid. [Trade only: solution 0.1% (10 mL).] ▶K ♀B ▶? $$$
NEDOCROMIL—OPHTHALMIC (*Alocril*) 1–2 gtts in each eye bid. [Trade only: solution 2% (5 mL).] ▶L ♀B ▶? $$$
PEMIROLAST (*Alamast*) 1–2 gtts in each eye qid. [Trade only: solution 0.1% (10 mL).] ▶? ♀C ▶? $$$

Antibacterials—Aminoglycosides

GENTAMICIN—OPHTHALMIC (*Garamycin, Genoptic, Gentak, ✚Diogent*) 1–2 gtts q2–4h; ½ inch ribbon of oint bid-tid. [Generic/Trade: solution 0.3% (5, 15 mL), ointment 0.3% (3.5 g tube).] ▶K ♀C ▶? $
TOBRAMYCIN—OPHTHALMIC (*Tobrex*) 1–2 gtts q1–4h or ½ inch ribbon of ointment q3–4h or bid-tid. [Generic/Trade: solution 0.3% (5 mL), ointment 0.3% (3.5 g tube).] ▶K ♀B ▶- $

Antibacterials—Fluoroquinolones

CIPROFLOXACIN—OPHTHALMIC (*Ciloxan*) 1–2 gtt q1–6h or ½ inch ribbon ointment bid-tid. [Generic/Trade: solution 0.3% (2.5,5,10 mL). Trade only: ointment 0.3% (3.5 g tube).] ▶LK ♀C ▶? $$
GATIFLOXACIN—OPHTHALMIC (*Zymar*) 1–2 gtts q2h while awake up to 8 times/d on d 1 & 2, then 1–2 gtts q4h up to 4 times/d on d 3–7. [Trade only: solution 0.3%.] ▶
LEVOFLOXACIN—OPHTHALMIC (*Iquix, Quixin*) Quixin: 1–2 gtts q2h while awake up to 8 times/d on d 1 & 2, then 1–2 gtts q4h up to 4 times/d on d 3–7.

(cont.)

Iquix: 1–2 gtts q30 min to 2h while awake and q4–6h overnight on d 1–3, then 1–2 gtts q1–4h while awake on d 4 to completion of therapy. [Trade only: solution 0.5% (Quixin, 5 mL), 1.5% (Iquix, 5 mL).] ▶KL ♀C ▶? $$$

MOXIFLOXACIN—OPHTHALMIC (*Vigamox*) 1 gtt tid × 7 d. [Trade only: solution 0.5% (5 mL).] ▶LK ♀C ▶? $$$

OFLOXACIN—OPHTHALMIC (*Ocuflox*) 1–2 gtts q1–6h × 7–10 d. [Generic/Trade: solution 0.3% (5, 10 mL).] ▶LK ♀C ▶? $$

Antibacterials—Other

AZITHROMYCIN—OPHTHALMIC (*Azasite*) 1 gtt bid × 2 d, then 1 gtt daily × 5 more d. [Trade only: solution 1% (2.5 mL).] ▶L ♀B ▶? $$$

BACITRACIN—OPHTHALMIC (*AK Tracin*) Apply ¼-½ inch ribbon of ointment q3–4h or bid-qid. [Generic/Trade: ointment 500 units/g (3.5 g tube) ▶Minimal absorption ♀C ▶? $

ERYTHROMYCIN—OPHTHALMIC (*Ilotycin, AK-Mycin*) ½ inch ribbon of ointment q3–4h or 2–8 times/d. [Generic only: ointment 0.5% (1, 3.5 g tube).] ▶L ♀B ▶+ $

NEOSPORIN OINTMENT—OPHTHALMIC (*neomycin + bacitracin + polymyxin*) ½ inch ribbon of ointment q3–4h × 7–10 d or ½ inch ribbon 2–3 times/d for mild-moderate infection. [Generic only: ointment. (3.5 g tube).] ▶K ♀C ▶? $

NEOSPORIN SOLUTION—OPHTHALMIC (*neomycin + polymyxin + gramicidin*) 1–2 gtts q1–6h × 7–10 d. [Generic/Trade: solution (10 mL) ▶KL ♀C ▶? $$

POLYSPORIN—OPHTHALMIC (*polymyxin + bacitracin*) ½ inch ribbon of ointment q3–4h × 7–10 d or ½ inch ribbon bid-tid for mild-moderate infection. [Generic only: ointment (3.5 g tube).] ▶K ♀C ▶? $$

POLYTRIM—OPHTHALMIC (*polymyxin + trimethoprim*) 1–2 gtts q3–6h × 7–10d, max 6 gtts/d. [Generic/Trade: solution (10 mL).] ▶KL ♀C ▶? $

SULFACETAMIDE—OPHTHALMIC (*Bleph-10, Sulf-10*) 1–2 gtts q2–6h × 7–10d or ½ inch ribbon of ointment q3–8h × 7–10d. [Generic/Trade: solution 10% (15 mL), ointment 10% (3.5 g tube). Generic only: solution 30% (15 mL).] ▶K ♀C ▶- $

Antiviral Agents

TRIFLURIDINE—OPHTHALMIC (*Viroptic*) Herpes: 1 gtt q2–4h × 7–14d, max 9 gtts/d, 21 d. [Generic/Trade solution 1% (7.5 mL).] ▶Minimal absorption ♀C ▶- $$$

Corticosteroid & Antibacterial Combinations

NOTE *Recommend that only ophthalmologists or optometrists prescribe due to infection, cataract, corneal/scleral perforation, and glaucoma risk from prolonged use. Monitor intraocular pressure.*

BLEPHAMIDE (*prednisolone—ophthalmic + sulfacetamide*) 1–2 gtts q1–8h or ½ inch ribbon of ointment daily-qid. [Generic/Trade: solution/susp (5,10 mL), Trade only: ointment (3.5 g tube).] ▶KL ♀C ▶? $

CORTISPORIN—OPHTHALMIC (*neomycin + polymyxin + hydrocortisone—ophthalmic*) 1–2 gtts or ½ inch ribbon of ointment q3–4h or more frequently prn. [Generic/Trade: susp (7.5 mL). Generic only: ointment (3.5 g tube).] ▶LK ♀C ▶? $

FML-S LIQUIFILM (*prednisolone—ophthalmic + sulfacetamide*) 1–2 gtts q1–8h or ½ inch ribbon of ointment daily-qid. [Trade only: susp (10 mL).] ▶KL ♀C ▶? $$

MAXITROL (*dexamethasone—ophthalmic + neomycin + polymyxin*) 1–2 gtts q1–8h or ½ -1 inch ribbon of ointment daily-qid. [Generic/Trade: susp (5 mL), ointment (3.5 g tube).] ▶KL ♀C ▶? $

PRED G (*prednisolone—ophthalmic + gentamicin*) 1–2 gtts q1–8h daily-qid or ½ inch ribbon of ointment bid-qid. [Trade only: susp (2,5,10 mL), ointment (3.5 g tube).] ▶KL ♀C ▶? $$

TOBRADEX (*tobramycin + dexamethasone—ophthalmic*) 1–2 gtts q2–6h or ½ inch ribbon of ointment bid-qid. [Trade only: susp (2.5,5,10 mL), ointment (3.5 g tube).] ▶L ♀C ▶? $$$

VASOCIDIN (*prednisolone—ophthalmic + sulfacetamide*) 1–2 gtts q1–8h or ½ inch ribbon of ointment daily-qid. [Generic only: solution (5,10 mL)] ▶KL ♀C ▶? $

ZYLET (*loteprednol + tobramycin*) 1–2 gtts q1–2h × 1–2 d then 1–2 gtts q4–6h. [Trade only: susp 0.5% loteprednol + 0.3% tobramycin (2.5, 5, 10 mL). ▶LK ♀C ▶? $$$

Corticosteroids

NOTE *Recommend that only ophthalmologists or optometrists prescribe due to infection, cataract, corneal/scleral perforation, and glaucoma risk. Monitor intraocular pressure.*

DIFLUPREDNATE (*Durezol*) 1 gtt into affected eye qid, beginning 24 h after surgery × 2 wk, then 1 gtt into affected eye bid × 1 wk, then taper based on response. [Ophthalmic emulsion 0.05% (2.5, 5 mL).] ▶Not absorbed ♀C ▶? ?

FLUOROMETHOLONE (*FML, FML Forte, Flarex*) 1–2 gtts q1–12h or ½ inch ribbon of ointment q4–24h. [Trade only: susp 0.1% (5,10,15 mL), 0.25% (2,5,10,15 mL), ointment 0.1% (3.5 g tube). ▶L ♀C ▶? $$

LOTEPREDNOL (*Alrex, Lotemax*) 1–2 gtts qid. [Trade only: susp 0.2% (Alrex 5,10 mL), 0.5% (Lotemax 2.5, 5,10,15 mL).] ▶L ♀C ▶? $$$

PREDNISOLONE—OPHTHALMIC (*Pred Forte, Pred Mild, Inflamase Forte, Econopred Plus, ✦AK Tate, Diopred*) Solution: 1–2 gtts up to q1h during d and q2h at night, when response observed, then 1 gtt q4h, then 1 gtt tid-qid. Susp: 1–2 gtts bid-qid. [Generic/Trade: solution & susp 1% (5,10,15 mL). Trade only (Pred Mild): susp 0.12% (5,10 mL), susp (Pred Forte) 1% (1 mL).] ▶L ♀C ▶? $$$

RIMEXOLONE (*Vexol*) 1–2 gtts q1–6h. [Trade only: susp 1% (5,10 mL).] ▶L ♀C ▶? $$

Glaucoma Agents—Beta Blockers   (Use caution in cardiac conditions and asthma.)

BETAXOLOL—OPHTHALMIC (*Betoptic, Betoptic S*)   1–2 gtts bid. [Trade only: susp 0.25% (5,10,15 mL). Generic only: solution 0.5% (5,10,15 mL).] ▶LK ♀C ▶? $$

CARTEOLOL—OPHTHALMIC (*Ocupress*)   1 gtt bid. [Generic only: solution 1% (5,10,15 mL).] ▶KL ♀C ▶? $

LEVOBUNOLOL (*Betagan*)   1–2 gtts daily bid. [Generic/Trade: solution 0.25% (5,10 mL) 0.5% (5,10,15 mL - Trade only 2 mL).] ▶? ♀C ▶- $$

METIPRANOLOL (*Optipranolol*)   1 gtt bid. [Generic/Trade: solution 0.3% (5,10 mL).] ▶? ♀C ▶? $

TIMOLOL—OPHTHALMIC (*Betimol, Timoptic, Timoptic XE, Istalol, Timoptic Ocudose*)   1 gtt bid. Timoptic XE, Istalol: 1 gtt daily. [Generic/Trade: solution 0.25 & 0.5% (5,10,15 mL), preservative free solution* 0.25% (0.2 mL), gel forming solution^ 0.25 & 0.5% (2.5, 5 mL). Note: *Timoptic Ocudose ^Timoptic XE.] ▶LK ♀C ▶+ $$

Glaucoma Agents—Carbonic Anhydrase Inhibitors

NOTE *Sulfonamide derivatives; verify absence of sulfa allergy before prescribing.*

BRINZOLAMIDE (*Azopt*)   1 gtt tid. [Trade only: susp 1% (5,10,15 mL).] ▶LK ♀C ▶? $$$

DORZOLAMIDE (*Trusopt*)   1 gtt tid. [Trade only: solution 2% (5, 10 mL).] ▶KL ♀C ▶- $$$

METHAZOLAMIDE (*Neptazane*)   25–50 mg PO daily-tid. [Generic only: Tabs 25, 50 mg.] ▶LK ♀C ▶? $$

Glaucoma Agents—Miotics

PILOCARPINE—OPHTHALMIC (*Pilopine HS, Isopto Carpine, ✦Diocarpine, Akarpine*)   1–2 gtts tid-qid up to 6 times/d or ½ inch ribbon of gel qhs. [Generic only: solution 0.5%(15 mL), 1%(2 mL), 2%(2 mL), 3% (15 mL), 4%(2 mL), 6%(15 mL). Generic/Trade: solution 1% (15 mL), 2% (15 mL), 4% (15 mL). Trade only (Pilopine HS): gel 4% (4 g tube).] ▶Plasma ♀C ▶? $

Glaucoma Agents—Prostaglandin Analogs

BIMATOPROST (*Lumigan*)   1 gtt qhs. [Trade only: solution 0.03% (2.5, 5, 7.5 mL).] ▶LK ♀C ▶? $$$

LATANOPROST (*Xalatan*)   1 gtt qhs. [Trade only: solution 0.005% (2.5 mL).] ▶LK ♀C ▶? $$$

TRAVOPROST (*Travatan, Travatan Z*)   1 gtt qhs. [Trade only: solution (Travatan) & benzalkonium chloride-free (Travatan Z) 0.004% (2.5, 5 mL).] ▶L ♀C ▶? $$$

Glaucoma Agents—Sympathomimetics

BRIMONIDINE (*Alphagan P, ◆Alphagan*) 1 gtt tid. [Trade only: solution 0.1% (5,10,15 mL). Generic/Trade: solution 0.15% (5,10,15 mL). Generic only: 0.2% solution (5,10,15 mL).] ▶L ♀B ▶? $$

Glaucoma Agents—Combinations and Other

COMBIGAN (*brimonidine + timolol*) 1 gtt q12h. [Trade only: solution brimonidine 0.2% + timolol 0.5% (5,10 mL).] ▶LK ♀C ▶- $$$
COSOPT (*dorzolamide + timolol*) 1 gtt bid. [Trade only: solution dorzolamide 2% + timolol 0.5% (5, 10 mL).] ▶LK ♀D ▶- $$$

Mydriatics & Cycloplegics

ATROPINE—OPHTHALMIC (*Isopto Atropine, Atropine Care*) 1–2 gtts before procedure or daily-qid, 1/8–1/4 inch ointment before procedure or daily-tid. Cycloplegia may last up to 5–10 d and mydriasis may last up to 7–14 d. [Generic/Trade: solution 1% (2, 5,15 mL) Generic only: ointment 1% (3.5 g tube).] ▶L ♀C ▶+ $
CYCLOPENTOLATE (*AK-Pentolate, Cyclogyl, Pentolair*) 1–2 gtts × 1–2 doses before procedure. Cycloplegia may last 6–24 h; mydriasis may last 1 d. [Generic/Trade: solution 1% (2,15 mL). Trade only (Cyclogyl): 0.5% (15 mL), 1% (5 mL) and 2% (2,5,15 mL).] ▶? ♀C ▶? $
HOMATROPINE (*Isopto Homatropine*) 1–2 gtts before procedure or bid-tid. Cycloplegia & mydriasis lasts 1–3 d. [Trade only: solution 2% (5 mL), 5% (5 mL). Generic/Trade: solution 5% (5 mL)] ▶? ♀C ▶? $
PHENYLEPHRINE—OPHTHALMIC (*AK-Dilate, Altafrin, Mydfrin, Refresh*) 1–2 gtts before procedure or tid-qid. No cycloplegia; mydriasis may last up to 5 h. [Rx Generic/Trade: solution 2.5% (2,3,5,15 mL),10% (5 mL). OTC Trade only (Altafrin & Refresh): solution 0.12% (15 mL).] ▶Plasma, L ♀C ▶? $
TROPICAMIDE (*Mydriacyl, Tropicacyl*) 1–2 gtts before procedure. Mydriasis may last 6 h. [Generic/Trade: solution 0.5% (15 mL), 1% (3,15 mL). Generic only: solution 1% (2 mL).] ▶? ♀? ▶? $

Nonsteroidal Anti-Inflammatories

BROMFENAC—OPHTHALMIC (*Xibrom*) 1 gtt bid × 2 wk. [Trade only: solution 0.09% (2.5, 5 mL).] ▶Minimal absorption ♀C, D (3rd trimester) ▶? $$$$
DICLOFENAC—OPHTHALMIC (*Voltaren, ◆Voltaren Ophtha*) 1 gtt up to qid. [Generic/Trade: solution 0.1% (2.5, 5 mL).] ▶L ♀B, D (3rd trimester) ▶? $$$
KETOROLAC—OPHTHALMIC (*Acular, Acular LS*) 1 gtt qid. [Trade only: solution Acular LS 0.4% (5 mL), Acular 0.5% (3, 5, 10 mL), preservative free Acular 0.5% unit dose (0.4 mL).] ▶L ♀C ▶? $$$
NEPAFENAC (*Nevanac*) 1 gtt tid × 2 wk. [Trade only: susp 0.1% (3 mL).] ▶Minimal absorption ♀C ▶? $$$

Other Ophthalmologic Agents

ARTIFICIAL TEARS (*Tears Naturale, Hypotears, Refresh Tears, GenTeal, Systane*) 1–2 gtts tid-qid prn. [OTC Generic/Trade: solution (15, 30 mL among others).] ▶Minimal absorption ♀A ▶+ $

CYCLOSPORINE—OPHTHALMIC (*Restasis*) 1 gtt in each eye q12h. [Trade only: emulsion 0.05% (0.4 mL single-use vials).] ▶Minimal absorption ♀C ▶? $$$$

HYDROXYPROPYL CELLULOSE (*Lacrisert*) Moderate-severe dry eyes: One insert in each eye daily. Some patients may require bid use. [Trade only: ocular insert 5 mg.] ▶Minimal absorption ♀+ ▶+ $$$

PETROLATUM (*Lacrilube, Dry Eyes, Refresh PM, ✦Duolube*) Apply ¼–½ inch ointment to inside of lower lid prn. [OTC Trade only: ointment (3.5 & 7 g) tube.] ▶Minimal absorption ♀A ▶+ $

PROPARACAINE (*Ophthaine, Ophthetic, ✦Alcaine*) Do not prescribe for unsupervised or prolonged use. Corneal toxicity and ocular infections may occur with repeated use. 1–2 gtts before procedure. [Generic/Trade: solution 0.5% (15 mL).] ▶L ♀C ▶? $

TETRACAINE—OPHTHALMIC (*Pontocaine*) Do not prescribe for unsupervised or prolonged use. Corneal toxicity and ocular infections may occur with repeated use. 1–2 gtts or ½–1 inch ribbon of ointment before procedure. [Generic only: solution 0.5% (15 mL), unit-dose vials (0.7 & 2 mL).] ▶Plasma ♀C ▶? $

NOTE for proparacaine and tetracaine above: *Do not prescribe for unsupervised or prolonged use. Corneal toxicity and ocular infections may occur with repeated use.*

PSYCHIATRY

Antidepressants—Heterocyclic Compounds

AMITRIPTYLINE (*Elavil*) Start 25–100 mg PO qhs; gradually increase to usual effective dose of 50–300 mg/d. Primarily inhibits serotonin reuptake. Demethylated to nortriptyline, which primarily inhibits norepinephrine reuptake. [Generic: Tabs 10, 25, 50, 75, 100,150 mg. Elavil brand name no longer available; has been retained in this entry for name recognition purposes only.] ▶L ♀C ▶+ $$$ ▶L ♀D ▶- $$

CLOMIPRAMINE (*Anafranil*) Start 25 mg PO qhs; gradually increase to usual effective dose of 150–250 mg/d. Max 250 mg/d. Primarily inhibits serotonin reuptake. [Generic/Trade: Caps 25, 50, 75 mg.]

DESIPRAMINE (*Norpramin*) Start 25–100 mg PO given once daily or in divided doses. Gradually increase to usual effective dose of 100–200 mg/d, max 300 mg/d. Primarily inhibits norepinephrine reuptake. [Generic/Trade: Tabs 10, 25, 50, 75, 100, 150 mg.] ▶L ♀C ▶+ $$

DOXEPIN (*Sinequan*) Start 75 mg PO qhs. Gradually increase to usual effective dose of 75–150 mg/d, max 300 mg/d. Primarily inhibits norepinephrine reuptake. [Generic/Trade: Caps 10, 25, 50, 75, 100, 150 mg. Oral concentrate 10 mg/mL.] ▶L ♀C ▶- $$

IMIPRAMINE (*Tofranil, Tofranil PM*) Depression: Start 75–100 mg PO qhs or in divided doses; gradually increase to max 300 mg/d. Enuresis: 25–75 mg PO qhs. [Generic/Trade: Tabs 10, 25, 50 mg. Trade only: Caps 75, 100, 125, 150 mg (as pamoate salt).] ▶L ♀D ▶- $$$

NORTRIPTYLINE (*Aventyl, Pamelor*) Start 25 mg PO given once daily or divided bid-qid. Usual effective dose is 75–100 mg/d, max 150 mg/d. Primarily inhibits norepinephrine reuptake. [Generic/Trade: Caps 10, 25, 50, 75 mg. Oral Solution 10 mg/5 mL.] ▶L ♀D ▶+ $$$

PROTRIPTYLINE (*Vivactil*) Depression: 15–40 mg/d PO divided tid-qid. Max 60 mg/d. [Trade only: Tabs 5, 10 mg.] ▶L ♀C ▶+ $$$$

Antidepressants—Monoamine Oxidase Inhibitors (MAOIs)

NOTE: *Must be on tyramine-free diet throughout treatment, and for 2 weeks after discontinuation. Numerous drug interactions; risk of hypertensive crisis and serotonin syndrome with many medications, including OTC. Allow ≥2 weeks wash-out when converting from an MAOI to an SSRI (6 weeks after fluoxetine), TCA, or other antidepressant.*

ISOCARBOXAZID (*Marplan*) Start 10 mg PO bid; increase by 10 mg q2–4 d. Usual effective dose is 20–40 mg/d. MAOI diet. [Trade only: Tabs 10 mg.] ▶L ♀C ▶? $$$

PHENELZINE (*Nardil*) Start 15 mg PO tid. Usual effective dose is 60–90 mg/d in divided doses. MAOI diet. [Trade only: Tabs 15 mg.] ▶L ♀C ▶? $$$

SELEGILINE—TRANSDERMAL (*Emsam*) Depression: start 6 mg/24 h patch q 24h. Max 12 mg/24 h. MAOI diet for doses ≥ 9 mg/d. [Trade only: Transdermal patch 6 mg/24 h, 9 mg/24 h, 12 mg/24 h.] ▶L ♀C ▶? $$$$$

TRANYLCYPROMINE (*Parnate*) Start 10 mg PO qam; increase by 10 mg/d at 1–3 wk intervals to usual effective dose of 10–40 mg/d divided bid. MAOI diet. [Generic/Trade: Tabs 10 mg.] ▶L ♀C ▶- $$

Antidepressants—Selective Serotonin Reuptake Inhibitors (SSRIs)

CITALOPRAM (*Celexa*) Depression: Start 20 mg PO daily; usual effective dose is 20–40 mg/d, max 60 mg/d. Suicidality. [Generic/Trade: Tabs 10, 20, 40 mg. Oral solution 10 mg/5 mL. Generic only: Oral disintegrating tab 10, 20, 40 mg.] ▶LK ♀C but - in 3rd trimester ▶- $$$

ESCITALOPRAM (*Lexapro, ✦Cipralex*) Depression, generalized anxiety disorder: Start 10 mg PO daily; max 20 mg/d. Suicidality. [Generic/Trade: Tabs 5, 10, 20 mg. Trade only: Oral solution 1 mg/mL.] ▶LK ♀C but - in 3rd trimester ▶- $$$

FLUOXETINE (*Prozac, Prozac Weekly, Sarafem*) Depression, OCD: Start 20 mg PO q am; usual effective dose is 20–40 mg/d, max 80 mg/d. Depression, maintenance: 20–40 mg/d (standard-release) or 90 mg PO once weekly (Prozac Weekly) starting 7 d after last standard-release dose. Bulimia: 60 mg PO daily; may need to titrate slowly, over several d. Panic disorder: Start 10 mg PO q am; titrate to 20 mg/d after one wk, max 60 mg/d. Premenstrual Dysphoric Disorder (Sarafem): 20 mg PO daily, given either throughout the menstrual cycle or for 14 d prior to menses; max 80 mg/d. Doses >20 mg/d can be divided bid (q am & q noon). Suicidality, many drug interactions. [Generic/Trade: Tabs 10 mg. Caps 10, 20, 40 mg. Oral solution 20 mg/5 mL. Caps (Sarafem) 10, 20 mg. Trade only: Tabs (Sarafem) 10, 15, 20 mg. Caps, delayed-release (Prozac Weekly) 90 mg. Generic only: Tabs 20, 40 mg.] ▶L ♀C but - in 3rd trimester ▶- $$$$

FLUVOXAMINE (Luvox, Luvox CR) OCD: Start 50 mg PO qhs; usual effective dose is 100–300 mg/d divided bid, max 300 mg/d. OCD and Social Anxiety Disorder (CR): Start 100 mg PO qhs; increase by 50 mg/d q wk prn to max 300 mg/d. OCD (children ≥8 yo): Start 25 mg PO qhs; usual effective dose is 50–200 mg/d divided bid, max 200 mg/d. Don't use with thioridazine, pimozide, alosetron, cisapride, tizanidine, tryptophan, or MAOIs; use caution with benzodiazepines, TCAs, theophylline, and warfarin. Suicidality. [Generic/Trade: Tabs 25, 50, 100 mg. Trade only: Caps, extended-release 100, 150 mg.] ▶L ♀C but - in 3rd trimester ▶- $$$$

PAROXETINE (Paxil, Paxil CR, Pexeva) Depression: Start 20 mg PO qam, max 50 mg/d. Depression, controlled-release: Start 25 mg PO qam, max 62.5 mg/d. OCD: Start 10–20 mg PO qam, max 60 mg/d. Social anxiety disorder: Start 10–20 mg PO qam, max 60 mg/d. Social anxiety disorder, controlled-release: Start 12.5 mg PO qam, max 37.5 mg/d. Generalized anxiety disorder: Start 20 mg PO qam, max 50 mg/d. Panic disorder: Start 10 mg PO qam, increase by 10 mg/d at intervals ≥1 wk to usual effective dose of 10–60 mg/d; max 60 mg/d. Panic disorder, controlled-release: Start 12.5 mg PO qam, max 75 mg/d. Posttraumatic stress disorder: Start 20 mg PO qam, max 50 mg/d. Premenstrual dysphoric disorder (PMDD), continuous dosing: Start 12.5 mg PO qam (controlled-release); may increase dose after 1 wk to max 25 mg qam. PMDD, intermittent dosing (given for 2 wk prior to menses): 12.5 mg PO qam (controlled-release), max 25 mg/d. Suicidality, many drug interactions. [Generic/Trade: Tabs 10, 20, 30, 40 mg. Oral Susp 10 mg/5 mL. Controlled-release tabs 12.5, 25 mg. Trade only: (Paxil CR) 37.5 mg.] ▶LK ♀D ▶? $$$

SERTRALINE (Zoloft) Depression, OCD: Start 50 mg PO daily; usual effective dose is 50–200 mg/d, max 200 mg/d. Panic disorder, post-traumatic stress disorder, social anxiety disorder: Start 25 mg PO daily, max 200 mg/d. Premenstrual dysphoric disorder (PMDD), continuous dosing: Start 50 mg PO daily, max 150 mg/d. PMDD, intermittent dosing (given for 14 d prior to menses): Start 50 mg PO daily × 3 d, then increase to 100 mg/d. Suicidality. [Generic/Trade: Tabs 25, 50, 100 mg. Oral concentrate 20 mg/mL (60 mL).] ▶LK ♀C but - in 3rd trimester ▶+ $$$

Antidepressants—Serotonin-Norepinephrine Reuptake Inhibitors (SNRIs)

DESVENLAFAXINE (Pristiq) 50 mg PO daily. Max 400 mg/d. [Trade only: Tabs, extended-release 50, 100 mg.] ▶LK ♀C ▶? $$$$

DULOXETINE (Cymbalta) Depression: 20 mg PO bid. Generalized anxiety disorder: Start 30–60 mg PO daily, max 120 mg/d. Diabetic peripheral neuropathic pain: 60 mg PO daily. Fibromyalgia: Start 30–60 mg PO daily, max 60 mg/d. Suicidality, hepatotoxicity, many drug interactions. [Trade only: Caps 20, 30, 60 mg.] ▶L ♀C ▶? $$$$

VENLAFAXINE (*Effexor, Effexor XR*) Depression/anxiety: Start 37.5–75 mg PO daily (Effexor XR) or 75 mg/d divided bid-tid (Effexor). Usual effective dose is 150–225 mg/d, max 225 mg/d (Effexor XR) or 375 mg/d (Effexor). Generalized anxiety disorder: Start 37.5–75 mg PO daily (Effexor XR), max 225 mg/d. Social anxiety disorder: Start 75 mg PO daily (Effexor XR). Panic disorder: Start 37.5 mg PO daily (Effexor XR), may titrate by 75 mg/d at weekly intervals to max 225 mg/d. Suicidality, seizures, hypertension. [Trade only: Caps, extended-release 37.5, 75, 150 mg. Generic/Trade: Tabs 25, 37.5, 50, 75, 100 mg. Generic only: Tabs, extended-release 37.5, 75, 150, 225 mg.] ▶LK ♀C but - in 3rd trimester ▶? $$$$

Antidepressants—Other

BUPROPION (*Wellbutrin, Wellbutrin SR, Wellbutrin XL, Aplenzin, Zyban, Buproban*) Depression: Start 100 mg PO bid (immediate-release tabs); can increase to 100 mg tid after 4–7 d. Usual effective dose is 300–450 mg/d, max 150 mg/dose and 450 mg/d. Sustained-release: Start 150 mg PO q am; may increase to 150 mg bid after 4–7 d, max 400 mg/d. Give last dose no later than 5 pm. Extended-release: Start 150 mg PO q am; may increase to 300 mg q am after 4 d, max 450 mg q am. Extended-release (Aplenzin): Start 174 mg PO q am; increase to target dose of 348 mg/d after ≥4 d. May increase to max dose of 522 mg/d after ≥4 wk. Seasonal affective disorder: Start 150 mg of extended release PO q am in autumn; can increase to 300 mg q am after 1 wk, max 300 mg/d. In the spring, decrease to 150 mg/d for 2 wk and then discontinue. Smoking cessation (Zyban, Buproban): Start 150 mg PO q am × 3 d, then increase to 150 mg PO bid × 7–12 wk. Max 150 mg PO bid. Give last dose no later than 5 pm. Seizures, suicidality. [Generic/Trade (for depression, bupropion HCl): Tabs 75,100 mg. Sustained release tabs 100, 150, 200 mg. Extended-release tabs 150, 300 mg (Wellbutrin XL). Generic/Trade (smoking cessation): Sustained-release tabs 150 mg (Zyban, Buproban). Trade only: extended release (Aplenzin, bupropion hydrobromide) tabs 174, 348, 522 mg.] ▶LK ♀C ▶- $$$$

MIRTAZAPINE (*Remeron, Remeron SolTab*) Start 15 mg PO qhs. Usual effective dose is 15–45 mg/d. Agranulocytosis in 0.1% of patients. Suicidality. [Generic/Trade: Tabs 15, 30, 45 mg. Tabs, orally disintegrating (SolTab) 15, 30, 45 mg. Generic only: Tabs 7.5 mg.] ▶LK ♀C ▶? $$

TRAZODONE Depression: Start 50–150 mg/d PO in divided doses; usual effective dose is 400–600 mg/d. Insomnia: 50–150 mg PO qhs. [Generic only: Tabs 50, 100, 150, 300 mg.] ▶L ♀C ▶- $

Antimanic (Bipolar) Agents

LAMOTRIGINE (*Lamictal, Lamictal CD*) Adults with bipolar disorder (maintenance): Start 25 mg PO daily, 50 mg PO daily if on enzyme-inducing drugs, or 25 mg PO qod if on valproate; titrate to 200 mg/d, 400 mg/d divided bid if on enzyme-inducing drugs, or 100 mg/d if on valproate. Potentially life-threatening rashes in 0.3% of adults and 0.8% of children; discontinue at first sign of rash. Drug interaction with valproic acid; see product information for adjusted dosing guidelines. [Generic/Trade: Chewable dispersible tabs 5, 25 mg. Trade only: Tabs 25, 100, 150, 200 mg.] ▶LK ♀C ▶- $$$$

LITHIUM (*Eskalith, Eskalith CR, Lithobid, ✦Lithane*)   Acute mania: Start 300–600 mg PO bid-tid; usual effective dose is 900–1,800 mg/d. Steady state is achieved in 5 d. Bipolar maintenance usually 900–1200 mg/d titrated to therapeutic trough level of 0.6–1.2 mEq/L. [Generic/Trade: Caps 300, Extended release tabs 300, 450 mg. Generic only: Caps 150, 600 mg, Tabs 300 mg, Syrup 300/5 mL.] ▶K ♀D ▶- $

TOPIRAMATE (*Topamax*)   Bipolar disorder (unapproved): Start 25–50 mg/d PO. Titrate prn to max 400 mg/d divided bid. [Trade only: Tabs 25, 50, 100, 200 mg. Sprinkle caps 15, 25 mg.] ▶K ♀C ▶? $$$$$

VALPROIC ACID (*Depakote, Depakote ER, Stavzor, Divalproex, ✦Epiject, Epival, Deproic*)   Mania: 250 mg PO tid (Depakote or Stavzor) or 25 mg/ kg once daily (Depakote ER); max 60 mg/kg/d. Hepatotoxicity, drug interactions, reduce dose in the elderly. [Generic/Trade: Caps 250 mg (Depakene), syrup (Depakene, valproic acid) 250 mg/5 mL. Trade only (Depakote): Caps, sprinkle 125 mg, delayed release tabs 125, 250, 500 mg; extended release tabs (Depakote ER) 250, 500 mg. Trade only (Stavzor): Delayed release caps 125, 250, 500 mg.] ▶L ♀D ▶+ $$$$

Antipsychotics—First Generation (Typical)

CHLORPROMAZINE (*Thorazine*)   Start 10–50 mg PO/IM bid-tid, usual dose 300–800 mg/d. [Generic only: Tabs 10, 25, 50, 100, 200 mg. Generic/Trade: Oral concentrate 30 mg/mL, 100 mg/mL. Trade only: Syrup 10 mg/5 mL. Suppositories 25, 100 mg.] ▶LK ♀C ▶- $$$

FLUPHENAZINE (*Prolixin, ✦Modecate, Modeten*)   1.25–10 mg/d IM divided q6–8h. Start 0.5–10 mg/d PO divided q6–8h. Usual effective dose 1–20 mg/d. Depot (fluphenazine decanoate/ enanthate): 12.5–25 mg IM/SC q3 wk = 10–20 mg/d PO fluphenazine. [Generic/Trade: Tabs 1, 2.5, 5, 10 mg. Elixir 2.5 mg/5 mL. Oral concentrate 5 mg/mL.] ▶LK ♀C ▶? $$$

HALOPERIDOL (*Haldol*)   2–5 mg IM. Start 0.5- 5 mg PO bid-tid, usual effective dose 6–20 mg/d. Therapeutic range 2–15 mg/mL. Depot haloperidol (haloperidol decanoate): 100–200 mg IM q4 wk = 10 mg/d oral haloperidol. [Generic only: Tabs 0.5, 1, 2, 5, 10, 20 mg. Oral concentrate 2 mg/ mL.] ▶LK ♀C ▶- $$$

PERPHENAZINE Start 4–8 mg PO tid or 8–16 mg PO bid-qid (*hospitalized patients*), max 64 mg/d PO. Can give 5–10 mg IM q6h, max 30 mg/d IM. [Generic only: Tabs 2, 4, 8, 16 mg. Oral concentrate 16 mg/5 mL.] ▶LK ♀C ▶? $$$

PIMOZIDE (*Orap*)   Tourette's: Start 1–2 mg/d PO in divided doses, increase q2 d to usual effective dose of 1–10 mg/d. [Trade only: Tabs 1, 2 mg.] ▶L ♀C ▶- $$$

THIORIDAZINE (*Mellaril, ✦Ridaril*)   Start 50–100 mg PO tid, usual dose 200–800 mg/d. Not first-line drug. Causes QTc prolongation, torsade de pointes, and sudden death. Contraindicated with SSRIs, propranolol, pindolol. Monitor baseline ECG and potassium. Pigmentary retinopathy with doses>800 mg/d. [Generic only: Tabs 10, 15, 25, 50, 100, 150, 200 mg. Oral concentrate 30, 100 mg/mL.] ▶LK ♀C ▶? $$

THIOTHIXENE (*Navane*)   Start 2 mg PO tid. Usual effective dose is 20–30 mg/d, max 60 mg/d PO. [Generic/Trade: Caps 1, 2, 5, 10. Oral concentrate 5 mg/mL. Trade only: Caps 20 mg.] ▶LK ♀C ▶? $$$

TRIFLUOPERAZINE (*Stelazine*) Start 2–5 mg PO bid. Usual effective dose is 15–20 mg/d. [Generic/Trade: Tabs 1, 2, 5, 10 mg. Trade only: Oral concentrate 10 mg/mL.] ▶LK ♀C ▶- $$$

Antipsychotics—Second Generation (Atypical)

ARIPIPRAZOLE (*Abilify, Abilify Discmelt*) Schizophrenia: Start 10–15 mg PO daily. Max 30 mg daily. Bipolar disorder: Start 15 mg PO daily. Max 30 mg/d. Agitation associated with schizophrenia or bipolar disorder: 9.75 mg IM recommended. May consider 5.25 to 15 mg if indicated. May repeat in >2 h up to max 30 mg/d. Depression, adjunctive therapy: Start 2–5 mg PO daily. Max 15 mg/d. [Trade only: Tabs 2, 5, 10, 15, 20, 30 mg. Oral solution 1 mg/mL (150 mL). Orally disintegrating tabs (Discmelt) 10, 15, 20, 30 mg.] ▶L ♀C ▶? $$$$$

CLOZAPINE (*Clozaril, FazaClo ODT*) Start 12.5 mg PO daily or bid. Usual effective dose is 300–450 mg/d divided bid, max 900 mg/d. Agranulocytosis 1–2%; check WBC and ANC q wk × 6 m, then q2 wk. Seizures, myocarditis, cardiopulmonary arrest. [Generic/Trade: Tabs 25, 100 mg. Generic only: Tabs 12.5, 50, 200 mg. Trade only: Orally disintegrating tab (Fazaclo ODT) 12.5, 25, 100 mg (scored).] ▶L ♀B ▶- $$$$$

OLANZAPINE (*Zyprexa, Zyprexa Zydis*) Agitation in acute bipolar mania or schizophrenia: Start 10 mg IM (2.5–5 mg in elderly or debilitated patients); may repeat in ≥2 h to max 30 mg/d. Psychotic disorders, oral therapy: Start 5–10 mg PO daily; usual effective dose is 10–15 mg/d. Bipolar disorder, maintenance treatment or monotherapy for acute manic or mixed episodes: Start 10–15 mg PO daily. Increase by 5 mg/d at intervals ≥24 h to usual effective dose of 5–20 mg/d, max 20 mg/d. Bipolar disorder, adjunctive for acute manic or mixed episodes: Start 10 mg PO daily; usual effective dose is 5–20 mg/d, max 20 mg/d. [Trade only: Tabs 2.5, 5, 7.5, 10, 15, 20 mg. Tabs, orally-disintegrating (Zyprexa Zydis) 5,10,15, 20 mg.] ▶L ♀C ▶- $$$$$

PALIPERIDONE (*Invega, 9-hydroxyrisperidone*) Schizophrenia: Start 6 mg PO qam. 3 mg/d may be sufficient in some. Max 12 mg/d. [Trade only: Extended-release tabs 3, 6, 9 mg. 12 mg strength not available in the USA or Canada.] ▶KL ♀C ▶- $$$$$

QUETIAPINE (*Seroquel, Seroquel XR*) Schizophrenia: Start 25 mg PO bid (regular tabs); increase by 25–50 mg bid-tid on d 2 and 3, and then to target dose of 300–400 mg/d divided bid-tid on d 4. Usual effective dose is 150–750 mg/d, max 800 mg/d. Schizophrenia, extended release tabs: Start 300 mg PO daily in evening, increase by up to 300 mg/d at intervals of >1 d to usual effective range of 400–800 mg/d. Acute bipolar mania: Start 50 mg PO bid on d 1, then increase to no higher than 100 mg bid on d 2, 150 mg bid on d 3, and 200 mg bid on d 4. May increase prn to 300 mg bid on d 5 and 400 mg bid thereafter. Usual effective dose is 400–800 mg/d, max 800 mg/d. Bipolar depression: 50 mg PO hs on d 1, 100 mg hs d 2, 200 mg hs d 3, and 300 mg hs d 4. May increase prn to 400 mg hs on d 5 and 600 mg hs on d 8. Eye exam for cataracts recommended q 6 mon. Bipolar maintenance: continue dose required to maintain symptom remission. [Trade only: Tabs 25, 50, 100, 200, 300, 400 mg. Extended-release tabs 50, 200, 300, 400 mg.] ▶LK ♀C ▶- $$$$$

ANTIPSYCHOTIC RELATIVE ADVERSE EFFECTS[a]

Generation	Antipsychotic	Anticholinergic	Sedation	Hypotension	Extrapyramidal Symptoms	Weight Gain	Diabetes/Hyperglycemia	Dyslipidemia
1st	chlorpromazine	+++	+++	++	++	++	?	?
1st	fluphenazine	++	+	+	++++	++	?	?
1st	haloperidol	+	+	+	++++	++	0	?
1st	loxapine	++	+	++	++	+	?	?
1st	molindone	++	++	+	++	+	?	?
1st	perphenazine	++	++	+	++	+	+/?	?
1st	pimozide	+	+	+	+++	?	?	?
1st	thioridazine	++++	+++	+++	+	+++	+/?	?
1st	thiothixene	+	++	++	+++	++	?	?
1st	trifluoperazine	++	+	+	+++	++	?	?
2nd	aripiprazole	++	+	0	0	0/+	0	0
2nd	clozapine	++++	+++	+++	0	+++	+	+
2nd	olanzapine	+++	++	+	0b	+++	+	+
2nd	risperidone	+	++	+	+b	++	?	?
2nd	quetiapine	+	+++	++	0	++	?	?
2nd	ziprasidone	+	+	0	0	0/+	0	0

[a]Risk of specific adverse effects is graded from 0 (absent) to ++++ (high). ? = Limited or inconsistent comparative data. [b]EPS (extrapyramidal symptoms) are dose-related and are more likely for risperidone >6-8 mg/d / olanzapine >20 mg/d. Akathisia risk remains unclear and may not be reflected in these ratings. There are limited comparative data for aripiprazole relative to other second generation antipsychotics.
References: Goodman & Gilman 11e p461-500, Applied Therapeutics 8e p78, APA schizophrenia practice guideline, Psychiatry Q 2002; 73:297, Diabetes Care 2004; 27:596.

RISPERIDONE (*Risperdal, Risperdal Consta*) Schizophrenia (adults): Start 2 mg/d PO given once daily or divided bid (0.5 mg bid in the elderly, debilitated, or with hypotension, severe renal or hepatic disease); increase by 1–2 mg/d (≤0.5 mg bid in elderly and debilitated) at intervals of ≥24 h to usual effective dose of 4–8 mg/d given once daily or divided bid, max 16 mg/d. Long-acting injection (Consta): Start 25 mg IM q 2 wk while continuing oral dose × 3 wk. May increase at 4 wk intervals to max 50 mg q 2 wk. Schizophrenia (13–17 yo): Start 0.5 mg PO daily; increase by 0.5–1.0 mg/d at intervals ≥24 h to target dose of 3 mg/d. Max 6 mg/d. Bipolar mania (adults): Start 2–3 mg PO daily; may increase by 1 mg/d at 24 h intervals to max 6 mg/d. Bipolar mania (10–17 yo): Start 0.5 mg PO daily; increase by 0.5–1.0 mg/d at intervals ≥24 h to recommended dose of 2.5 mg/d. Max 6 mg/d. Autistic disorder irritability (5–16 yo): Start 0.25 mg (<20 kg) or 0.5 mg (≥20 kg) PO daily. May increase after ≥4 d to 0.5 mg/d (<20 kg) or 1.0 mg/d (≥20 kg). Maintain ≥14 d. May then increase at ≥14 d intervals by increments of 0.25 mg/d (<20 kg) or 0.5 mg/d (≥20 kg) to max 1.0 mg/d (<20 kg), 2.5 mg/d (20–44 kg) or 3.0 mg/d
(cont.)

(>45 kg). [Trade only: Tabs 0.25, 0.5, 1, 2, 3, 4 mg. Orally disintegrating tabs (M-TAB) 0.5, 1, 2 mg. Oral solution 1 mg/mL (30 mL).] ▶LK ♀C ▶- $$$$$

ZIPRASIDONE (*Geodon*) Schizophrenia: Start 20 mg PO bid with food; may adjust at >2 d intervals to max 80 mg PO bid. Acute agitation: 10–20 mg IM, max 40 mg/d. Bipolar mania: Start 40 mg PO bid with food; may increase to 60–80 mg bid on d 2. Usual effective dose is 40–80 mg bid. [Trade only: Caps 20, 40, 60, 80 mg, Susp 10 mg/mL.] ▶L ♀C ▶- $$$$$

Anxiolytics / Hypnotics—Benzodiazepines— Long Half-Life (25–100 h)

BROMAZEPAM (◆LECTOPAM) Canada only. 6–18 mg/d PO in divided doses. [Generic/Trade: TABS 1.5, 3, 6 MG.] ▶L ♀D ▶- $

CHLORDIAZEPOXIDE (*Librium*) Anxiety: 5–25 mg PO or 25–50 mg IM/IV tid-qid. Acute alcohol withdrawal: 50–100 mg PO/IM/IV, repeat q3–4h prn up to 300 mg/d. Half-life 5–30 h. [Generic/Trade: Caps 5, 10, 25 mg.] ▶LK ♀D ▶- ©IV $$

CLONAZEPAM (*Klonopin, Klonopin Wafer, ◆Rivotril, Clonapam*) Panic disorder: Start 0.25–0.5 mg PO bid-tid, max 4 mg/d. Half-life 18- 50 h. Epilepsy: Start 0.5 mg PO tid. Max 20 mg/d. [Generic/Trade: Tabs 0.5, 1, 2 mg. Orally disintegrating tabs (approved for panic disorder only) 0.125, 0.25, 0.5, 1, 2 mg.] ▶LK ♀D ▶- ©IV $

CLORAZEPATE (*Tranxene, Tranxene SD*) Start 7.5–15 mg PO qhs or bid-tid, usual effective dose is 15–60 mg/d. Acute alcohol withdrawal: 60–90 mg/d on first d divided bid-tid, reduce dose to 7.5–15 mg/d over 5 d. [Generic/Trade: Tabs 3.75, 7.5, 15 mg. Trade only (Tranxene SD): Extended release Tabs 11.25, 22.5 mg.] ▶LK ♀D ▶- ©IV $

DIAZEPAM (*Valium, Diastat, Diastat AcuDial, ◆Vivol, E Pam, Diazemuls*) Active seizures: 5–10 mg IV q10–15 min to max 30 mg, or 0.2–0.5 mg/kg rectal gel PR. Skeletal muscle spasm, spasticity related to cerebral palsy, paraplegia, athetosis, stiff man syndrome: 2–10 mg PO/PR tid-qid. Anxiety: 2–10 mg PO bid-qid. Half-life 20–80 h. Alcohol withdrawal: 10 mg PO tid-qid × 24 h then 5 mg PO tid-qid prn. [Generic/Trade: Tabs 2, 5, 10 mg. Generic only: Oral solution 5 mg/5 mL. Oral concentrate (Intensol) 5 mg/mL. Trade only: Rectal gel (Diastat) 2.5, 5, 10, 15, 20 mg. Rectal gel (Diastat AcuDial) 10, 20 mg.] ▶LK ♀D ▶- ©IV $

FLURAZEPAM (*Dalmane*) 15–30 mg PO qhs. Half-life 70–90 h. [Generic/Trade: Caps 15, 30 mg.] ▶LK ♀X ▶- ©IV $

Anxiolytics / Hypnotics—Benzodiazepines—Medium Half-Life (10–15 h)

ESTAZOLAM (*ProSom*) 1–2 mg PO qhs. [Generic/Trade: Tabs 1, 2 mg.] ▶LK ♀X ▶- ©IV $$

LORAZEPAM (*Ativan*) Anxiety: 0.5–2 mg IV/IM/PO q6–8h, max 10 mg/d. Half-life 10–20 h. Status epilepticus: 4 mg IV over 2 min; may repeat in 10–15 min. Peds status epilepticus: 0.05–0.1 mg/kg (max 4 mg) IV over 2–5 min; may repeat 0.05 mg/kg × 1 in 10–15 min. [Generic/Trade: Tabs 0.5, 1, 2 mg. Generic only: Oral concentrate 2 mg/mL.] ▶LK ♀D ▶- ©IV $

TEMAZEPAM (*Restoril*)   7.5–30 mg PO qhs. Half-life 8–25 h. [Generic/Trade: Caps 15, 30 mg. Trade only: Caps 7.5, 22.5 mg.] ▶LK ♀X ▶- ©IV $

Anxiolytics / Hypnotics—Benzodiazepines—Short Half-Life (<12 h)

NOTE *To avoid withdrawal, gradually taper when discontinuing after prolonged use. Sedative-hypnotics have been associated with severe allergic reactions and complex sleep behaviors including sleep driving. Use caution and discuss with patients.*

ALPRAZOLAM (*Xanax, Xanax XR, Niravam*)   0.25–0.5 mg PO bid-tid. Half-life 12 h. Multiple drug interactions. [Trade only: Orally disintegrating tab (Niravam) 0.25, 0.5, 1, 2 mg. Generic/Trade: Tabs 0.25, 0.5, 1, 2 mg. Extended release tabs: 0.5, 1, 2, 3 mg. Generic only: Oral concentrate (Intensol) 1 mg/mL.] ▶LK ♀D ▶- ©IV $

OXAZEPAM (*Serax*)   10–30 mg PO tid-qid. Half-life 8 h. [Generic/Trade: Caps 10, 15, 30 mg. Trade only: Tabs 15 mg.] ▶LK ♀D ▶- ©IV $$$

TRIAZOLAM (*Halcion*)   0.125–0.5 mg PO qhs. 0.125 mg/d in elderly. Half-life 2–3 h. [Generic/Trade: Tabs 0.125, 0.25 mg.] ▶LK ♀X ▶- ©IV $

Anxiolytics / Hypnotics—Other

BUSPIRONE (*BuSpar, Vanspar*)   Anxiety: Start 15 mg "dividose" daily (7.5 mg PO bid), usual effective dose 30 mg/d. Max 60 mg/d. [Generic/Trade: Tabs 5, 10, Dividose Tabs 15, 30 mg (scored to be easily bisected or trisected). Generic only: Tabs 7.5 mg.] ▶K ♀B ▶- $$$

CHLORAL HYDRATE (*Aquachloral Supprettes, Somnote*)   25–50 mg/kg/d up to 1000 mg PO/PR. Many physicians use higher than recommended doses in children (eg, 75 mg/kg). [Generic only: Syrup 500 mg/5 mL, rectal suppositories 500 mg. Trade only: Caps 500 mg. Rectal suppositories: 325, 650 mg.] ▶LK ♀C ▶+ ©IV $

ESZOPICLONE (*Lunesta*)   2 mg PO qhs prn. Max 3 mg. Elderly: 1 mg PO qhs prn, max 2 mg. [Trade only: Tabs 1, 2, 3 mg.] ▶L ♀C ▶? ©IV $$$$

RAMELTEON (*Rozerem*)   Insomnia: 8 mg PO qhs. [Trade only: Tabs 8 mg.] ▶L ♀C ▶? $$$

ZALEPLON (*Sonata, ✦Starnoc*)   5–10 mg PO qhs prn, max 20 mg. Do not use for benzodiazepine or alcohol withdrawal. [Trade only: Caps 5, 10 mg.] ▶L ♀C ▶- ©IV $$$

ZOLPIDEM (*Ambien, Ambien CR*)   Insomnia: 10 mg PO qhs (standard tabs, short-term) or 12.5 mg PO qhs (controlled release tabs). Do not use for benzodiazepine or alcohol withdrawal. Start with 5 mg (standard tabs) or 6.25 mg (controlled release) in the elderly or debilitated. [Generic/Trade: Tabs 5, 10 mg. Trade only: Controlled release tabs 6.25, 12.5 mg.] ▶L ♀B ▶+ ©IV $$$$

ZOPICLONE, ✦IMOVANE ▶L ♀D ▶- $

Combination Drugs

SYMBYAX (*olanzapine + fluoxetine*)   Bipolar depression: Start 6/25 mg PO qhs. Max 18/75 mg/d. [Trade only: Caps (olanzapine/fluoxetine) 3/25, 6/25, 6/50, 12/25, 12/50 mg.] ▶LK ♀C ▶- $$$$$

Drug Dependence Therapy

ACAMPROSATE (*Campral*) Maintenance of abstinence from alcohol: 666 mg (2 tabs) PO tid. Start after alcohol withdrawal and when patient is abstinent. [Trade only: delayed-release tabs 333 mg.] ▶K ♀C ▶? $$$$

DISULFIRAM (*Antabuse*) Sobriety: 125–500 mg PO daily. Patient must abstain from any alcohol for ≥12 h before using. Metronidazole and alcohol in any form (cough syrups, tonics, etc.) contraindicated. [Trade only: Tabs 250, 500 mg.] ▶L ♀C ▶? $$$

NALTREXONE (*ReVia, Depade, Vivitrol*) Alcohol/opioid dependence: 25–50 mg PO daily. Avoid if recent ingestion of opioids (past 7–10 d). Hepatotoxicity with higher than approved doses. [Generic/Trade: Tabs 50 mg. Trade only (Vivitrol): extended-release injectable susp kits 380 mg.] ▶LK ♀C ▶? $$$$

NICOTINE GUM (*Nicorette, Nicorette DS*) Smoking cessation: Gradually taper 1 piece q1–2h × 6 wk, 1 piece q2–4h × 3 wk, then 1 piece q4–8h × 3 wk, max 30 pieces/d of 2 mg or 24 pieces/d of 4 mg. Use Nicorette DS 4 mg/piece in high cigarette use (>24 cigarettes/d). [OTC/Generic/Trade: gum 2, 4 mg.] ▶LK ♀C ▶- $$$$$

NICOTINE INHALATION SYSTEM (*Nicotrol Inhaler, ✚Nicorette inhaler*) 6–16 cartridges/d × 12 wk [Trade only: Oral inhaler 10 mg/cartridge (4 mg nicotine delivered), 42 cartridges/box.] ▶LK ♀D ▶- $$$$$

NICOTINE LOZENGE (*Commit*) Smoking cessation: In those who smoke <30 min from waking use 4 mg lozenge; others use 2 mg. Take 1–2 lozenges q1–2 h × 6 wk, then q2–4h in wk 7–9, then q4–8h in wk 10–12. Length of therapy 12 wk. [OTC Generic/Trade: lozenge 2, 4 mg in 48, 72 & 168-count packages.] ▶LK ♀D ▶- $$$$$

NICOTINE NASAL SPRAY (*Nicotrol NS*) Smoking cessation:1–2 doses each h, with each dose = 2 sprays, one in each nostril (1 spray = 0.5 mg nicotine). Minimum recommended: 8 doses/d, max 40 doses/d. [Trade only: nasal solution 10 mg/mL (0.5 mg/inhalation); 10 mL bottles.] ▶LK ♀D ▶- $$$$$

NICOTINE PATCHES (*Habitrol, NicoDerm CQ, ✚Prostep*) Smoking cessation: Start one patch (14–22 mg) daily, taper after 6 wk. Ensure patient has stopped smoking. [OTC/Rx/Generic/Trade: patches 11, 22 mg/ 24 h. 7, 14, 21 mg/ 24 h (Habitrol & NicoDerm). OTC/Trade: 15 mg/ 16 h (Nicotrol).] ▶LK ♀D ▶- $$$$

SUBOXONE (*buprenorphine + naloxone*) Treatment of opioid dependence: Maintenance: 16 mg SL daily. Can individualize to range of 4–24 mg SL daily. [Trade only: SL tabs 2/0.5 and 8/2 mg buprenorphine/naloxone.] ▶L ♀C ▶- ©III $$$$$

VARENICLINE (*Chantix*) Smoking cessation: Start 0.5 mg PO daily for d 1–3, then 0.5 mg bid d 4–7, then 1 mg bid thereafter. Take after meals with full glass of water. Start 1 wk prior to cessation and continue × 12 wk. [Trade only: Tabs 0.5, 1 mg.] ▶K ♀C ▶? $$$$

Stimulants / ADHD / Anorexiants

ADDERALL (*dextroamphetamine + amphetamine*) (*Adderall XR*) ADHD, standard-release tabs: Start 2.5 mg (3–5 yo) or 5 mg (≥6 yo) PO daily-bid,
(cont.)

increase by 2.5–5 mg every wk, max 40 mg/d. ADHD, extended-release caps (Adderall XR): If 6–12 yo, then start 5–10 mg PO daily to a max of 30 mg/d. If 13–17 yo, then start 10 mg PO daily to a max of 20 mg/d. If adult, then 20 mg PO daily. Narcolepsy, standard-release: Start 5–10 mg PO q am, increase by 5–10 mg q wk, max 60 mg/d. Avoid evening doses. Monitor growth and use drug holid when appropriate. [Generic/Trade: Tabs 5, 7.5, 10, 12.5, 15, 20, 30 mg. Trade only: Caps, extended release (Adderall XR) 5, 10, 15, 20, 25, 30 mg.] ▶L ♀C ▶ –©II $$$$

ARMODAFINIL (*Nuvigil*) Obstructive sleep apnea/hypopnea syndrome and narcolepsy: 150–250 mg PO q am. Inconsistent evidence for improved efficacy of 250 mg/d dose. Shift work sleep disorder: 150 mg PO 1 h prior to start of shift. [Trade only: tabs 50, 150, 250 mg.] ▶L ♀C ▶? ©IV ?

ATOMOXETINE (*Strattera*) ADHD: Children/adolescents >70 kg and adults: Start 40 mg PO daily, then increase after >3 d to target of 80 mg/d divided daily-bid. Max 100 mg/d. [Trade only: caps 10, 18, 25, 40, 60, 80, 100 mg.] ▶K ♀C ▶? $$$$$

CAFFEINE (*NoDoz, Vivarin, Caffedrine, Stay Awake, Quick-Pep, Cafcit*) 100–200 mg PO q3–4h prn. [OTC Generic/Trade: Tabs/Caps 200 mg. Oral solution caffeine citrate (Cafcit) 20 mg/mL. OTC Trade only: Extended-release tabs 200 mg. Lozenges 75 mg.] ▶L ♀B/C ▶? $

DEXMETHYLPHENIDATE (*Focalin, Focalin XR*) ADHD, extended release, not already on stimulants: 5 mg (children) or 10 mg (adults) PO q am. Immediate release, not already on stimulants: 2.5 mg PO bid. Max 20 mg/d for both. If taking racemic methylphenidate use conversion of 2.5 mg for each 5 mg of methylphenidate, max 20 mg/d. [Generic/Trade: Tabs, immediate-release 2.5, 5, 10 mg. Trade only: Extended release caps (Focalin XR) 5, 10, 15, 20 mg.] ▶LK ♀C ▶? ©II $$$

DEXTROAMPHETAMINE (*Dexedrine, Dextrostat*) Narcolepsy: Age 6–12 yo: start 5 mg PO qam, increase by 5 mg/d q wk. Age >12 yo: start 10 mg PO qam, increase by 10 mg/d q wk. Usual dose range 5–60 mg/d in divided doses (tabs) or daily (extended-release). ADHD: 2.5–5 mg PO qam, usual max 40 mg/d. Avoid evening doses. Monitor growth and use drug holidays when appropriate. [Generic/Trade: Caps, extended-release 5, 10, 15 mg. Generic only: Tabs 5, 10 mg. Oral soln 5 mg/5 mL.] ▶L ♀C ▶– ©II $$$

LISDEXAMFETAMINE (*Vyvanse*) ADHD adults and children ages 6–12 yo: Start 30 mg PO q am. May increase weekly by 10–20 mg/d to max 70 mg/d. Avoid evening doses. Monitor growth and use drug holidays when appropriate. [Trade: Caps 20, 30, 40, 50, 60, 70 mg.] ▶L ♀C ▶? ©II $$$$

METHYLPHENIDATE (*Ritalin, Ritalin LA, Ritalin SR, Methylin, Methylin ER, Metadate ER, Metadate CD, Concerta, Daytrana, ✦Biphentin*) ADHD/Narcolepsy: 5–10 mg PO bid-tid or 20 mg PO qam (sustained and extended release), max 60 mg/d. Or 18–36 mg PO qam (Concerta), max 72 mg/d. Avoid evening doses. Monitor growth and use drug holid when appropriate. [Trade only: tabs 5, 10, 20 mg (Ritalin, Methylin, Metadate). Sustained-release tabs 10, 20 mg (Methylin ER, Metadate ER). Extended release tabs 18, 27, 36, 54 mg (Concerta). Extended release caps 10, 20, 30, 40, 50, 60 mg (Metadate CD) May be sprinkled on food. Sustained-release tabs 20 mg (Ritalin SR).

BODY MASS INDEX*	Heights are in feet and inches; weights are in pounds					
BMI	*Class.*	*4' 10"*	*5' 0"*	*5' 4"*	*5' 8"*	*6' 0"*	*6' 4"*
<19	Underweight	<91	<97	<110	<125	<140	<156
19–24	Healthy Weight	91–119	97–127	110–144	125–163	140–183	156–204
25–29	Overweight	120–143	128–152	145–173	164–196	184–220	205–245
30–40	Obese	144–191	153–204	174–233	197–262	221–293	246–328
>40	Very Obese	>191	>204	>233	>262	>293	>328

*BMI = kg/m² = (weight in pounds)(703)/(height in inches)². Anorectants appropriate if BMI ≥30 (with comorbidities ≥27); surgery an option if BMI >40 (with comorbidities 35–40). www.nhlbi.nih.gov

Extended release caps 10, 20, 30, 40 mg (Ritalin LA). Chewable tabs 2.5, 5, 10 mg (Methylin). Oral soln 5 mg/5 mL, 10 mg/5 mL (Methylin). Transdermal patch (Daytrana) 10 mg/9 h, 15 mg/9 h, 20 mg/9 h, 30 mg/9 h. Generic only: tabs 5, 10, 20 mg, extended release tabs 10, 20 mg, sustained-release tabs 20 mg.] ▶LK ♀C ▶? ©II $$

MODAFINIL (Provigil, ✦Alertec) Narcolepsy and sleep apnea/hypopnea: 200 mg PO qam. Shift work sleep disorder: 200 mg PO one h before shift. [Trade only: Tabs 100, 200 mg.] ▶L ♀C ▶? ©IV $$$$$

PHENTERMINE (Adipex-P, Ionamin, Pro-Fast) 8 mg PO tid or 15–37.5 mg/d q am or 10–14 h before retiring. For short-term use. [Generic/Trade: Caps 15, 30, 37.5 mg. Tabs 37.5 mg. Trade only: Caps, extended release 15, 30 mg (Ionamin). Generic only (Pro-Fast): Caps 18.75 mg, Tabs 8 mg.] ▶KL ♀C ▶- ©IV $$

SIBUTRAMINE (Meridia) Start 10 mg PO q am, max 15 mg/d. Monitor pulse and BP. [Trade only: Caps 5, 10, 15 mg.] ▶KL ♀C ▶- ©IV $$$$

PULMONARY

Beta Agonists—Short Acting

ALBUTEROL (AccuNeb, Ventolin HFA, Proventil, Proventil HFA, ProAir HFA, VoSpire ER, ✦Airomir, Asmavent, salbutamol) MDI 2 puffs q4–6h prn. 0.5 mL of 0.5% soln (2.5 mg) nebulized tid-qid. One 3 mL unit dose (0.083%) nebulized tid-qid. Caps for inhalation 200–400 mcg q4–6h. 2–4 mg PO tid-qid or extended release 4–8 mg PO q12h up to 16 mg PO q12h. Children 2–5 yo: 0.1–0.2 mg/kg/dose PO tid up to 4 mg tid; 6–12 yo: 2–4 mg or extended release 4 mg PO q12h. Prevention of exercise-induced bronchospasm: MDI: 2 puffs 15–30 min before exercise. [Generic/Trade: MDI 90 mcg/actuation, 200 metered doses/canister. "HFA" inhalers use hydrofluoroalkane propellant instead of CFCs but are otherwise equivalent. Soln for inhalation 0.042% (AccuNeb) and 0.083% (Proventil) in 3 mL vial, 0.5% (5 mg/mL) in 20 mL with dropper (Proventil). Soln extended-release 4, 8 mg (VoSpire ER). Soln for inhalation 0.021% in 3 mL vial (AccuNeb). Generic only: Syrup 2 mg/5 mL. Tabs immediate-release 2, 4 mg.] ▶L ♀C ▶? $$

FENOTEROL (✦*Berotec*) Canada only. 1–2 puffs prn tid-qid. Nebulizer: up to 2.5 mg q6 h. [Trade only: MDI 100 mcg/actuation. Soln for inhalation: 20 mL bottles of 1 mg/mL (*with preservatives that may cause bronchoconstriction in those with hyperreactive airways*).] ▶L ♀C ▶? $

LEVALBUTEROL (*Xopenex, Xopenex HFA*) MDI 2 puffs q4–6h prn. 0.63–1.25 mg nebulized q6–8h. 6–11 yo: 0.31 mg nebulized tid. [Generic/Trade: Soln for inhalation 0.31, 0.63, 1.25 mg in 3 mL and 1.25 mg in 0.5 mL unit-dose vials. Trade only: HFA MDI 45 mcg/actuation, 15 g 200/canister. "HFA" inhalers use hydrofluoroalkane propellant.] ▶L ♀C ▶? $$$

METAPROTERENOL (*Alupent, ✦Orciprenaline*) MDI 2–3 puffs q3–4h: 0.2–0.3 mL 5% soln nebulized q4h. 20 mg PO tid-qid >9 yo, 10 mg PO tid-qid if 6–9 yo, 1.3–2.6 mg/kg/d divided tid-qid if 2–5 yo. [Trade only: MDI 0.65 mg/actuation, 14 g 200/canister. Generic/Trade: Soln for inhalation 0.4% & 0.6% in 2.5 mL unit-dose vials. Generic only: Syrup 10 mg/5 mL, Tabs 10 & 20 mg.] ▶L ♀C ▶? $$

PIRBUTEROL (*Maxair Autohaler*) MDI: 1–2 puffs q4–6h. [Trade only: MDI 200 mcg/actuation, 14 g 400/canister.] ▶L ♀C ▶? $$$$

Beta Agonists—Long Acting

ARFORMOTEROL (*Brovana*) COPD: 15 mcg nebulized bid. [Trade only: Solution for inhalation 15 mcg in 2 mL vial.] ▶L ♀C ▶? $$$$$

FORMOTEROL (*Foradil, Perforomist, ✦Oxeze Turbuhaler*) 1 puff bid. Nebulized: 20 mcg q12h. Not for acute bronchospasm. Use only in combination with corticosteroids. [Trade only: DPI 12 mcg, 12 & 60 blisters/pack (Foradil). Soln for inhalation: 20 mcg in 2 mL vial (Perforomist). Canada only (Oxeze): DPI 6 & 12 mcg 60 blisters/pack.] ▶L ♀C ▶? $$$

SALMETEROL (*Serevent Diskus*) 1 puff bid. Not for acute bronchospasm. Use only in combination with corticosteroids. [Trade only: DPI (Diskus): 50 mcg, 60 blisters.] ▶L ♀C ▶? $$$$

Combinations

ADVAIR (*fluticasone—inhaled + salmeterol*) (*Advair HFA*) Asthma: DPI: 1 puff bid (all strengths). MDI: 2 puffs bid (all strengths). COPD: DPI: 1 puff bid (250/50 only). [Trade only: DPI: 100/50, 250/50, 500/50 mcg fluticasone/salmeterol per actuation; 60 doses/DPI. Trade only (Advair HFA): MDI 45/21, 115/21, 230/21 mcg fluticasone/salmeterol per actuation; 120 doses/canister.] ▶L ♀C ▶? $$$$$

COMBIVENT (*albuterol + ipratropium*) 2 puffs qid, max 12 puffs/d. Contraindicated with soy or peanut allergy. [Trade only: MDI: 90 mcg albuterol/18 mcg ipratropium per actuation, 200/canister.] ▶L ♀C ▶? $$$$

DUONEB (*albuterol + ipratropium, ✦Combivent inhalation solution*) One unit dose qid. [Generic/Trade: Unit dose: 2.5 mg albuterol/0.5 mg ipratropium per 3 mL vial, premixed; 30 & 60 vials/carton.] ▶L ♀C ▶? $$$$$

SYMBICORT (*budesonide + formoterol*) Asthma: 2 puffs bid (both strengths). [Trade only: MDI: 80/4.5 & 160/4.5 mcg budesonide/formoterol per actuation; 120 doses/canister.] ▶L ♀C ▶? $$$$

Inhaled Steroids

NOTE See Endocrine-Corticosteroids when oral steroids necessary.

BECLOMETHASONE—INHALED (*QVAR*) 1–4 puffs bid (40 mcg). 1–2 puffs bid (80 mcg). [Trade only: HFA MDI: 40 mcg & 80 mcg/actuation, 7.3 g 100 actuations/canister.] ▶L ♀C ▶? $$$

BUDESONIDE—INHALED (*Pulmicort Respules, Pulmicort Flexhaler*) 1–2 puffs daily-bid. [Trade only: DPI: (Flexhaler) 90 & 180 mcg powder/actuation 60 & 120 doses respectively/canister. Respules: 0.25, 0.5, & 1 mg/2 mL unit dose.] ▶L ♀B ▶? $$$$

CICLESONIDE—INHALED (*Alvesco*) 80 mcg/puff: 1–4 puffs bid. 160 mcg/ puff: 1–2 puffs bid. [Trade only: 80 mcg/actuation, 60 per canister. 160 mcg/ actuation, 60 & 120 per canister.] ▶L ♀C ▶? $$$$

FLUNISOLIDE—INHALED (*AeroBid, AeroBid-M, Aerospan*) 2–4 puffs bid. [Trade only: MDI: 250 mcg/actuation, 100 metered doses/canister. AeroBid-M (AeroBid + menthol flavor). Aerospan HFA MDI: 80 mcg/actuation, 60 & 120 metered doses/canister.] ▶L ♀C ▶? $$$

FLUTICASONE—INHALED (*Flovent HFA, Flovent Diskus*) MDI: 2–4 puffs bid. [Trade only: HFA MDI: 44, 110, 220 mcg/actuation 120/canister. DPI (Diskus): 50, 100, 250 mcg/actuation delivering 44, 88, 220 mcg respectively.] ▶L ♀C ▶? $$$$

MOMETASONE—INHALED (*Asmanex Twisthaler*) 1–2 puffs q pm or 1 puff bid. If prior oral corticosteroid therapy: 2 puffs bid. [Trade only: DPI: 220 mcg/ actuation, 30, 60 & 120/canister.] ▶L ♀C ▶? $$$$

TRIAMCINOLONE—INHALED (*Azmacort*) 2 puffs tid-qid or 4 puffs bid; max dose 16 puffs/d. [Trade only: MDI: 75 mcg/actuation, 240/canister. Built-in spacer.] ▶L ♀D ▶? $$$$

Leukotriene Inhibitors

MONTELUKAST (*Singulair*) Adults: 10 mg PO daily. Children 6–14 yo: 5 mg PO daily. 2–5 yo: 4 mg PO daily. 12–23 mo (asthma): 4 mg (oral granules) PO daily. 6–23 mo (allergic rhinitis): 4 mg (oral granules) PO daily. Prevention of exercise-induced bronchoconstriction: 10 mg PO 2 h before exercise. [Trade only: Tabs 10 mg. Oral granules 4 mg packet, 30/box. Chewable tabs (cherry flavored) 4 & 5 mg.] ▶L ♀B ▶? $$$$

PREDICTED PEAK EXPIRATORY FLOW (liters/min)   *Am Rev Resp Dis* 1963; 88:644

Age (yr)	Women *(height in inches)*					Men *(height in inches)*					Child *(height in inches)*	
	55″	60″	65″	70″	75″	60″	65″	70″	75″	80″		
20 yr	390	423	460	496	529	554	602	649	693	740	44″	160
30 yr	380	413	448	483	516	532	577	622	664	710	46″	187
40 yr	370	402	436	470	502	509	552	596	636	680	48″	214
50 yr	360	391	424	457	488	486	527	569	607	649	50″	240
60 yr	350	380	412	445	475	463	502	542	578	618	52″	267
70 yr	340	369	400	432	461	440	477	515	550	587	54″	293

INHALED STEROIDS: ESTIMATED COMPARATIVE DAILY DOSES*

Drug	Form	≥12 yo & ADULTS			CHILDREN (5–11 yo)		
		Low Dose	Medium Dose	High Dose	Low Dose	Medium Dose	High Dose
beclomethasone HFA MDI	40 mcg/puff	2–6	6–12	>12	2–4	4–8	>8
	80 mcg/puff	1–3	3–6	>6	1–2	2–4	>4
budesonide DPI	90 mcg/dose	2–6	6–13	>13	2–4	4–9	>9
	180 mcg/dose	1–3	3–7	>7	1–2	2–4	>4
budesonide	soln for nebs	–	–	–	0.5 mg 0.25–0.5 mg (0–4 yo)	1 mg >0.5–1 mg (0–4 yo)	2 mg >1 mg (0–4 yo)
flunisolide MDI	250 mcg/puff	2–4	4–8	>8	2–3	4–5	>5
flunisolide HFA MDI	80 mcg/puff	4	5–8	>8	2	4	>8
fluticasone HFA MDI	44 mcg/puff	2–6	6–10	>10	2–4 (0–11 yo)	4–8 (0–11 yo)	>8 (0–11 yo)
	110 mcg/puff	1–2	2–4	>4	1–2 (0–11 yo)	2–3 (0–11 yo)	>4 (0–11 yo)
	220 mcg/puff	1	1–2	>2	n/a	1–2 (0–11 yo)	>2 (0–11 yo)
fluticasone DPI	50 mcg/dose	2–6	6–10	>10	2–4	4–8	>8
	100 mcg/dose	1–3	3–5	>5	1–2	2–4	>4
	250 mcg/dose	1	2	>2	n/a	1	>1
mometasone DPI	220 mcg/dose	1	2	>2	n/a	n/a	n/a
triamcinolone MDI	75 mcg/puff	4–10	10–20	>20	4–8	8–12	>12

*HFA = Hydrofluoroalkane (propellant). MDI = metered dose inhaler. DPI = dry powder inhaler. All doses in puffs (MDI) or inhalations (DPI) Reference: http://www.nhlbi.nih.gov/guidelines/asthma/asthsumm.pdf

ZAFIRLUKAST (*Accolate*) 20 mg PO bid. Peds 5–11 yo, 10 mg PO bid. Take 1 h ac or 2 h pc. Potentiates warfarin & theophylline. [Trade only: Tabs 10, 20 mg.] ▶L ♀B ▶– $$$

ZILEUTON (*Zyflo CR*) 1200 mg PO bid. Hepatotoxicity, potentiates warfarin, theophylline, & propranolol. [Trade only: Tabs, extended release 600 mg.] ▶L ♀C ▶? $$$$$

Other Pulmonary Medications

ACETYLCYSTEINE—INHALED (*Mucomyst*) Mucolytic: 3–5 mL of 20% or 6–10 mL of 10% soln nebulized tid-qid. [Generic/Trade: Soln for inhalation 10 & 20% in 4, 10 & 30 mL vials.] ▶L ♀B ▶? $

AMINOPHYLLINE (♣*Phyllocontin*) Acute asthma: loading dose: 6 mg/kg IV over 20–30 min. Maintenance 0.5–0.7 mg/kg/h IV. [Generic only: Tabs 100 & 200 mg. Oral liquid 105 mg/5 mL. Canada Trade only: Tabs controlled release (*12 h*) 225, 350 mg, scored.] ▶L ♀C ▶? $

CROMOLYN—INHALED (*Intal, Gastrocrom, ♣Nalcrom*) Asthma: 2–4 puffs qid or 20 mg nebs qid. Prevention of exercise-induced bronchospasm: 2 puffs 10–15 min prior to exercise. Mastocytosis: Oral concentrate 200 mg PO qid for adults, 100 mg qid in children 2–12 yo. [Trade only: MDI 800 mcg/actuation, 112 & 200/canister. Oral concentrate 100 mg/5 mL in 8 amps/foil pouch (Gastrocrom). Generic/Trade: Soln for nebs: 20 mg/2 mL.] ▶LK ♀B ▶? $$$

DORNASE ALFA (*Pulmozyme*) Cystic fibrosis: 2.5 mg nebulized daily-bid. [Trade only: soln for inhalation: 1 mg/mL in 2.5 mL vials.] ▶L ♀B ▶? $$$$$

EPINEPHRINE RACEMIC (*S-2, ♣Vaponefrin*) Severe croup: 0.05 mL/kg/dose diluted to 3 mL w/NS. Max dose 0.5 mL. [Trade only: soln for inhalation: 2.25% epinephrine in 15 & 30 mL.] ▶Plasma ♀C ▶– $

IPRATROPIUM—INHALED (*Atrovent, Atrovent HFA*) 2 puffs qid, or one 500 mcg vial neb tid-qid. Contraindicated with soy or peanut allergy (Atrovent MDI only). [Trade only: Atrovent HFA MDI: 17 mcg/actuation, 200/canister. Generic/Trade: Soln for nebulization: 0.02% (500 mcg/vial) in unit dose vials.] ▶Lung ♀B ▶? $$$

KETOTIFEN (♣*Zaditen*) Canada only. 6 mo to 3 yo: 0.05 mg/kg PO bid. Children >3 yo: 1 mg PO bid. [Generic/Trade: Tabs 1 mg. Syrup 1 mg/5 mL.] ▶L ♀C ▶– $$

INHALER COLORS (Body then cap—Generics may differ)

Advair:	purple	Atrovent HFA:	clear/ green	Proventil HFA:	yellow/ orange
Advair HFA:	purple/light purple				
		Azmacort:	white/white	Pulmicort:	white/brown
Aerobid:	grey/purple	Combivent:	clear/ orange	QVAR 40 mcg:	beige/grey
Aerobid-M:	grey/green			QVAR 80 mcg:	mauve/grey
Aerospan:	purple/grey	Flovent HFA:	orange/ peach	Serevent	green
Alupent:	clear/blue			Diskus:	
Alvesco 80 mcg:	brown/red	Foradil:	grey/beige	Spiriva:	grey
		Intal:	white/blue	Tilade:	white/white
Alvesco 160 mcg:	purple/grey	Maxair:	white/white	Ventolin HFA:	light blue/ navy
		Maxair Autohaler:	white/white		
Asmanex:	white/white	ProAir HFA:	red/white	Xopenex HFA:	blue/red

THEOPHYLLINE (*Elixophyllin, Uniphyl, Theo-24, T-Phyl, ✦Theo-Dur, Theolair*) 5–13 mg/kg/d PO in divided doses. Max dose 900 mg/d. Peds dosing variable. [Generic/Trade: Elixir 80 mg/15 mL. Trade only: Caps - Theo-24: 100, 200, 300, 400 mg. T-Phyl - 12 Hr SR tabs 200 mg. Theolair - tabs 125, 250 mg. Generic only: 12 Hr tabs 100, 200, 300, 450 mg, 12 Hr caps 125, 200, 300 mg.] ▶L ♀C ▶+ $

TIOTROPIUM (*Spiriva*) COPD: Handihaler: 18 mcg inhaled daily. [Trade only: Cap for oral inhalation 18 mcg. To be used with "Handihaler" device only. Packages of 5, 30, 90 caps with Handihaler device.] ▶K ♀C ▶- $$$$

TOXICOLOGY

ACETYLCYSTEINE (*N-acetylcysteine, Mucomyst, Acetadote, ✦Parvolex*) Contrast nephropathy prophylaxis: 600 mg PO bid on the d before and on the d of contrast. Acetaminophen toxicity: Mucomyst — loading dose 140 mg/kg PO or NG, then 70 mg/kg q4h × 17 doses. May be mixed in water or soft drink diluted to a 5% solution. Acetadote — loading dose 150 mg/kg in 200 mL of D5W infused over 60 min; maintenance dose 50 mg/kg in 500 mL of D5W infused over 4 h followed by 100 mg/kg in 1000 mL of D5W infused over 16 h. [Generic/Trade: solution 10%, 20%. Trade only: IV (Acetadote) ▶L ♀B ▶? $$$$

CHARCOAL (*activated charcoal, Actidose-Aqua, CharcoAid, EZ-Char, ✦Charcodate*) 25–100 g (1–2 g/kg or 10 times the amount of poison ingested) PO or NG as soon as possible. May repeat q1–4h prn at doses equivalent to 12.5 g/h. When sorbitol is coadministered, use only with the first dose if repeated doses are to be given. [OTC/Generic/Trade: Powder 15,30,40,120,240 g. Solution 12.5 g/60 mL, 15 g/75 mL, 15 g/120 mL, 25 g/120 mL, 30 g/120 mL, 50 g/240 mL. Susp 15 g/120 mL, 25 g/120 mL, 30 g/150 mL, 50 g/240 mL. Granules 15 g/120 mL.] ▶Not absorbed ♀+ ▶+ $

CYANIDE ANTIDOTE KIT (*amyl nitrite + sodium nitrite + sodium thiosulfate*) Induce methemoglobinemia with inhaled amyl nitrite 0.3 mL followed by sodium nitrite 300 mg IV over 2–4 min. Then administer sodium thiosulfate 12.5 g IV. [Package contains amyl nitrite inhalant (0.3 mL), sodium nitrite (300 mg/10 mL), sodium thiosulfate (12.5 g/50 mL).] ▶? ♀- ▶? $$$$$

DEFERASIROX (*Exjade*) Chronic iron overload: 20 mg/kg PO daily; adjust dose q3–6 mo based on ferritin trends. Max 30 mg/kg/d. [Trade only: Tabs for dissolving into oral susp 125, 250, 500 mg.] ▶L ♀B ▶? $$$$$

DEFEROXAMINE (*Desferal*) Chronic iron overload: 500–1000 mg IM daily and 2 g IV infusion (≤15 mg/kg/h) with each unit of blood or 1–2 g SC daily (20–40 mg/kg/d) over 8–24 h via continuous infusion pump. Acute iron toxicity: IV infusion up to 15 mg/kg/h (consult poison center). ▶K ♀C ▶? $$$$

FLUMAZENIL (*Romazicon*) Benzodiazepine sedation reversal: 0.2 mg IV over 15 sec, then 0.2 mg q1 min prn up to 1 mg total dose. Overdose reversal: 0.2 mg IV over 30 sec, then 0.3–0.5 mg q30 second prn up to 3 mg total dose. Contraindicated in mixed drug OD or chronic benzodiazepine use. ▶LK ♀C ▶? $$$

HYDROXOCOBALAMIN (*Cyanokit*) Cyanide poisoning: 5 g IV over 15 min; may repeat prn. ▶K ♀C ▶? $$$$$

ANTIDOTES

Toxin	Antidote/Treatment	Toxin	Antidote/Treatment
acetaminophen	N-acetylcysteine	ethylene glycol	fomepizole
antidepressants*	bicarbonate	heparin	protamine
arsenic, mercury	dimercaprol (BAL)	iron	deferoxamine
benzodiazepine	flumazenil	lead	EDTA, succimer
beta blockers	glucagons	methanol	fomepizole
calcium channel blockers	calcium chloride, glucagons	methemoglobin	methylene blue
cyanide	hydroxocobalamin	opioids	naloxone
		organophosphates	atropine+pralidoxime
digoxin	dig immune Fab	warfarin	vitamin K, FFP

*cyclic

IPECAC SYRUP Emesis: 30 mL PO for adults, 15 mL if 1–12 yo. [Generic only (*OTC*): syrup.] ▶Gut ♀C ▶? $

METHYLENE BLUE (*Methblue 65, Urolene blue*) Methemoglobinemia: 1–2 mg/kg IV over 5 min. Dysuria: 65–130 mg PO tid after meals with plenty of water. May turn urine/contact lenses blue. [Trade only: Tab 65 mg.] ▶K ♀C ▶? $$

PRALIDOXIME (*Protopam, 2-PAM*) Organophosphate poisoning; consult poison center: 1–2 g IV infusion over 15–30 min or slow IV injection ≥5 min (max rate 200 mg/min). May repeat dose after 1 h if muscle weakness persists. Peds: 20–50 mg/kg/dose IV over 15–30 min.] ▶K ♀C ▶? $$$

SUCCIMER (*Chemet*) Lead toxicity in children ≥1 yo: Start 10 mg/kg PO or 350 mg/m2 q8h × 5 d, then reduce the frequency to q12h × 2 wk. [Trade only: Caps 100 mg.] ▶K ♀C ▶? $$$$$

UROLOGY

Benign Prostatic Hyperplasia

ALFUZOSIN (*UroXatral, ✦Xatral*) BPH: 10 mg PO daily after a meal. [Trade only: Extended-release tab 10 mg.] ▶KL ♀B ▶- $$$

DUTASTERIDE (*Avodart*) BPH: 0.5 mg PO daily. [Trade only: Cap 0.5 mg.] ▶L ♀X ▶- $$$$

FINASTERIDE (*Proscar, Propecia*) Proscar: 5 mg PO daily alone or in combination with doxazosin to reduce the risk of symptomatic progression of BPH. Propecia: Androgenetic alopecia in men: 1 mg PO daily. [Generic/Trade: Tabs 1 mg (Propecia), 5 mg (Proscar).] ▶L ♀X ▶- $$$

TAMSULOSIN (*Flomax*) 0.4 mg PO daily, 30 min after a meal. Max 0.8 mg/d. [Trade only: Cap 0.4 mg.] ▶LK ♀B ▶- $$$

Bladder Agents—Anticholinergics & Combinations

DARIFENACIN (*Enablex*) Overactive bladder with symptoms of urinary urgency, frequency and urge incontinence: 7.5 mg PO daily. May increase to max dose 15 mg PO daily in 2 wk. Max dose 7.5 mg PO daily with moderate liver

(cont.)

impairment or when coadministered with potent CYP3A4 inhibitors (ketoconazole, itraconazole, ritonavir, nelfinavir, clarithromycin & nefazodone). [Trade only: Extended-release tabs 7.5, 15 mg]. ▶LK ♀C ▶- $$$$

OXYBUTYNIN (*Ditropan, Ditropan XL, Oxytrol, ✦Oxybutyn, Uromax*) Bladder instability: 2.5–5 mg PO bid-tid, max 5 mg PO qid. Extended release tabs: 5–10 mg PO daily, increase 5 mg/d q wk to 30 mg/d. Oxytrol: 1 patch twice weekly on abdomen, hips or buttocks. [Generic/Trade: Tab 5 mg. Syrup 5 mg/5 mL. Extended release tabs 5, 10, 15 mg. Trade only: Transdermal (Oxytrol) 3.9 mg/d.] ▶LK ♀B ▶? $

PROSED/DS (*methenamine + phenyl salicylate + methylene blue + benzoic acid + hyoscyamine*) 1 tab PO qid with liberal fluids. May turn urine/contact lenses blue. [Trade only: Tab (methenamine 81.6 mg/phenyl salicylate 36.2 mg/methylene blue 10.8 mg/benzoic acid 9.0 mg/hyoscyamine sulfate 0.12 mg). Prosed EC = enteric coated form.] ▶KL ♀C ▶? $$$

SOLIFENACIN (*VESIcare*) Overactive bladder with symptoms of urinary urgency, frequency or urge incontinence: 5 mg PO daily. Max dose: 10 mg daily (5 mg daily if CrCl<30 mL/min, moderate hepatic impairment, or concurrent ketoconazole or other potent CYP3A4 inhibitors). [Trade only: Tabs 5, 10 mg.] ▶LK ♀C ▶- $$$$

TOLTERODINE (*Detrol, Detrol LA, ✦Unidet*) Overactive bladder: 1–2 mg PO bid (Detrol) or 2–4 mg PO daily (Detrol LA). [Trade only: Tabs 1, 2 mg. Caps, extended release 2, 4 mg]. ▶L ♀C ▶- $$$$

TROSPIUM (*Sanctura, Sanctura XR, ✦Trosec*) Overactive bladder with urge incontinence: 20 mg PO bid; give 20 mg qhs if CrCl <30 mL/min. If ≥75 yo may taper down to 20 mg daily. Extended release: 60 mg PO q am, 1 h before food. [Trade only: Tab 20 mg, Cap, extended release, 60 mg.] ▶LK ♀C ▶? $$$$

URISED (*methenamine + phenyl salicylate + atropine + hyoscyamine + benzoic acid + methylene blue*) (*Usept*) Dysuria: 2 tabs PO qid. May turn urine/contact lenses blue, don't use with sulfa. [Trade only: Tab (methenamine 40.8 mg/phenyl salicylate 18.1 mg/atropine 0.03 mg/hyoscyamine 0.03 mg/4.5 mg benzoic acid/5.4 mg methylene blue).] ▶K ♀C ▶? $$$$

UTA (*methenamine + sodium phosphate + phenyl salicylate + methylene blue + hyoscyamine*) 1 cap PO qid with liberal fluids. [Trade only: Cap (methenamine 120 mg/sodium phosphate 40.8 mg/phenyl salicylate 36 mg/methylene blue 10 mg/hyoscyamine 0.12 mg).] ▶KL ♀C ▶? $$$

UTIRA-C (*methenamine + sodium phosphate + phenyl salicylate + methylene blue + hyoscyamine*) 1 cap PO qid with liberal fluids. [Trade only: Tab (methenamine 81.6 mg/sodium phosphate 40.8 mg/phenyl salicylate 36.2 mg/methylene blue 10.8 mg/hyoscyamine 0.12 mg). ▶KL ♀C ▶? $$

Bladder Agents—Other

BETHANECHOL (*Urecholine, Duvoid, ✦Myotonachol*) Urinary retention: 10–50 mg PO tid-qid. [Generic/Trade: Tabs 5, 10, 25, 50 mg.] ▶L ♀C ▶? $

PHENAZOPYRIDINE (*Pyridium, Azo-Standard, Urogesic, Prodium, Pyridiate, Urodol, Baridium, UTI Relief, ✦Phenazo*) Dysuria: 200 mg PO tid × 2 d. May turn urine/contact lenses orange. [OTC Generic/Trade: Tabs 95, 97.2 mg. Rx Generic/Trade: Tabs 100, 200 mg.] ▶K ♀B ▶? $

Erectile Dysfunction

ALPROSTADIL (*Muse, Caverject, Caverject Impulse, Edex, Prostin VR Pediatric, prostaglandin E1, ✚Prostin VR*) 1 intraurethral pellet (Muse) or intracavernosal injection (Caverject, Edex) at lowest dose that will produce erection. Onset of effect is 5–20 min. [Trade only: Syringe system (Edex) 10, 20, 40 mcg. (Caverject) 5, 10, 20 mcg. (Caverject Impulse) 10, 20 mcg. Pellet (Muse) 125, 250, 500, 1000 mcg. Intracorporeal injection of locally-compounded combination agents (many variations): "Bi-mix" can be 30 mg/mL papaverine + 0.5 to 1 mg/mL phentolamine, or 30 mg/mL papaverine + 20 mcg/mL alprostadil in 10 mL vials. "Tri-mix" can be 30 mg/mL papaverine + 1 mg/mL phentolamine + 10 mcg/mL alprostadil in 5, 10 or 20 mL vials.] ▶L ♀- ▶- $$$$

SILDENAFIL (*Viagra, Revatio*) Erectile dysfunction: Start 50 mg PO 0.5–4 h prior to intercourse. Max 1 dose/d. Usual effective range 25–100 mg. Start at 25 mg if >65 yo or liver/renal impairment. Pulmonary hypertension: 20 mg PO tid. Contraindicated with nitrates. [Trade only (Viagra): Tabs 25, 50, 100 mg. Unscored tab but can be cut in half. Revatio: Tabs 20 mg.] ▶LK ♀B ▶- $$$$

TADALAFIL (*Cialis*) 2.5–5 mg PO daily without regard to timing of sexual activity. As needed dosing: Start 10 mg PO ≥30–45 min prn prior to sexual activity. May increase to 20 mg or decrease to 5 mg prn. Max 1 dose/d. Start 5 mg (max 1 dose/d) if CrCl 31–50 mL/min. Max 5 mg/d if CrCl <30 mL/min on dialysis. Max 10 mg/d if mild to moderate hepatic impairment; avoid in severe hepatic impairment. Max 10 mg once in 72 h if concurrent potent CYP3A4 inhibitors. Contraindicated with nitrates & alpha-blockers (except tamsulosin 0.4 mg daily). Not FDA approved for women. [Trade only: Tabs 2.5, 5, 10, 20 mg.] ▶L ♀B ▶- $$$$

VARDENAFIL (*Levitra*) Start 10 mg PO 1 h before sexual activity. Usual effective dose range 5–20 mg. Max 1 dose/d. Use lower dose (5 mg) if ≥65 yo or moderate hepatic impairment (max 10 mg). Contraindicated with nitrates and alpha-blockers. Not FDA-approved in women. [Trade only: Tabs 2.5, 5, 10, 20 mg.] ▶LK ♀B ▶- $$$$

YOHIMBINE (*Yocon, Yohimex*) Erectile dysfunction (not FDA approved): 5.4 mg PO tid. [Generic/Trade: Tab 5.4 mg.] ▶L ♀- ▶- $

Nephrolithiasis

CITRATE (*Polycitra-K, Urocit-K, Bicitra, Oracit, Polycitra, Polycitra-LC*) Urinary alkalinization: 1 packet in water/juice PO tid-qid. [Trade only: Polycitra-K packet (potassium citrate): 3300 mg. Oracit oral solution: 5 mL = sodium citrate 490 mg. Generic/Trade: Urocit-K wax (potassium citrate) Tabs 5, 10 mEq. Generic only: Polycitra-K oral solution (5 mL = potassium citrate 1100 mg), Bicitra oral solution (5 mL = sodium citrate 500 mg), Polycitra-LC oral solution (5 mL = potassium citrate 550 mg/sodium citrate 500 mg), Polycitra oral syrup (5 mL = potassium citrate 550 mg/sodium citrate 550 mg).] ▶K ♀C ▶? $$$

APPENDIX

ADULT EMERGENCY DRUGS (selected)

ALLERGY	diphenhydramine (*Benadryl*): 50 mg IV/IM. epinephrine: 0.1-0.5 mg IM (1:1000 solution), may repeat after 20 minutes. methylprednisolone (*Solu-Medrol*): 125 mg IV/IM.
HYPERTENSION	esmolol (*Brevibloc*): 500 mcg/kg IV over 1 minute, then titrate 50-200 mcg/kg/minute fenoldopam (*Corlopam*): Start 0.1 mcg/kg/min, titrate up to 1.6 mcg/kg/min labetalol (*Normodyne*): Start 20 mg slow IV, then 40-80 mg IV q10 min prn up to 300 mg total cumulative dose nitroglycerin (*Tridil*): Start 10-20 mcg/min IV infusion, then titrate prn up to 100 mcg/minute nitroprusside (*Nipride*): Start 0.3 mcg/kg/min IV infusion, then titrate prn up to 10 mcg/kg/minute
DYSRHYTHMIAS / ARREST	adenosine (*Adenocard*): PSVT (not A-fib): 6 mg rapid IV & flush, preferably through a central line or proximal IV. If no response after 1-2 minutes then 12 mg. A third dose of 12 mg may be given prn. amiodarone (*Cordarone, Pacerone*): V-fib or pulseless V-tach: 300 mg IV/IO; may repeat 150 mg just once. Life-threatening ventricular arrhythmia: Load 150 mg IV over 10 min, then 1 mg/min x 6h, then 0.5 mg/min x 18h. atropine: 0.5 mg IV, repeat prn to maximum of 3 mg. diltiazem (*Cardizem*): Rapid A-fib: bolus 0.25 mg/kg or 20 mg IV over 2 min. May repeat 0.35 mg/kg or 25 mg 15 min after 1st dose. Infusion 5-15 mg/h. epinephrine: 1 mg IV/IO q3-5 minutes for cardiac arrest. [1:10,000 solution] lidocaine (*Xylocaine*): Load 1 mg/kg IV, then 0.5 mg/kg q8-10min prn to max 3 mg/kg. Maintenance 2g in 250ml D5W (8 mg/ml) at 1-4 mg/min drip (7-30 ml/h).
PRESSORS	dobutamine (*Dobutrex*): 2-20 mcg/kg/min. 70 kg: 5 mcg/kg/min with 1 mg/mL concentration (eg, 250 mg in 250 mL D5W) = 21 mL/h. dopamine (*Intropin*): Pressor: Start at 5 mcg/kg/min, increase prn by 5-10 mcg/kg/min increments at 10 min intervals, max 50 mcg/kg/min. 70 kg: 5 mcg/kg/min with 1600 mcg/mL concentration (eg, 400 mg in 250 ml D5W) = 13 mL/h. Doses in mcg/kg/min: 2-4 = (traditional renal dose, apparently ineffective) dopaminergic receptors; 5-10 = (cardiac dose) dopaminergic and beta1 receptors; >10 = dopaminergic, beta1, and alpha1 receptors. norepinephrine (*Levophed*): 4 mg in 500 ml D5W (8 mcg/ml) at 2-4 mcg/min. 22.5 ml/h = 3 mcg/min. phenylephrine (*Neo-Synephrine*): 50 mcg boluses IV. Infusion for hypotension: 20 mg in 250ml D5W (80 mcg/ml) at 40-180 mcg/min (35-160ml/h).
INTUBATION	etomidate (*Amidate*): 0.3 mg/kg IV. methohexital (*Brevital*): 1-1.5 mg/kg IV. propofol (*Diprivan*): 2.0-2.5 mg/kg IV. rocuronium (*Zemuron*): 0.6-1.2 mg/kg IV. succinylcholine (*Anectine*): 1 mg/kg IV. Peds (<5 yo): 2 mg/kg IV. thiopental (*Pentothal*): 3-5 mg/kg IV.
SEIZURES	diazepam (*Valium*): 5-10 mg IV, or 0.2-0.5 mg/kg rectal gel up to 20 mg PR. fosphenytoin (*Cerebyx*): Load 15-20 "phenytoin equivalents" per kg either IM, or IV no faster than 100-150 mg/min. lorazepam (*Ativan*): 0.05-0.15 mg/kg up to 3-4 mg IV/IM. phenobarbital: 200-600 mg IV at rate ≤60 mg/min; titrate prn up to 20 mg/kg phenytoin (*Dilantin*): 15-20 mg/kg up to 1000 mg IV no faster than 50 mg/min.

CARDIAC DYSRHYTHMIA PROTOCOLS (for adults and adolescents)

Chest compressions ~100/minute. Ventilations 8-10/minute if intubated; otherwise 30:2 compression/ventilation ratio. Drugs that can be administered down ET tube (use 2-2.5 x usual dose): epinephrine, atropine, lidocaine, vasopressin, naloxone.

V-Fib, Pulseless V-Tach
Airway, oxygen, CPR until defibrillator ready
Defibrillate 360 J (old monophasic), 120-200 J (biphasic), or with AED
Resume CPR x 2 minutes (5 cycles)
Repeat defibrillation if no response
Vasopressor during CPR:
- Epinephrine 1 mg IV/IO q3-5 minutes, or
- Vasopressin 40 units IV to replace 1st or 2nd dose of epinephrine
Rhythm/pulse check every ~2 minutes
Consider antiarrhythmic during CPR:
- Amiodarone 300 mg IV/IO; may repeat 150 mg just once
- Lidocaine 1.0-1.5 mg/kg IV/IO, then repeat 0.5-0.75 mg/kg to max 3 doses or 3 mg/kg
- Magnesium 1-2 g IV/IO if suspect torsade de pointes

Asystole or Pulseless Electrical Activity (PEA)
Airway, oxygen, CPR
Vasopressor (when IV/IO access):
- Epinephrine 1 mg IV/IO q3-5 minutes, or
- Vasopressin 40 units IV/IO to replace 1st or 2nd dose of epinephrine
Consider atropine 1 mg IV/IO for asystole or slow PEA. Repeat q3-5 min up to 3 doses.
Rhythm/pulse check every ~2 minutes
Consider 6 H's: hypovolemia, hypoxia, H+ acidosis, hyper / hypokalemia, hypoglycemia, hypothermia
Consider 5 T's: Toxins, tamponade-cardiac, tension pneumothorax, thrombosis (coronary or pulmonary), trauma

Bradycardia, <60 bpm and Inadequate Perfusion
Airway, oxygen, IV
Prepare for transcutaneous pacing; don't delay if advanced heart block
Consider atropine 0.5 mg IV; may repeat to max 3 mg
Consider epinephrine (2-10 mcg/min) or dopamine (2-10 mcg/kg/min)
Prepare for transvenous pacing

Tachycardia with Pulses
Airway, oxygen, IV
If unstable and heart rate >150 bpm, then synchronized cardioversion
If stable narrow-QRS (<120 ms):
- Regular: Attempt vagal maneuvers. If no success, then adenosine 6 mg IV, then 12 mg prn up to twice.
- Irregular: Control rate with diltiazem or beta blocker (caution in CHF or pulmonary disease).
If stable wide-QRS (>120 ms):
- Regular and suspect V-tach: Amiodarone 150 mg IV over 10 min; repeat prn to max 2.2 g/24h. Prepare for elective synchronized cardioversion.
- Regular and suspect SVT with aberrancy: adenosine as per narrow-QRS above.
- Irregular and A-fib: Control rate with diltiazem or beta blocker (caution in CHF/pulmonary disease).
- Irregular and A-fib with pre-excitation (WPW): Avoid AV nodal blocking agents; consider amiodarone 150 mg IV over 10 minutes.
- Irregular and torsade de pointes: magnesium 1-2 g IV load over 5-60 minutes, then infusion.

bpm=beats per minute; CPR=cardiopulmonary resuscitation; ET=endotracheal; IO=intraosseous; J=Joules; ms=milliseconds; WPW=Wolf-Parkinson-White. Source *Circulation* 2005; 112, suppl IV.

INDEX

To facilitate speed of use, index entries are shown with page number and approximate position on the page ("t" is top; "m" is middle; "b" is bottom). Although the PDA edition of the *Tarascon Pocket Pharmacopoeia* contains more than 6000 drug names, it is physically impossible to include all in pocket-sized manuals. Therefore, rarely used or specialized drugs appear in the PDA only (noted as "PDA" in the index) or in both the PDA and Deluxe edition (noted as "D" in the index).

153
Index
t = top of page
m = middle of page
b = bottom of page
D,PDA = see page 152

156
Index

t = top of page
m = middle of page
b = bottom of page
D,PDA = see page 152

157
Index

t = top of page
m = middle of page
b = bottom of page
D,PDA = see page 152

158

Index

t = top of page
m = middle of page
b = bottom of page
D,PDA = see page 152

160
Index

t = top of page
m = middle of page
b = bottom of page
D,PDA = see page 152

162
Index

t = top of page
m = middle of page
b = bottom of page
D,PDA = see page 152

164

Index

t = top of page
m = middle of page
b = bottom of page
D,PDA = see page 152

165

Index

t = top of page
m = middle of page
b = bottom of page
D,PDA = see page 152

170

Index

t = top of page
m = middle of page
b = bottom of page
D,PDA = see page 152

171
Index
t = top of page
m = middle of page
b = bottom of page
D,PDA = see page 152

175
Index
t = top of page
m = middle of page
b = bottom of page
D,PDA = see page 152

177
Index
t = top of page
m = middle of page
b = bottom of page
D,PDA=see page 152